Respiratory Disease Series: Diagnostic Tools and Disease Managements

Series editors
Hiroyuki Nakamura
Department of Respiratory Medicine, Tokyo Medical University Ibaraki Medical Center, Ibaraki, Japan

Kazutetsu Aoshiba
Department of Respiratory Medicine, Tokyo Medical University Ibaraki Medical Center, Ibaraki, Japan

This book series cover a variety of topics in respiratory diseases, with each volume providing an overview of the current state of knowledge, recent discoveries and future prospects for each disease. In each chapter the editors pose critical questions, which are often unresolved clinical issues. These are then discussed by the authors, providing insights and suggestions as to which developments need to be addressed. The series offers new information, which will inspire innovative ideas to further develop respiratory medicine. This collection of monographs is aimed at benefiting patients across the globe suffering from respiratory disease.

Edited by established authorities in the field and written by pioneering experts, this book series will be valuable to those researchers and physicians working in respiratory medicine. The series is aimed at a broad readership, and the books will also be a valuable resource for radiologists, emergency medicine physicians, pathologists, pharmacologists and basic research scientists.

More information about this series at http://www.springer.com/series/15152

Hiroyuki Nakamura • Kazutetsu Aoshiba
Editors

Chronic Obstructive Pulmonary Disease

A Systemic Inflammatory Disease

Springer

Editors
Hiroyuki Nakamura
Department of Respiratory Medicine
Tokyo Medical University Ibaraki Medical Center
Ibaraki, Japan

Kazutetsu Aoshiba
Department of Respiratory Medicine
Tokyo Medical University Ibaraki Medical Center
Ibaraki, Japan

ISSN 2509-5552 ISSN 2509-5560 (electronic)
Respiratory Disease Series: Diagnostic Tools and Disease Managements
ISBN 978-981-10-0838-2 ISBN 978-981-10-0839-9 (eBook)
DOI 10.1007/978-981-10-0839-9

Library of Congress Control Number: 2016956541

Printed on acid-free paper

This Springer imprint is published by Springer Nature
The registered company is Springer Science+Business Media Singapore Pte Ltd.

Preface

Chronic obstructive pulmonary disease (COPD) is a chronic inflammatory disease of the lung mainly caused by long-term smoking and aging. The number of COPD patients is increasing worldwide and the World Health Organization (WHO) estimates that COPD will be the third most common cause of death after ischemic heart disease and cerebrovascular disease by 2020. Particularly in Japan, the smoking rate is still high compared with that of Western countries, and currently population aging is rapidly progressing in a manner unlike any other in the world. Therefore, taking measures against COPD s an urgent issue.

Worldwide, the National Heart, Lung, and Blood Institute (NHLBI)/WHO joint workshop, the Global Initiative for Chronic Obstructive Lung Disease (GOLD), established guidelines for the management of COPD in 2001. Subsequently, the guidelines have been repeatedly revised. The combined assessment of COPD, a new classification of COPD severity based on current symptoms, and future exacerbation risk, were proposed in 2011 [1], and this classification method was successively incorporated in the 2015 revision [2]. However, it is necessary to verify the validity of this classification in the future.

In addition, in Japan, a large-scale epidemiological study [Nippon COPD Epidemiology (NICE) study] estimated that there were at least 5 million COPD patients, but only approximately 10 % of the patients had been actually diagnosed with COPD [3], indicating that COPD is very poorly recognized generally and that additional educational activities are required. Furthermore, because another epidemiological study showed large individual differences in symptoms and disease progression rates among COPD patients [4] and, in addition, individual COPD patients have various pathological conditions, emphasis is given to the heterogeneity and complexity of COPD.

Many studies have so far been conducted on genetic factors of COPD. Many gene polymorphisms susceptible to COPD, such as those in SERPINE [5], glutathione S-transferase (GST), heme oxygenase-1 (HO-1), matrix metalloproteinase (MMP), Toll-like receptor (TLR), and surfactant protein D (SP-D) [6], have been reported in Japan.

Because COPD is caused by smoking in many cases, it is self-evident that, first of all, smoking cessation is necessary. Why airway inflammation persists after smoking cessation has not been elucidated.

So far, protease–antiprotease imbalance and oxidative stress [7], among other factors, have been considered as mechanisms of COPD development. Furthermore, theories explaining COPD development from the standpoint of cellular senescence [8], apoptosis [9], and autophagy have also recently been proposed.

Although COPD is a chronic inflammatory disease of the lung, it has recently been shown to be important to understand COPD as a systemic inflammatory disease not limited to the lung. Therefore, the management of systemic comorbidities is considered to be an extremely important task [10].

Treatment during the stable phase is largely divided into non-drug therapy and drug therapy, and it is important to comprehensively administer these therapies. Exercise therapy, nutritional therapy, home oxygen therapy, and so on, are provided as non-drug therapeutic approaches, and further development is expected in the future.

Bronchodilators are mainly used for drug therapy, and the use of multiple drugs concurrently according to the severity of COPD is recommended. However, bronchodilators merely treat the symptoms of COPD, and therefore it is desirable to develop new drugs that fundamentally inhibit inflammation in COPD. In addition, inhaled corticosteroids are used in severe patients with repeated exacerbations. However, at present, it has not been concluded whether inhaled corticosteroids inhibit pulmonary and systemic inflammation.

In addition, it has been revealed that the exacerbation of COPD worsens the prognosis, and how to take measures against such exacerbation is also a problem [11, 12].

Furthermore, COPD is often complicated by other respiratory diseases. In particular, we have encountered many cases of asthma–COPD overlap syndrome (ACOS), combined pulmonary fibrosis and emphysema (CPFE), and combined COPD and lung cancer, and it is also necessary to promptly take measures against these complications.

So far, there have been a small number of textbooks dealing with COPD, but these books are uniformly organized in the conventional style. Therefore, the books have shortcomings in that it is difficult to understand what the problems are at present and how to cope with those problems. In the present volume, the authors are all authorities in the field in Japan who have long been engaged in clinical practice and research regarding COPD. Each chapter in this book takes an issue about which readers often have questions and presents it as a subtitle in the form of a clinical question. Each author will provide up-to-date information on each issue and describe his or her thoughts and future perspectives in response to the clinical question, based on such information. Thus, by offering the most recent knowledge, presented as clinical questions with answers and commentary, this book will allow readers not only to obtain cutting-edge information on COPD, but also will allow the readers to understand what the authors really think and what their future perspectives are—sure to satisfy the intellectual curiosity of the readers.

Considering the nature of this project, useful information will be provided not only to those who are studying COPD for the first time, but also to physicians in clinical practice, instructors, and many researchers engaged in basic research.

I am convinced that this information, transmitted from Japanese researchers to physicians in practice and researchers worldwide, will further deepen the understanding of this intractable disease. Furthermore, I expect that awareness concerning the pathogenesis of COPD will be further strengthened, leading to the development of innovative treatments. It will please me immensely if this book can be helpful for the many patients suffering from COPD.

Ibaraki, Japan Hiroyuki Nakamura

References

1. National Institute of Health, national Heart, Lung, and Blood Institute: global strategy for the diagnosis, management, and prevention of chronic obstructive pulmonary disease. NHLBI/WHO Workshop Report Updated 2011.
2. National Institute of Health, national Heart, Lung, and Blood Institute: global strategy for the diagnosis, management, and prevention of chronic obstructive pulmonary disease. NHLBI/WHO Workshop Report Updated 2015.
3. Fukuchi Y, Nishimura M, Ichinose M, et al. COPD in Japan: the Nippon COPD Epidemiology study. Respirology. 2004;9:458–65.
4. Nishimura M, Makita H, Nagai K, et al. Annual change in pulmonary function and clinical phenotype in chronic obstructive pulmonary disease. Am J Respir Crit Care Med. 2012;185:44–52.
5. Fujimoto K, Ikeda S, Arai T, et al. Polymorphism of SERPINE2 gene is associated with pulmonary emphysema in consecutive autopsy cases. BMC Med Genet. 2010;11:159.
6. Ishii T, Hagiwara K, Kamio K, et al. Involvement of surfactant protein D in emphysema revealed by genetic association study. Eur J Hum Genet. 2012;20:230–5.
7. Suzuki M, Betsuyaku T, Ito Y, et al. Down-regulated NF-E2-related factor 2 in pulmonary macrophages of aged smokers and patients with chronic obstructive pulmonary disease. Am J Respir Cell Mol Biol. 2008;39:673–82.
8. Tsuji T, Aoshiba K, Nagai A. Alveolar cell senescence in patients with pulmonary emphysema. Am J Respir Crit Care Med. 2006;174:886–93.
9. Aoshiba K, Yokohori N, Nagai A. Alveolar wall apoptosis causes lung destruction and emphysematous changes. Am J Respir Cell Mol Biol. 2003;28:555–62.
10. Iwamoto H, Yokoyama A, Kitahara Y, et al. Airflow limitation in smokers is associated with subclinical atherosclerosis. Am J Respir Crit Care Med. 2009;179:35–40.
11. Tanabe N, Muro S, Hirai T, et al. Impact of exacerbations on emphysema progression in chronic obstructive pulmonary disease. Am J Respir Crit Care Med. 2011;183:1653–9.
12. Yamaya M, Azuma A, Takizawa H, et al. Macrolide effects on the prevention of COPD exacerbations. Eur Respir J. 2012;40:485–94.

Contents

Part I
Definition and Epidemiology

Chapter 1
Definition of Chronic Obstructive Pulmonary Disease (COPD): Is the Latest GOLD Classification of Severity Still Valid?

Kazuhisa Asai and Kazuto Hirata

Abstract Chronic obstructive pulmonary disease (COPD) is characterized by persistent airflow limitation that is usually progressive and associated with an enhanced chronic inflammatory response evoked by the presence of noxious particles or gases in the airways. The progression of airflow limitation has a tremendous impact on disease severity and overall prognosis. However, other factors, such as symptoms, exacerbations, or comorbidities, also have a considerable impact on individual COPD patients. The Global Initiative for Chronic Obstructive Lung Disease (GOLD) Scientific Committee launched a joint project between the World Health Organization and the National Heart, Lung, and Blood Institute. The initial report of the GOLD guideline for COPD was published in 2001. Since then, the GOLD Scientific Committee has kept the GOLD guideline updated by revising it on the basis of the latest scientific evidence. Although the GOLD classification was initially based on the severity of airflow limitation, the classification of symptoms, breathlessness, and risk of exacerbations as well as spirometry results was recently included because of the accumulated scientific evidence. In this chapter, we will define COPD and discuss the latest GOLD classification.

Keywords Chronic obstructive pulmonary disease (COPD) • The Global Initiative for Chronic Obstructive Lung Disease (GOLD)

1.1 Introduction

Chronic obstructive pulmonary disease (COPD) is characterized by a persistent airflow limitation that is usually progressive and associated with an enhanced chronic inflammatory response in the airways. Most surveys on COPD conducted worldwide have reported a disease prevalence of approximately 10 %. Fukuchi

---

K. Asai • K. Hirata (✉)
Department of Respiratory Medicine, Graduate School of Medicine, Osaka City University, 1-4-3, Asahi-machi, Abeno-ku, Osaka 545-8585, Japan
e-mail: kazutoh@msic.med.osaka-cu.ac.jp

H. Nakamura, K. Aoshiba (eds.), *Chronic Obstructive Pulmonary Disease*, Respiratory Disease Series: Diagnostic Tools and Disease Managements,
DOI 10.1007/978-981-10-0839-9_1

et al. conducted the Nippon COPD Epidemiology study to determine the prevalence of COPD in Japan [1]. For this purpose, more than 2300 subjects aged more than 40 years and representative of the total population of Japan were screened via spirometry, and the prevalence of COPD in Japan was estimated at 8.6 %, which corresponds to approximately 5.3 million people aged more than 40 years or approximately 2.1 million people aged more than 70 years. The survey conducted by the World Health Organization (WHO) in 2004 indicates that COPD is the fourth most important cause of death worldwide and is expected to become the third largest cause of death until 2020. Chronic airflow limitation in COPD is caused by several factors, including small airway disease (obstructive bronchiolitis) and parenchymal destruction (emphysema), and the relative contribution of these factors varies on an individual basis (Fig. 1.1). Previous definitions of COPD have emphasized the terms "emphysema" and "chronic bronchitis," which were not included in the GOLD definition. Emphysema, which is the destruction of the alveolar surfaces involved in gas exchange, is a pathological term and is often diagnosed in patients with COPD. On the other hand, chronic bronchitis, which is characterized by cough and the production of sputum for at least 3 months for 2 consecutive years, is a strictly clinical and epidemiological term. Chronic cough, production of sputum, and chronic bronchitis may precede the development of airflow limitation and obstructive bronchiolitis. Two important elements of COPD—small airway disease (obstructive bronchiolitis) and parenchymal destruction (emphysema)—were identified before the creation of the GOLD guidelines. The chronic inflammation caused by small airway disease evokes structural changes and narrowing of the small airways. The destruction of the lung parenchyma by inflammatory processes, oxidative stress, or protease/antiprotease imbalance decreases the number of alveolar attachments on the small airways, decreases lung elastic recoil, and limits airflow. Since the 1950s, the diseases that cause obstructive ventilatory impairment have attracted much interest because of the development of respiratory tests and the elucidation of respiratory physiology and pathology. In the UK, obstructive ventilatory impairment was primarily diagnosed as "chronic bronchitis" from the symptomatic point of view. The definition of chronic bronchitis was "the occurrence of cough and the production of sputum for at least 3 months for 2 consecutive years." However, in the United States, obstructive ventilatory impairment was primarily diagnosed as "pulmonary emphysema" from the pathological point of view. Pulmonary emphysema is characterized

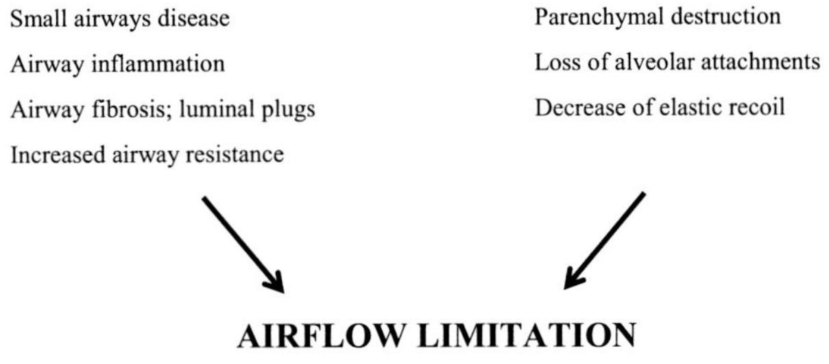

Fig. 1.1 Mechanisms underlying airflow limitation in COPD

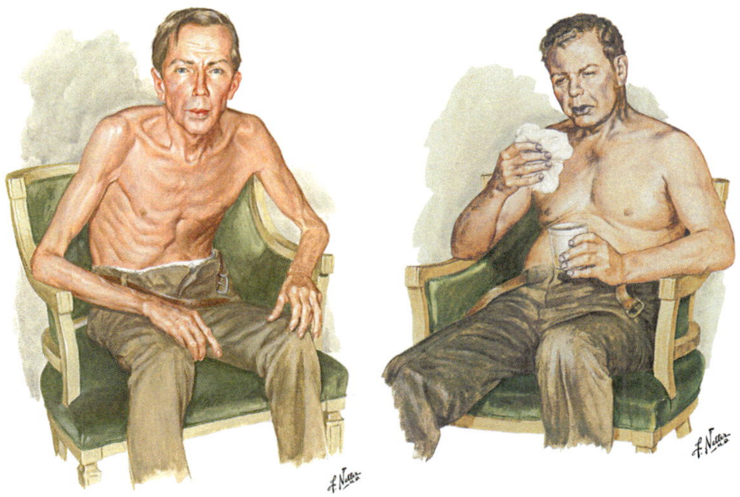

Fig. 1.2 Pink puffer and blue bloater (Netter illustration used with permission of Elsevier, Inc. All rights reserved www.netterimages.com)

by the destruction of the lung parenchyma. The similarities and differences between the two disease entities have been discussed extensively. Fletcher, Burrows et al. defined the concept of obstructive ventilatory impairment and named the group of diseases that caused obstructive ventilatory impairment as chronic obstructive lung disease (COLD) [2, 3]. At that time, the presence of subtypes was assumed. Later, Burrow et al. classified COLD into type A (emphysema type), type B (bronchitis type), and type X (intermediate form between types A and B) [3]. On the other hand, Filley et al. classified COLD into type PP (pink puffer) and type BB (blue bloater) (Fig. 1.2) [4]. Another problem in the differentiation between COPD and bronchial asthma is that both diseases are characterized by obstructive ventilatory impairment, and the underlying complication is airway inflammation.

1.2 Historical Transition of the Concept of COPD

After the increased interest in infectious diseases and in pneumoconiosis as a respiratory disease, the diseases that caused obstructive ventilatory impairment attracted much interest in the 1950s, after the World War II, because of the development of respiratory tests. In the UK, obstructive ventilatory impairment was primarily diagnosed as "chronic bronchitis" from the symptomatic point of view whereas, in the United States, it was primarily diagnosed as "pulmonary emphysema" from the pathological point of view. The similarities and differences between the two disease entities have been discussed extensively. The landmark meeting conducted in 1959—the CIBA Guest Symposium—and the concept of chronic nonspecific lung disease (CNSLD) helped elucidate the two disease concepts [5]. Fletcher, in the UK, and Burrows, in the United States, defined the concept of obstructive ventilatory impairment and named the group of diseases that caused obstructive ventilatory impairment as chronic obstructive lung disease (COLD) [6]. COLD is characterized by chronic and irreversible airway obstruction. Airflow obstruction is characterized by the narrowing of the airway lumen and reservoir of secretion in lumen due to chronic inflammation of the airways and by the decrease in the lung elastic recoil due to the alveolar destruction. The narrowing of the airway lumen defines chronic bronchitis, whereas the decrease in the lung elastic recoil defines emphysema. Burrow et al. classified COLD into type A (emphysema type), type B (bronchitis type), and type X (intermediate form between types A and B) [3]. On the other hand, Filley et al. classified COLD into type PP (pink puffer) and type BB (blue bloater) [4]. Hogg et al. revealed that the distal airways, which are defined as airways with an inner diameter of 2 mm or less, contributed much more to the total airway resistance in subjects with COLD but contributed less than 20 % in healthy subjects [7]. This observation allowed us to hypothesize that the dysfunction of the distal airways is key for the early diagnosis of COLD. Later, the physiology of the distal airways was investigated. Various parameters in the flow volume curve, such as V25, V50, single-breath nitrogen washout for measuring the closing volume, and the frequency dependence of lung compliance, have been diligently studied to help elucidate the pathophysiology of COLD. However, these attempts failed to reach the initial goal to diagnose COLD earlier because of insufficient sensitivity and specificity due to large variations in the test values and overlap with values from healthy subjects. Therefore, forced expiratory volume in one second (FEV1) or forced expiratory volume in one second % (FEV1/forced vital capacity (FVC)) was used for the diagnosis of COPD. In 1987, the American Thoracic Society changed the name of the disease from COLD to COPD and redefined its concept. Therefore, COPD was redefined as a disease characterized by emphysema, chronic bronchitis, and distal airway dysfunction and was caused by nonreversible airflow obstruction. Following this definition, the GOLD guidelines were published in 2001. Several revisions were made in these guidelines on the basis of the accumulated scientific evidence, and GOLD was last updated in 2016.

1.3 Difference Between COPD and Bronchial Asthma

Both COPD and bronchial asthma are characterized by obstructive ventilatory impairment, and the underlying condition is airway inflammation. In 1961, Orie et al. hypothesized that chronic bronchitis and emphysema, both of which are now considered COPDs, and bronchial asthma were only phenotypes of the same disease, which was caused by inflammation of the airways, and therefore these conditions should be considered the same disease. The hypothesis was that different environmental factors, including allergens, tobacco, and air pollutants, affected the underlying genetic predisposition for atopic constitution and airway hyperresponsiveness and produced different phenotypes, including bronchial asthma and COPD. This was later referred to as the Dutch hypothesis, and the concept of CNSLD was proposed. Although the most common cause of COPD is smoking, not all of the smokers necessarily develop COPD. The Dutch hypothesis states that the susceptibility for developing COPD in smokers is due to genetic predisposition for atopy. The basis for this hypothesis was that airway hyperresponsiveness, high peripheral blood eosinophilia, and high IgE levels were observed in COPD, and the number of eosinophils in sputum was correlated with an obstructive ventilatory impairment similar to that observed in bronchial asthma. COPD itself sometimes has asthma-like characteristics, and it is known that the development of COPD together with asthma is frequent. A new concept on the development of the asthma COPD overlap syndrome was proposed. In addition to the Dutch hypothesis, the British hypothesis considered that the excessive secretion associated with respiratory tract infection was the leading cause of obstructive ventilatory impairment. The Dutch and British hypotheses were confirmed in studies on bronchial asthma and COPD and helped elucidate the pathogenesis of these diseases.

1.4 Chronic Bronchitis and Pulmonary Emphysema

In the COPD guideline of the Japanese Respiratory Society, COPD is diagnosed using FEV1. However, this guideline also indicates the presence of two phenotypes, distal airway disease and emphysema lesions, which act jointly at various levels and cause airflow limitation. Filley et al. suggest the presence of two different phenotype groups in COPD, i.e., type PP (pink puffer) and type BB (blue bloater) COPD [4]. Pink puffers have a pink complexion and dyspnea. Emphysema-type COPD (in which emphysema lesions are the predominant type) is equivalent to PP-type COPD. PP-type COPD involves severe emphysema, increased residual lung capacity and volume, decreased elastic recoil, decreased diffusing capacity, and a ventilator/perfusion mismatch secondary to emphysema-associated destruction of blood vessels. Arterial blood gas (ABG) is usually near normal owing to compensatory hyperventilation, PaO_2 levels are normal, and $PaCO_2$ levels are low to normal. Pink puffers have increased tidal volume and retraction of accessory respiratory muscles for compensation. The amount of energy required for respiration causes an imbalance between energy intake and energy consumption. Although subjects with BB-type COPD tend to be normal weight or overweight, those with PP-type COPD tend to be underweight (Fig. 1.2). It has been reported that PP-type COPD is more common than BB-type COPD in Japan. Blue bloaters have cyanosis and right heart failure. Non-emphysema-type COPD (in which distal airway disease is the predominant type) is equivalent to BB-type COPD. Patients with BB-type COPD have cyanosis and chronic bronchitis, normal to low lung capacity, increased residual volume with air trapping, and characteristic ABG, i.e., decreased PaO_2 and increased $PaCO_2$, although the diffusion capacity is normal. Subjects with BB-type COPD tend to be overweight.

1.5 Global Initiative for Chronic Obstructive Lung Disease (GOLD)

The GOLD program was initiated in 1998 to provide recommendations for the management of COPD on the basis of the best scientific information available. The first report, the Global Strategy for Diagnosis, Management, and Prevention of COPD, was issued in 2001. This report was widely translated into many languages and distributed worldwide and served as a global guideline. The GOLD Scientific Committee launched a joint project between the WHO and the National Heart, Lung, and Blood Institute (NHLBI) in 2002. Its members are recognized leaders in COPD research and clinical practice, with the scientific credentials to review published research on COPD management and prevention, to evaluate the impact of this research on the recommendations proposed in the GOLD guidelines related to management and prevention, and to provide yearly updates on the GOLD website. A complete revision was prepared in 2006, 2011, and 2016 on the basis of published research. With regard to the classification and severity of COPD, a new combined assessment was introduced in 2011 (Fig. 1.3). In the 2011 report, the GOLD Scientific Committee recommends the assessment of COPD on the basis of a combination of factors, including the patient level of symptoms, the future risk of exacerbations, and the severity of the spirometric abnormality; however, the severity of the spirometric abnormality should not be used alone. A previous spirometric classification divided airflow limitation into four grades using the fixed ratio (FEV1/FVC), and airflow limitation was defined as a post-bronchodilator FEV1/FVC < 0.7 (Table 1.1). It has been recognized that the use of the fixed ratio might

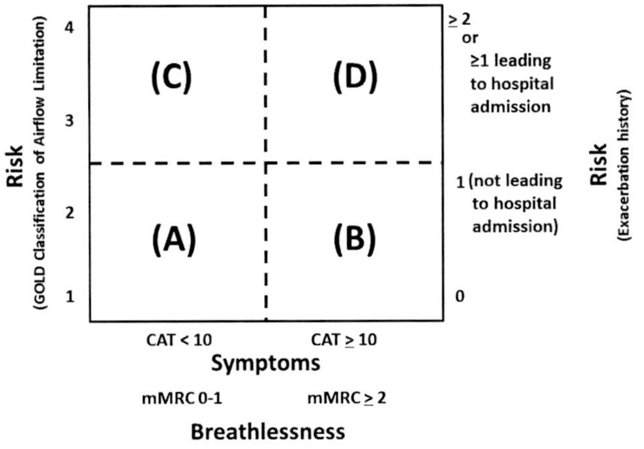

Fig. 1.3 Assessment using symptoms, breathlessness, spirometric classification, and risk of exacerbations

Table 1.1 Classification of severity of airflow limitation in COPD (Based on post-bronchodilator FEV1)

In patients with $FEV_1/FVC < 0.70$:		
GOLD 1:	Mild	$FEV_1 \geq 80\,\%$ predicted
GOLD 2:	Moderate	$50\,\% \leq FEV_1 < 80\,\%$ predicted
GOLD 3:	Severe	$30\,\% \leq FEV_1 < 50\,\%$ predicted
GOLD 4:	Very severe	$FEV_1 < 30\,\%$ predicted

lead to more frequent diagnoses of COPD in the older population with mild COPD—because the normal aging process affects lung volume and flow—but might lead to underdiagnosis in younger populations. Similarly, the use of the spirometric classification of airflow limitation might lead to the classification of COPD as more severe in older populations and less severe in younger populations. Moreover, the frequent presence of the exacerbation phenotype has been reported [8]. Although acute exacerbations are key events in COPD progression, the determinants of their frequency are poorly understood. Using a large observational cohort, the Evaluation of COPD Longitudinally to Identify Predictive Surrogate Endpoints (ECLIPSE) study revealed that acute exacerbations are independent of spirometric severity. Although acute exacerbations become more frequent and more severe as the severity of COPD increases, the single best predictor of exacerbations across all GOLD stages is the history of exacerbations, not the severity of COPD (Fig. 1.4). The frequent exacerbation phenotype appeared to be relatively preserved over a period of 3 years (Fig. 1.4). Proper COPD treatment is based on an accurate assessment of the severity of COPD, its impact on the patient's health status, and the risk of future events such as acute exacerbations, hospital admissions, and death. In the GOLD 2011 assessment, severity alone was not used to achieve proper treatment, but other aspects of COPD were considered separately, including the current level of patient symptoms, severity of the spirometric abnormality, risk of exacerbations, and presence of comorbidities. Several validated questionnaires are available to assess symptoms in patients with COPD. For symptoms, GOLD recommends the use of two well-known questionnaires, the modified British Medical Research Council (mMRC) questionnaire and the COPD Assessment Test (CAT) [9]. Although the mMRC questionnaire only assesses disability due to breathlessness, CAT can assess other measures of health status and predict future mortality risk better than airflow limitation [10]. The CAT provides a broader coverage of the impact of COPD on the patient's quality of life (QOL). The CAT was developed and validated by Jones et al. [9]. The CAT is an 8-item unidimensional measure of the impairment of the health status in COPD; it has been applied worldwide and its translation has been validated in several languages. Previously used disease-specific questionnaires, such as the St George's Respiratory Questionnaire (SGRQ) [11], Chronic Respiratory Disease Questionnaire [12], and the COPD Clinical Questionnaire [13], are reliable, validated, and widely used in clinical trials or in clinical practice. However, some of these instruments are lengthy and have highly complex scoring algorithms for routine use in clinical practice. A brief questionnaire that is easy to complete and interpret

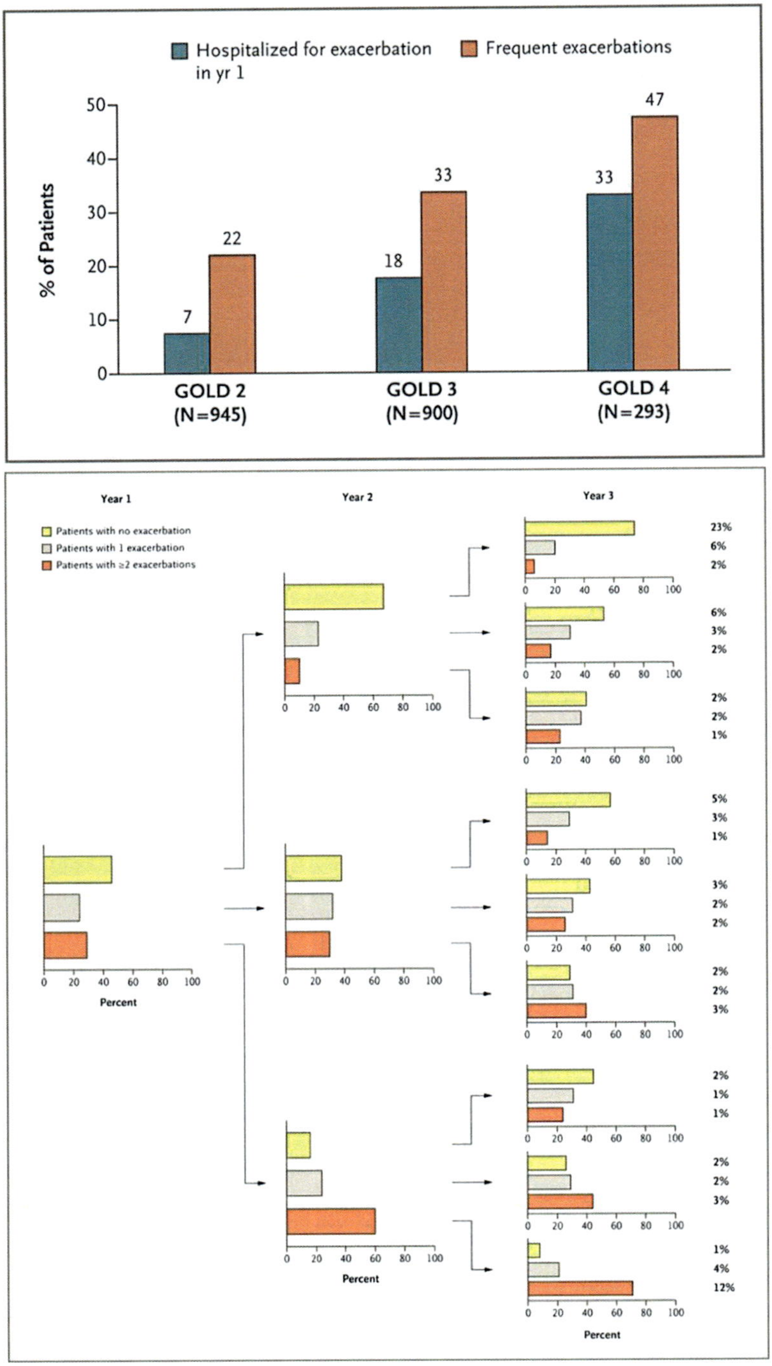

Fig. 1.4 The frequent exacerbation phenotype in COPD (Reproduced with permission from Hurst et al. [8])

is necessary for routine use, and the CAT was developed for this purpose. Eight items of the CAT were identified out of 21 candidate items using the psychometric and Rasch analysis, and the correlation (r) with the COPD-specific version of the SGRQ was 0.80 and the internal consistency was excellent [9]. The score ranges from 0 to 40 and can be correlated with the SGRQ scoring. The CAT also performs spirometric assessments to classify airflow limitation severity in patients with COPD. For this purpose, specific spirometric cut points are used for simplicity and the cut-point values are the same as those used previously. To minimize variability, spirometry should be performed after the administration of an adequate dose of a short-acting inhaled bronchodilator. However, there is only a weak correlation between FEV1 and the COPD symptoms that impair the patient's QOL. For this reason, both symptomatic assessment and spirometric assessment are required.

The acute exacerbations of COPD may lead to hospital admissions or death and are closely associated with the patient's QOL. The assessment of the risk of exacerbation and the prevention of future exacerbation are important tactics. Acute exacerbations of COPD are acute events characterized by a worsening of the patient's respiratory symptoms to levels that are lower than the normal variations, and the worsened status leads to a change in medication [14–16]. These exacerbations are serious events in the clinical course of COPD because of their negative effects on symptoms and lung function, and the patient recovery from exacerbation takes several weeks [17] and impairs the patient's QOL [18]. Moreover, these exacerbations accelerate the rate of decline of lung function [19] and are associated with significant mortality, particularly in patients who require hospitalization. Both the mortality rate during hospitalization and the all-cause mortality 3 years after hospitalization were increased [20, 21]. Not only the proper treatment but also the early detection and prevention of these exacerbations are essential to improve COPD prognosis. The patients with two or more exacerbations of COPD per year are often defined as "frequent exacerbators," and this phenotype appears stable over time [8]. The risks of exacerbation can be evaluated in the combined assessment. The frequency of acute exacerbations varies among patients [22]. The best predictor of frequent exacerbations (two or more exacerbations per year) is the history of previously treated events [8]. In addition, the worsening of airflow limitation is associated with the increased prevalence of exacerbations and risk of death. A large body of evidence has been accumulated for patients evaluated in previous GOLD spirometric classifications.

Prospectively collected data from large clinical trials such as ECLIPSE [8], UPLIFT [23], and TORCH [24] have indicated that worsening of airflow limitation leads to an increased risk of exacerbations, hospitalization, and death. These data are not precise estimates and do not apply to every patient but clearly indicate the increased risk of exacerbations and death between distinct spirometric levels. Although even patients classified as GOLD 2 (with moderate airflow limitation) may experience frequent exacerbations that require treatment with antibiotics and/or systemic corticosteroids, the risk of exacerbations significantly increases in patients classified as GOLD 3 (severe) and GOLD 4 (very severe). Because acute exacerbations increase the decline of lung function, deteriorate the health status, and increase the risk of death, the assessment of the exacerbation risk can be used to assess outcomes in general.

1.6 Combined COPD Assessment

In the GOLD 2011, the combined COPD assessment was introduced to understand the impact of COPD on individual patients. It combines the assessment of symptoms with the patient's spirometric classification and/or the risk of exacerbations. This combined approach is shown in Fig. 1.3. Symptoms are shown in the X-axis and the exacerbation risk is shown in the Y-axis. The mMRC questionnaire and CAT scale are recommended for assessing symptoms, and an mMRC grade $\geq$2 or a CAT score $\geq$10 indicate a high level of symptoms (the CAT score is preferred because it provides a more comprehensive assessment of the impact of symptoms on the disease; in the absence of this score, mMRC scores provide an assessment of the impact of dyspnea. However, it is unnecessary to use more than one scale). Two classification can be used to assess the exacerbation risk. The first classification is a population-based estimation using the GOLD spirometric classification, such that GOLD 3 or GOLD 4 categories indicate high risk. The second classification involves the estimation of individual patient's history of exacerbations, such that two or more exacerbations in the preceding year indicate high risk (in cases of discrepancies between the spirometric classification and the number of exacerbations in the preceding year, the assessment that indicates the highest risk should be used).

To use the classification shown in Fig. 1.3, first assess symptoms (X-axis) with the mMRC or CAT scale to determine the symptom category. The patients who belong to the left half side of the box (mMRC grade 0–1 or CAT $<$ 10) have fewer symptoms, whereas the patients who belong to the right half side of the box (mMRC grade $\geq$ 2 or CAT $\geq$ 10) have more symptoms. Subsequently, assess the risk of exacerbations (Y-axis) using the GOLD spirometric classification or the number of exacerbations in the preceding year to determine the exacerbation risk category. The patients who belong to the lower part of the box are at low risk for exacerbations, whereas those who belong to the upper part of the box are at high risk for exacerbations. This classification can be done using either of two methods: (1) use spirometry to determine the GOLD grade of airflow limitation (GOLD 1 and GOLD 2 indicate low risk whereas GOLD 3 and GOLD 4 indicate high risk) or (2) assess the number of exacerbations the patient experienced within the previous 12 months (0 or 1 indicates low risk whereas two or more exacerbations indicate high risk). In some patients, these two classification will not indicate the same level of risk; in this case, the risk should be determined using the method that indicates the highest risk. In summary, patient group A is low risk, with fewer symptoms; this group is typically GOLD 1 or GOLD 2 (mild or moderate airflow limitation), with none or one exacerbation per year, and mMRC grade 0–1 or CAT score $<$ 10. Patient group

B is low risk, with more symptoms, typically GOLD 1 or GOLD 2 (mild or moderate airflow limitation), with none or one exacerbation per year, and mMRC grade ≥ 2 or CAT score ≥ 10. Patient group C is high risk, with fewer symptoms, typically GOLD 3 or GOLD 4 (severe or very severe airflow limitation), with two or more exacerbations per year, and mMRC grade 0–1 or CAT score < 10. Patient group D is high risk, with more symptoms, typically GOLD 3 or GOLD 4 (severe or very severe airflow limitation), with two or more exacerbations per year, and mMRC grade ≥ 2 or CAT score ≥ 10.

After the GOLD 2011 combined assessment of COPD was introduced in clinical practice, patients with COPD were assessed and classified into subcategories A to D and managed according to the GOLD guidelines. The combined assessment of COPD was introduced to improve COPD management. Acute exacerbations of COPD are critical events in the clinical course of COPD, and the management of these exacerbations is key to improve disease management. It is important to classify patients with COPD in advance and prevent future exacerbations. However, a previously used spirometric classification of COPD is not a good predictor of acute exacerbation and prognosis. The multidimensional combined assessment of COPD by classifying the disease into categories A to D provides a better diagnostic classification because it identifies more individuals at high risk of exacerbations than a previous classification based solely on the spirometric value [25]. However, contrary to expectations, hospital admissions due to COPD or all causes were higher in group B than in group C [25]. Moreover, survival in group C (high risk, poor lung function, and fewer symptoms) with more severe COPD was higher than in group B (low risk, better lung function, more symptoms) with less severe COPD (Fig. 1.5) [25]. GOLD groups C and D are heterogeneous and composed of phenotypes with variable risk of exacerbations or death. Symptoms (X-axis) were defined by two different scores, CAT and mMRC, and the kappa agreement between CAT and mMRC ranged between 0.13 and 0.77 [26]. The use of CAT allowed the classification of most patients as having more symptoms (GOLD B or D), whereas mMRC provided a more homogeneous distribution

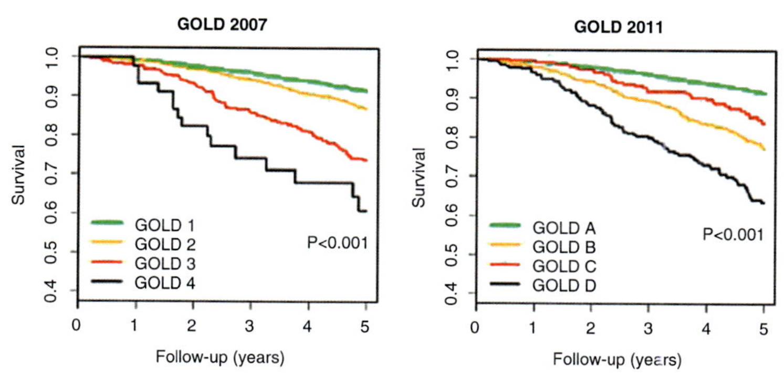

Fig. 1.5 Survival curves of COPD patients in spirometric GOLD2007 classification and combined assessment of GOLD2011 (Reproduced with permission from Ref. [25])

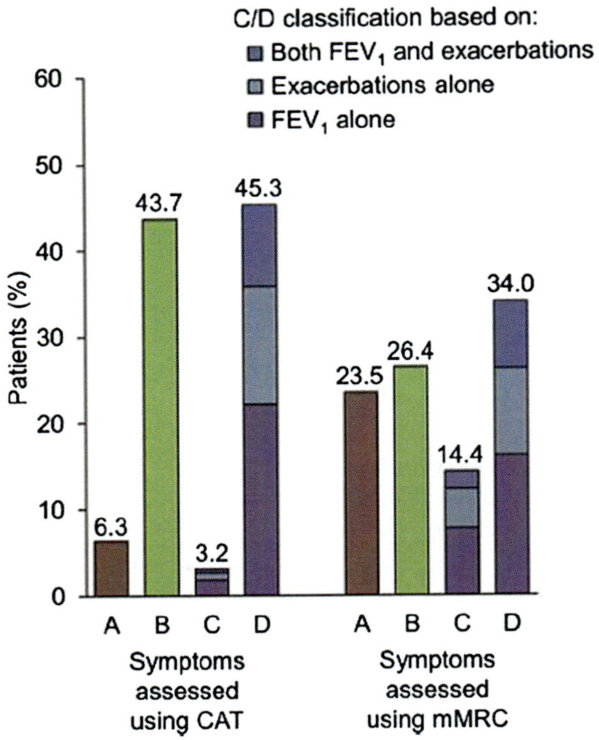

Fig. 1.6 Distribution of COPD severity assessed according to GOLD2011 by using CAT and mMRC (Reproduced with permission from Ref. [27])

(Fig. 1.6) [27]. Patients with COPD often present various comorbidities, such as cardiovascular disease, skeletal muscle dysfunction, metabolic syndrome, osteoporosis, depression, and lung cancer. These comorbidities can occur in patients with mild, moderate, or severe airflow limitation and influence hospitalization and mortality [28]. This discordance between groups B and C is most likely caused by the heterogeneous distribution of comorbidities, in particular cardiovascular disease [25]. In addition, poorer prognosis could be caused by cardiovascular disease or cancer. This result has also been confirmed in an ongoing, longitudinal, noninterventional study within the German COPD National Prospective Registry [27]. Although the GOLD guideline recommends paying attention to comorbidities, diagnosing them routinely, and treating them appropriately, the comorbid status was not included in the combined assessment of COPD (Fig. 1.3). The latest GOLD guideline was published in 2016 [29]. Although some parts of this report were partially changed, there were no drastic changes in the chapter on the diagnosis and assessment of COPD. Therefore, individual assessments that consider comorbidities should be developed. Moreover, several variables, including FEV1, exercise tolerance assessed by walking distance or peak oxygen consumption, weight loss, and reduction in arterial oxygen tension, can help identify patients at increased risk for mortality. The BODE index provides a composite score (for body mass index, obstruction, dyspnea, and exercise) that is a better predictor of subsequent survival than any component score in isolation [30], and other composite scores are being validated. Composite scores such as the BODE index may complement the current GOLD classification of severity independently or can be integrated into the GOLD classification of severity.

1.7 Conclusion

Since 2011, the combined assessment of COPD has been used to assess the severity of COPD. The predictivity of the combined assessment for exacerbation is better than that of previously used severity assessments that were based exclusively on spirometry values. The therapeutic option to control symptoms and prevent exacerbations is based on the combined assessment of COPD, and the latest GOLD classification of severity, based on this assessment, is still valid. However, the predictivity of the combined assessment for prognosis is not very precise because of other influencing factors such as comorbidities. Therefore, a revised classification of severity in future GOLD guidelines should take into consideration other factors.

References

1. Fukuchi Y, Nishimura M, Ichinose M, et al. COPD in Japan: the Nippon COPD Epidemiology study. Respirology. 2004;9(4):458–65.
2. Tsukamura M. Chronic obstructive lung disease. A statement of the committee on therapy. Am Rev Respir Dis. 1965;92:513–8.
3. Burrows B, Fletcher CM, Heard BE, et al. The emphysematous and bronchial types of chronic airways obstruction. A clinicopathological study of patients in London and Chicago. Lancet. 1966;1(7442):830–5.
4. Filley GF, Beckwitt HJ, Reeves JT, et al. Chronic obstructive bronchopulmonary disease. II. Oxygen transport in two clinical types. Am J Med. 1968;44(1):26–38.
5. Orie NG, Sluiter HJ, De Vries K, et al. The host factor in bronchitis. In: Orie NG, Sluiter HJ, editors. Bronchitis. Assen: Royal Van Gorcum; 1961. p. 43–59.
6. American Thoracic Society. A statement of the committee on therapy; Chronic obstructive lung disease. Am Rev Respir Dis. 1965;92:513–8.
7. Hogg JC, Macklem PT, Thurlbeck WM. Site and nature of airway obstruction in chronic obstructive lung disease. N Engl J Med. 1968;278(25):1355–60.
8. Hurst JR, Vestbo J, Anzueto A, et al. Susceptibility to exacerbation in chronic obstructive pulmonary disease. N Engl J Med. 2010;363(12):1128–38.
9. Jones PW, Harding G, Berry P, et al. Development and first validation of the COPD Assessment Test. Eur Respir J. 2009;34(3):648–54.
10. Nishimura K, Izumi T, Tsukino M, et al. Dyspnea is a better predictor of 5-year survival than airway obstruction in patients with COPD. Chest. 2002;121(5):1434–40.
11. Jones PW, Quirk FH, Baveystock CM. The St George's Respiratory Questionnaire. Respir Med. 1991;85:Suppl. B:25–31.
12. Larson JL, Covey MK, Berry JK, et al. Reliability and validity of the Chronic Respiratory Disease Questionnaire. Am Rev Respir Dis. 1993;147:A530.

13. van der Molen T, Willemse BW, Schokker S, et al. Development, validity and responsiveness of the Clinical COPD Questionnaire. Health Qual Life Outcomes. 2003;1:13.
14. Rodriguez-Roisin R. Toward a consensus definition for COPD exacerbations. Chest. 2000;117:398S–401.
15. Burge S, Wedzicha JA. COPD exacerbations: definitions and classifications. Eur Respir J Suppl. 2003;41:46s–53.
16. Celli BR, Barnes PJ. Exacerbations of chronic obstructive pulmonary disease. Eur Respir J. 2007;29:1224–38.
17. Seemungal TA, Donaldson GC, Bhowmik A, et al. Time course and recovery of exacerbations in patients with chronic obstructive pulmonary disease. Am J Respir Crit Care Med. 2000;161:1608–13.
18. Kessler R, Stahl E, Vogelmeier C, et al. Patient understanding, detection, and experience of COPD exacerbations: an observational, interview-based study. Chest. 2006;130:133–42.
19. Donaldson GC, Seemungal TA, Bhowmik A, et al. Relationship between exacerbation frequency and lung function decline in chronic obstructive pulmonary disease. Thorax. 2002;57:847–52.
20. Connors Jr AF, Dawson NV, Thomas C, et al. Outcomes following acute exacerbation of severe chronic obstructive lung disease. The SUPPORT investigators (Study to understand prognoses and preferences for outcomes and risks of treatments). Am J Respir Crit Care Med. 1996;154:959–67.
21. Gunen H, Hacievliyagil SS, Kosar F, et al. Factors affecting survival of hospitalized patients with COPD. Eur Respir J. 2005;26:234–41.
22. Agusti A, Calverley PM, Celli B, et al. Characterizations of COPD heterogeneity in the ECLIPSE cohort. Respir Res. 2010;11:122.
23. Decramer M, Celli B, Kesten S, et al. Effect of tiotropium on outcomes in patients with moderate chronic obstructive pulmonary disease (UPLIFT): a prespecified subgroup analysis of a randomized controlled trial. Lancet. 2009;374:1171–8.
24. Jenkins CR, Jones PW, Calverley PM, et al. Efficacy of salmeterol/fluticasone propionate by GOLD stage of chronic obstructive pulmonary disease: analysis from the randomized, placebo-controlled TORCH study. Respir Res. 2009;10:59.
25. Lange P, Marott JL, Vestbo J, et al. Prediction of the clinical course of chronic obstructive pulmonary disease, using the new GOLD classification: a study of the general population. Am J Respir Crit Care Med. 2012;186(10):975–81.
26. Karloh M, Mayer AF, Maurici R, et al. The COPD Assessment Test: what do we know so far?: a systematic review and meta-analysis about clinical outcomes prediction and classification of patients into GOLD stages. Chest. 2016;149(2):413–25.
27. Worth H, Buhl R, Criée CP, et al. The 'real-life' COPD patient in Germany: the DACCORD study. Respir Med. 2016;111:64–71.
28. Mannino DM, Thorn D, Swensen A, et al. Prevalence and outcomes of diabetes, hypertension and cardiovascular disease in COPD. Eur Respir J. 2008;32(4):962–9.
29. Global strategy for the diagnosis, management, and prevention of chronic obstructive pulmonary disease. http://www.goldcopd.org/guidelines-global-strategy-for-diagnosis-management.html.
30. Celli BR, Cote CG, Marin JM, et al. The body-mass index, airflow obstruction, dyspnea, and exercise capacity index in chronic obstructive pulmonary disease. N Engl J Med. 2004;350:1005–12.

Chapter 2
Epidemiology of COPD: Why Is the Disease So Poorly Recognized?

Yoko Shibata

Abstract COPD is currently ranked third in the cause of death around the world. The habit of smoking cigarettes is obviously related to occurrence of COPD, and many cases of COPD are caused by heavy cigarette smoking. However, besides cigarette smoking, occupational exposure to airborne particulates and pollutants are also known to be risk factors for developing COPD. Particularly, the indoor use of biomass fuel has been pointed out as one of the major risk factors for the occurrence COPD in developing countries. COPD develops after a long period of exposure to cigarette smoke; thus, it is characterized by a gradual progression of symptoms. Many patients are not diagnosed with COPD until their symptoms have considerably worsened or acute exacerbation due to respiratory inflammation. Health damage by COPD has a great impact on society as well as on the individual patient; hence, it is important to make a diagnosis early and prevent patients from exposure to risk factors.

Keywords Epidemiology • Incidence • Prevalence • Decline in FEV1 • Cigarette smoking • Biomass fuel

2.1 Introduction

COPD is a lifestyle-related disease developed due to damage in airway and alveoli after toxic particle inhalation, including long-term cigarette smoke. Chronic airway inflammation by cigarette smoking causes peripheral airway wall thickening and increase of airway secretions, moreover, destruction of the alveolar wall leading to, especially, elastic fiber fragmentation. This causes a loss of alveolar attachment in the peripheral airways, resulting in the reduction of elasticity of the alveolar wall itself. A series of these changes increases peripheral airway resistance, and then causes airflow obstruction upon expiration. This airflow obstruction leads to a

Y. Shibata (✉)
Department of Cardiology, Pulmonology and Nephrology, Yamagata University School of Medicine, 2-2-2 Iida-Nishi, Yamagata City, Yamagata 990-9585, Japan
e-mail: shibata@med.id.yamagata-u.ac.jp

H. Nakamura, K. Aoshiba (eds.), *Chronic Obstructive Pulmonary Disease*, Respiratory Disease Series: Diagnostic Tools and Disease Managements, DOI 10.1007/978-981-10-0839-9_2

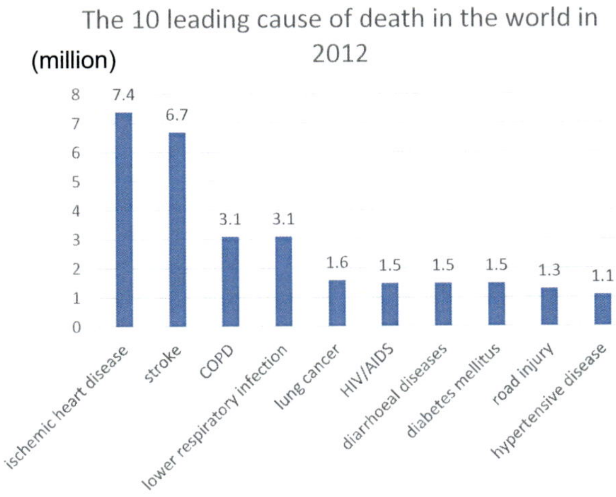

Fig. 2.1 Top 10 cause of death in the world in 2012 (World Health Organization reported COPD as top 3 cause of death in the world in 2012 http://www.who.int/mediacentre/factsheets/fs310/en/)

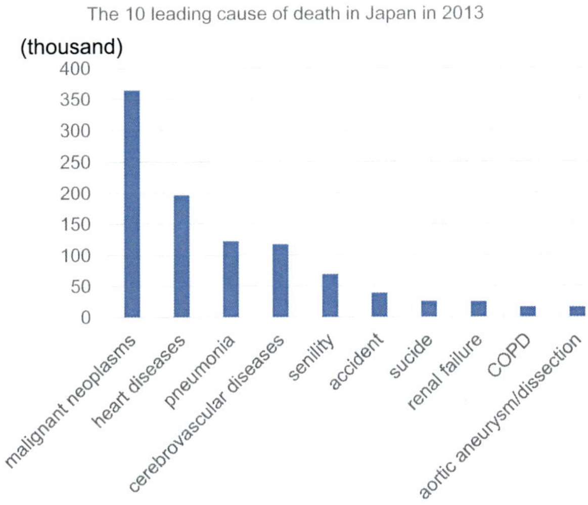

Fig. 2.2 Top 10 cause of death in Japan in 2013 (Japanese Ministry of Health, Labour and Welfare reported COPD as top 9 cause of death in Japan in 2013. http://www.mhlw.go.jp/toukei/saikin/hw/jinkou/kakutei13/dl/10_h6.pdf)

symptom of dyspnea through air trapping in the lung. In COPD, inflammation as well as chronic airway inflammation spills over throughout the body causing various concomitant diseases and, then finally, exacerbates patient health conditions [1].

According to a WHO report, COPD is currently ranked third in the cause of death around the world (Fig. 2.1). In Japan, it is the seventh cause of death in men and sixteenth in women and the ninth for the overall population (Fig. 2.2). The association between cigarette smoking and COPD is clear. It is known that the increase in mortality rate of COPD was 30 years behind the increase in the cigarette smoking rate. As the cigarette smoking rate in Japan is still high compared to

Western countries, the impact of COPD on society is assumed to continue for the time being.

2.2 Risk Factors of COPD

2.2.1 Cigarette Smoking

It is known that pulmonary function in patients with COPD declines over time due to cigarette smoking [2]. In a recently conducted Framingham cohort study, decline over time in forced expiratory volume in one second (FEV1) was 38.2 mL/year [95 % confidence interval (CI), 33.9–42.6] in male smokers and 23.9 mL/year (95 % CI, 20.9–27.0) in female smokers, while it was 19.6 (95 % CI, 17.1–22.1) and 17.6 (95 % CI, 13.8–21.4) mL/year, respectively, in male and female nonsmokers [3]. In many clinical studies, FEV1 reduction over time was often 50–60 mL/year in untreated patients with COPD [4]. In short, it can be readily assumed that early identification of COPD and early achievement of smoking cessation are critical in individuals with high risk of COPD.

2.2.2 Other Risk Factors

A recent review article indicated that almost half of COPD cases had causes other than cigarette smoking [5]. In addition, an epidemiological study conducted in the USA, the UK, and Spain reported that the prevalence of COPD was about 23 % in nonsmokers [5]. In a regional epidemiological study conducted in Takahata in Yamagata Prefecture, airflow obstruction (FEV1/forced vital capacity (FVC) under 70 %) was found in 10 % overall, 16 % of male, and 6 % of female adults over 40 years old, while nonsmokers accounted for 6 % overall, 8 % of males, and 5 % of females [6]. Although a high percentage of nonsmokers was observed in especially women with airflow obstruction, in fact, almost half of men with airflow obstruction were also nonsmokers. Risk factors for COPD other than habitual cigarette smoking may include genetic predisposition, environmental factors, and social status.

2.2.2.1 Genetic Factors

As for genetically developing COPD, an α1-antitrypsin deficiency is a factor that is well known. However, it is less frequent in Japan, and so it is not sufficient to explain many cases of COPD development in nonsmokers. Recently, results of a genome-wide association study highlighted several disease candidate genes

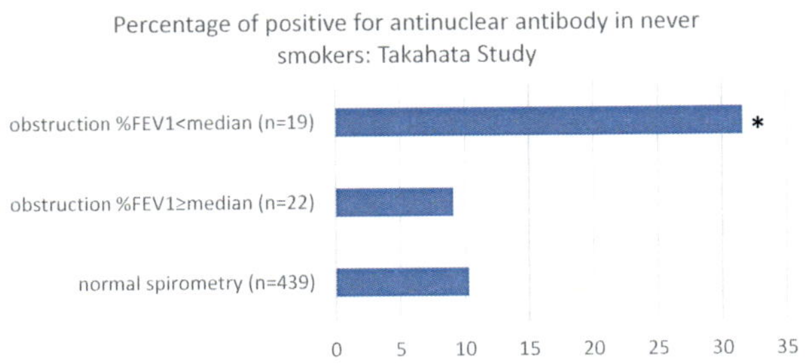

Fig. 2.3 Percentage of positive for antinuclear antibody in male never-smokers: Takahata study (Antinuclear antibody levels were determined by MESACUP ANA EIA kit which can measure antibodies to several connective tissue disease antigens (ACTDA). An ACTDA index $\geq$20.0 was defined as positive [9]) (*$P < 0.05$ Chi-square test)

[7]. However, odds ratio having risk allele for developing COPD is not high enough, and a causal relation between disease candidate genes and the development of COPD is far from proven. Thus, disease candidate genes should be considered as one risk factor.

The association of advanced airway hypersensitivity to COPD is also known. In a cohort study conducted in the USA among 3099 subjects over 20 years, patients with asthma had 10 times higher likelihood of symptoms of chronic bronchiolitis and 17 times higher likelihood of progression to pulmonary emphysema [5].

Recently, the contribution of autoimmunity to COPD pathology was reported [8]. The Takahata study investigated the proportion of subjects testing positive for antinuclear antibodies in a regional population [9]. In males, a negative correlation between antinuclear antibodies and FEV1 was observed, and a positive rate of antinuclear antibodies was significantly higher in the severe airflow obstruction group than in the no/weak airflow obstruction group in male nonsmokers (Fig. 2.3). In other words, upregulated autoimmunity was suggested to be a risk factor for developing COPD.

2.2.2.2 Environmental Factors

Occupational Airborne Particles

Occupational exposure to airborne particles can occur in various occupations. Some particles are considered to have a higher risk of developing COPD than cigarette smoking. In addition to tunnel excavation and mining-related inhalation of metallic substances, plastics, rubber, leather, and food may be the source of occupational airborne particles [10].

Air Pollution

Air pollution is roughly divided into indoor and outdoor air pollutants.

Indoor Air Pollutants

When biomass fuel is used, indoor air pollutant levels are much higher than that of the air outside. The indoor use of biomass fuel is less frequent in developed countries, while more than 90 % of individuals in rural areas use biomass fuel in developing countries; thus, half of the world population is burning biomass fuel [11]. The prevalence rate of COPD due to biomass fuel smoke in Turkish women is reported to be 23 % [5].

Wood, charcoal, and coal are used as biomass fuel, resulting in the production of hazardous substances including particulate matter (PM), carbon monoxide, nitrogen dioxide, sulfur dioxide, formaldehyde, polycyclic organic compounds, and acrolein [11]. In one meta-analysis, risk of COPD due to exposure to biomass fuel smoke was 2.44 times higher (95 % CI, 1.9–3.33) in the overall population, 4.30 times higher (95 % CI, 1.85–10.01) in males, 2.73 times higher (95 % CI, 2.28–3.28) in females, 2.31 times higher (95 % CI, 1.41–3.78) in Asian subjects, and 2.56 times higher (95 % CI, 1.71–3.83) in non-Asian subjects [12]. Smoking cigarettes further increases the risk more than 4 times [13]. The use of biomass fuel is associated with an increase in the number of individuals with respiratory symptoms, decrease of pulmonary function, and progression of COPD, and this effect is related to the magnitude of exposure to smoke and the duration of exposure [13].

As for other indoor air-polluting substances, secondary cigarette smoke, nitrogen dioxide, and mold are also reported to be associated with COPD. An increase in passive smoke exposure is associated with increased risk of COPD [14]. In a recent report from Sweden, the prevalence of COPD in nonsmokers was 4.2 % in subjects without passive cigarette smoke exposure, 8.0 % in subjects breathing passive cigarette smoke at home, 8.3 % in subjects with cigarette smoke exposure at their previous workplace, and 14.7 % in subjects with cigarette smoke exposure at home and at both previous and current workplaces [15].

Outdoor Air Pollution

Air-polluting substances are produced with the use of biomass fuel at home, industrial gases, and the exhaust from motor vehicles. Nitrogen dioxide, ozone, and PM are typical substances [16]. Recently, fine PM ($PM_{2.5}$) blowing in from China has drawn attention as an environmental issue, and its harmful effect on the health of Japanese citizens is concerning. Causality between air pollution and COPD has not been fully elucidated; thus, air pollution is considered to be one of the risk factors for developing COPD. In a cohort study conducted among individuals without diagnosed COPD in Vancouver, Canada, elevation in black carbon concentrations in ambient air was associated with an increase in COPD hospitalizations and COPD mortality during the follow-up period, and exposure to higher levels of wood smoke pollution was associated with an increase in COPD hospitalizations [17]. Moreover, it was reported that in women living less than 100 m from a busy road, COPD was 1.79 times more likely than for women living farther away, as epidemiological data suggesting an association between air pollutants from motor vehicles and COPD [16].

2.2.2.3 Low Socioeconomic Status

Prevalence of COPD patients caused by extreme malnutrition, low intake of antioxidant-rich food, and poor living environment are currently not fully assessed in Japan. It is hard to evaluate this, because groups that have a lower socioeconomic status are less likely to visit medical institutions, and they are more frequently exposed to cigarette smoke.

2.3 Decline in FEV1 in Patients with COPD

A large-scale clinical study reported a greater decline in pulmonary function in patients with COPD in the early stages of airflow obstruction [18]. In addition, a greater decline in pulmonary function was indicated in subjects with milder airflow obstruction in a recent clinical study conducted in subjects with an average age of about 60 years [19]. On the other hand, a clinical study conducted in subjects with an average age of about 50 years revealed a greater decline in pulmonary function in subjects with severe airflow obstruction [20]. This may be because, in natural history of COPD development, a rapid decline in pulmonary function occurs in earlier stage of the disease, and then this decline is slowed once a certain age has been reached partly due to cessation of smoking or reduction of cigarette inhalation per day.

Nishimura et al. reported a decline in pulmonary function in patients with COPD in a Hokkaido COPD cohort study (Japan) [21]. This study indicated that patients with COPD consisted of "pulmonary function sustainers" whose pulmonary function was less likely to deteriorate over time and "pulmonary function decliners" whose pulmonary function did deteriorate over time. In other words, deterioration over time of pulmonary function in patients with COPD may not be uniform. A recent report from Lange et al. also indicated that not all COPD developed because of a rapid decline in FEV1, but individuals whose pulmonary function declined originally in their youth developed COPD through a slow decline in FEV1 due to persistent smoking [22].

2.4 Incidence of COPD

Although the investigative method varies widely among studies, the prevalence rate of COPD is reported to be between 2.8 and 15.7 (1000 person-years) [23]. A report from Japan identified that the prevalence rate per 1000 person-years was 8.1 (95 % CI, 7.3–8.9) in males and 3.1 (95 % CI, 2.4–3.8) in females despite there being few epidemiological studies investigating COPD prevalence rates in Japan [24].

2.5 Prevalence of COPD

The COPD prevalence rate is high globally. The PLATINO study and the BOLD study are studies representative of COPD. In the former study, a positive rate of airflow obstruction after inhalation of a bronchodilator was investigated in several cities in Latin American countries, and positive rates were reported as 7.8–19.4 % [25]. The latter study examined the prevalence rate of stage II or higher COPD in the criteria of Global Initiative for Chronic Obstructive Lung Disease (GOLD) in subjects 40 years or older in Western countries and reported that the prevalence rate was 16.4 %, 8.5 %, and 10.4 % in men, women, and the overall population [26].

In Japan, a positive rate of airflow obstruction in subjects 40 years or older was investigated in the NICE study between September and December 2000 without inhaling bronchodilator. In this study, randomly selected general citizens were enrolled to conform to the population rate by age structure in Japan, and spirometry was performed in 2343 subjects in 35 medical facilities in 18 prefectures. As a result, airflow obstruction was indicated in 16.4 %, 5.0 %, and 10.9 % of males, females, and the overall population [27]. When excluding airflow obstruction due to asthma, the COPD prevalence rate was 8.6–10.9 %.

There are only a few studies reporting prevalence rate of airflow obstruction in regional general populations in Japan. Osaka et al. reported that spirometry (without the use of a bronchodilator) was performed in a regional annual health check in Takahata (hereafter referred to as the Takahata study) from 2004 to 2006 [6]. The Takahata study indicated that the FEV1 percentage predicted decreased with age in cigarette smokers in both males and females (Fig. 2.4). Airflow obstruction was observed in 16.4 % in males, 5.8 % in females, and 10.6 % in overall subjects 40 years or older participating in the regional annual health check [6]. As shown in Fig. 2.5, the prevalence of airflow obstruction increased with age. Airflow obstruction was observed especially in approximately 25 % of males 70 years or older [6]. The prevalence of airflow obstruction in males 70 years or older increased to approximately 35 % when they were former/current smokers [6]. Moreover, the number of patients with moderate to severe airflow obstruction rapidly increased in subjects 50 years or older [6].

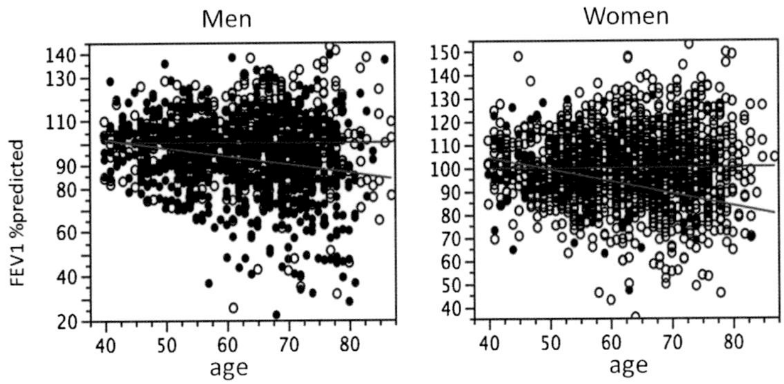

Fig. 2.4 Relationship between forced expiratory volume in 1 s (FEV1) and age in never-smokers and smokers: Takahata study (Correlation of age and FEV1 % predicted are shown. Both in males (*left panel*) and females (*right panel*), FEV1 in smokers were reduced according to the age elevation.) (*Open circle* never-smoker, *closed* past or active smokers, *red line* regression line of never-smokers, *blue line* regression line of past or active smokers [6])

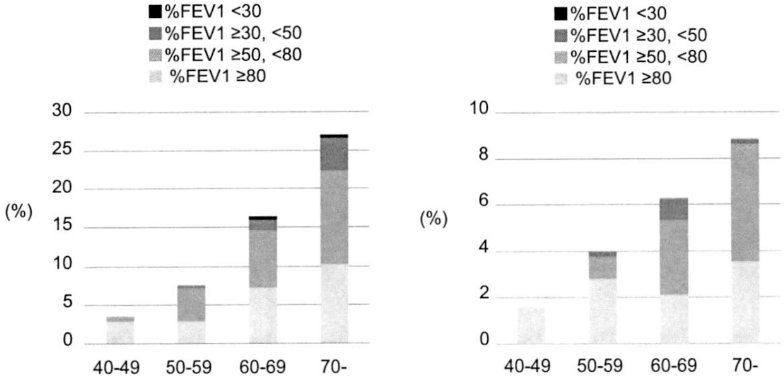

Fig. 2.5 Prevalence rate of airflow obstruction according to age (The prevalence rate of airflow obstruction increased with age. *Left panel* males, *right panel* females [6])

2.6 Undiagnosed COPD

The COPD prevalence in the abovementioned NICE study suggested that more than five million patients with COPD potentially exist in Japan; however, the number of outpatients with COPD was reported to be approximately 200,000 in a patient survey conducted by the Ministry of Health, Labour and Welfare. Therefore, COPD may have not been appropriately diagnosed in Japan. In NICE study, only 9.4 % cases with airflow limitation reported a previous diagnosis of COPD [27]. It is indicated that underdiagnosis of COPD is not an issue unique to Japan but is present around the world. In 20,050 patients analyzed in the NHANES III, spirometry detected impaired pulmonary function in 6.8 %, and 63.3 % of these had never been diagnosed with obstructive lung disease [28]. Lamprecht et al. integrated data from the BOLD, PLATINO, EPI-SCAN, and PREPOCOL studies and reported that 81.4 % of patients with COPD who were diagnosed using spirometry had not previously been diagnosed as COPD [29].

COPD is a chronic disease which progresses through changes in lung tissues and pathology over a long time period due to long-term exposure to cigarette smoke [30]. Because of its slow progression, it is often hard for patients with COPD to recognize that they "have a disease" based on their symptoms. For example, undiagnosed patients with COPD may not think they have a lung disease even though they have chronic symptoms such as cough or sputum production, because they often think those symptoms were caused by smoking [31]. In addition, although they have exertional dyspnea, they often do not think they have lung disease because they think that their exertional dyspnea was caused by aging. In many cases, they finally visited a medical institution when exertional dyspnea had considerably worsened, or they were diagnosed with COPD with acute exacerbation that is triggered by respiratory inflammation. Balcells et al. reported that one third of patients hospitalized for the first time for acute exacerbation of COPD had not been previously diagnosed with COPD before hospitalization [32].

2.7 Impact of COPD on Health Status in the General Population

Worldwide deaths from COPD show a tendency toward increase. The total mortality of COPD continued to increase, exceeding 16,000 deaths (12,669 deaths in males and 3606 deaths in females) in 2010 in Japan as well due to aging. The crude death rate by COPD also exceeded 13.2 per 100,000 population in 2011. COPD itself can be a cause of death; however, it is accompanied by various comorbidities which have an impact on health conditions that result in death in some cases. COPD is ranked high on the list of cause of life lost in the disability-adjusted life year [DALY: designed as a composite indicator to quantify the burden of disease and damage on each health problem, calculated as the sum of the years of life lost due to premature mortality (YLL) and the years lost due to disability (YLD)] and is predicted to rank fifth in 2020.

COPD can be accompanied by various diseases, and concomitant COPD is reported to cause an increase of the length of hospital stay in patients with each disease. In the Lung Health Study which enrolled patients with COPD suffering from moderate to severe airflow obstruction, an analysis of death revealed that lung cancer, cardiovascular disease, and respiratory failure were the main causes of death [33]. In the abovementioned Hokkaido cohort study, lung cancer and respiratory failure were main causes of death, showing relatively fewer cardiovascular deaths compared to the Lung Health studies conducted in Western countries [21]. We performed a pulmonary function test in approximately 3000 regional

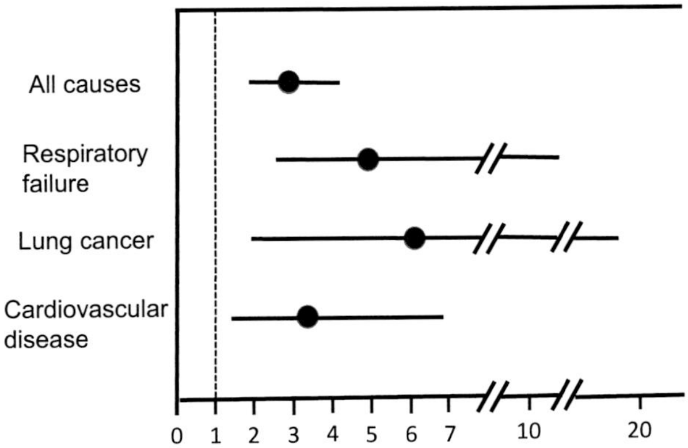

Fig. 2.6 Increase in relative risk of death with airflow obstruction (References were the mortality risk of the subjects without airflow obstruction [34])

subjects and performed follow-up for 7 years, and about 120 subjects had died. In the group consisting of subjects with airflow obstruction suggesting COPD, a majority of the causes of death included pneumonia, lung cancer, and cardiovascular diseases [34] (Fig. 2.6).

2.8 Conclusions

Health damage by COPD has a great impact on society as well as on the individual patient. However, many patients with COPD remain undiagnosed all over the world. Thus, those patients continue to smoke cigarettes despite their developing disease. The early diagnosis and provision of antismoking education to prevent patients from exposure to risk factors are necessary to reduce health damage due to COPD. However, it is reported that many cigarette smokers do not give serious consideration to giving up smoking, and screening such as that for pulmonary function is not necessarily associated with success in quitting. This issue may not be solved by mere medical intervention alone, in which disease is detected in the early stages and antismoking education is provided. Social intervention or establishing stricter regulations on smoking such as raising the tax rate on cigarettes may be required.

References

1. Barnes PJ, Celli BR. Systemic manifestations and comorbidities of COPD. Eur Respir J. 2009;33:1165–85.
2. Fletcher C, Peto R. The natural history of chronic airflow obstruction. Br Med J. 1977;1:1645–8.

3. Kohansal R, Martinez-Camblor P, Agusti A, Buist AS, Mannino DM, Soriano JB. The natural history of chronic airflow obstruction revisited: an analysis of the Framingham offspring cohort. Am J Respir Crit Care Med. 2009;180:3–10.
4. Calverley PM, Anderson JA, Celli B, Ferguson GT, Jenkins C, Jones PW, Yates JC, Vestbo J. Salmeterol and fluticasone propionate and survival in chronic obstructive pulmonary disease. N Engl J Med. 2007;356:775–89.
5. Salvi SS, Barnes PJ. Chronic obstructive pulmonary disease in non-smokers. Lancet. 2009;374:733–43.
6. Osaka D, Shibata Y, Abe S, Inoue S, Tokairin Y, Igarashi A, Yamauchi K, Kimura T, Sato M, Kishi H, Takabatake N, Sata M, Watanabe T, Konta T, Kawata S, Kato T, Kubota I. Relationship between habit of cigarette smoking and airflow limitation in healthy Japanese individuals: the Takahata study. Intern Med. 2010;49:1489–99.
7. Todd JL, Goldstein DB, Ge D, Christie J, Palmer SM. The state of genome-wide association studies in pulmonary disease: a new perspective. Am J Respir Crit Care Med. 2011;184:873–80.
8. Curtis JL, Freeman CM, Hogg JC. The immunopathogenesis of chronic obstructive pulmonary disease: insights from recent research. Proc Am Thorac Soc. 2007;4:512–21.
9. Nakano H, Shibata Y, Inoue S, Igarashi A, Yamauchi K, Abe S, Sato M, Aida Y, Nunomiya K, Kimura T, Nemoto T, Watanabe T, Konta T, Ueno Y, Kato T, Kayama T, Kubota I. Relationships between values of antibodies to several connective tissue disease autoantigens and pulmonary function in a Japanese general population: the Takahata Study. PLoS One. 2013;8, e81678.
10. Hulin M, Simoni M, Viegi G, Annesi-Maesano I. Respiratory health and indoor air pollutants based on quantitative exposure assessments. Eur Respir J. 2012;40:1033–45.
11. Laumbach RJ, Kipen HM. Respiratory health effects of air pollution: update on biomass smoke and traffic pollution. J Allergy Clin Immunol. 2012;129:3–11; quiz 12–13.
12. Hu G, Zhou Y, Tian J, Yao W, Li J, Li B, Ran P. Risk of COPD from exposure to biomass smoke: a metaanalysis. Chest. 2010;138:20–31.
13. Diette GB, Accinelli RA, Balmes JR, Buist AS, Checkley W, Garbe P, Hansel NN, Kapil V, Gordon S, Lagat DK, Yip F, Mortimer K, Perez-Padilla R, Roth C, Schwaninger JM, Punturieri A, Kiley J. Obstructive lung disease and exposure to burning biomass fuel in the indoor environment. Glob Heart. 2012;7:265–70.
14. Jordan RE, Cheng KK, Miller MR, Adab P. Passive smoking and chronic obstructive pulmonary disease: cross-sectional analysis of data from the Health Survey for England. BMJ Open. 2011;1, e000153.
15. Hagstad S, Bjerg A, Ekerljung L, Backman H, Lindberg A, Ronmark E, Lundback B. Passive smoking exposure is associated with increased risk of COPD in never-smokers. Chest. 2013;145(6):1298–304.
16. Ko FW, Hui DS. Air pollution and chronic obstructive pulmonary disease. Respirology. 2012;17:395–401.
17. Gan WQ, FitzGerald JM, Carlsten C, Sadatsafavi M, Brauer M. Associations of ambient air pollution with chronic obstructive pulmonary disease hospitalization and mortality. Am J Respir Crit Care Med. 2013;187:721–7.
18. Tashkin DP, Celli B, Senn S, Burkhart D, Kesten S, Menjoge S, Decramer M. A 4-year trial of tiotropium in chronic obstructive pulmonary disease. N Engl J Med. 2008;359:1543–54.
19. Mohamed Hoesein FA, Zanen P, Boezen HM, Groen HJ, van Ginneken B, de Jong PA, Postma DS, Lammers JW. Lung function decline in male heavy smokers relates to baseline airflow obstruction severity. Chest. 2012;142:1530–8.
20. Drummond MB, Hansel NN, Connett JE, Scanlon PD, Tashkin DP, Wise RA. Spirometric predictors of lung function decline and mortality in early chronic obstructive pulmonary disease. Am J Respir Crit Care Med. 2012;185:1301–6.
21. Nishimura M, Makita H, Nagai K, Konno S, Nasuhara Y, Hasegawa M, Shimizu K, Betsuyaku T, Ito YM, Fuke S, Igarashi T, Akiyama Y, Ogura S. Annual change in pulmonary

function and clinical phenotype in chronic obstructive pulmonary disease. Am J Respir Crit Care Med. 2012;185:44–52.
22. Lange P, Celli B, Agusti A, Boje Jensen G, Divo M, Faner R, Guerra S, Marott JL, Martinez FD, Martinez-Camblor P, Meek P, Owen CA, Petersen H, Pinto-Plata V, Schnohr P, Sood A, Soriano JB, Tesfaigzi Y, Vestbo J. Lung-function trajectories leading to chronic obstructive pulmonary disease. N Engl J Med. 2015;373:111–22.
23. Rycroft CE, Heyes A, Lanza L, Becker K. Epidemiology of chronic obstructive pulmonary disease: a literature review. Int J Chron Obstruct Pulmon Dis. 2012;7:457–94.
24. Kojima S, Sakakibara H, Motani S, Hirose K, Mizuno F, Ochiai M, Hashimoto S. Incidence of chronic obstructive pulmonary disease, and the relationship between age and smoking in a Japanese population. J Epidemiol. 2007;17:54–60.
25. Menezes AM, Perez-Padilla R, Jardim JR, Muino A, Lopez MV, Valdivia G, Montes de Oca M, Talamo C, Hallal PC, Victora CG. Chronic obstructive pulmonary disease in five Latin American cities (the PLATINO study): a prevalence study. Lancet. 2005;366:1875–81.
26. Buist AS, McBurnie MA, Vollmer WM, Gillespie S, Burney P, Mannino DM, Menezes AM, Sullivan SD, Lee TA, Weiss KB, Jensen RL, Marks GB, Gulsvik A, Nizankowska-Mogilnicka E. International variation in the prevalence of COPD (the BOLD Study): a population-based prevalence study. Lancet. 2007;370:741–50.
27. Fukuchi Y, Nishimura M, Ichinose M, Adachi M, Nagai A, Kuriyama T, Takahashi K, Nishimura K, Ishioka S, Aizawa H, Zaher C. COPD in Japan: the Nippon COPD Epidemiology study. Respirology. 2004;9:458–65.
28. Mannino DM, Gagnon RC, Petty TL, Lydick E. Obstructive lung disease and low lung function in adults in the United States: data from the National Health and Nutrition Examination Survey, 1988–1994. Arch Intern Med. 2000;160:1683–9.
29. Lamprecht B, Soriano JB, Studnicka M, Kaiser B, Vanfleteren LE, Gnatiuc L, Burney P, Miravitlles M, Garcia-Rio F, Akbari K, Ancochea J, Menezes AM, Perez-Padilla R, Montes de Oca M, Torres-Duque CA, Caballero A, Gonzalez-Garcia M, Buist S. Determinants of underdiagnosis of COPD in national and international surveys. Chest. 2015;148:971–85.
30. Decramer M, Cooper CB. Treatment of COPD: the sooner the better? Thorax. 2010;65:837–41.
31. Santos SR, Lizzi ES, Vianna EO. Characteristics of undiagnosed COPD in a senior community center. Int J Chron Obstruct Pulmon Dis. 2014;9:1155–61.
32. Balcells E, Gimeno-Santos E, de Batlle J, Ramon MA, Rodriguez E, Benet M, Farrero E, Ferrer A, Guerra S, Ferrer J, Sauleda J, Barbera JA, Agusti A, Rodriguez-Roisin R, Gea J, Anto JM, Garcia-Aymerich J. Characterisation and prognosis of undiagnosed chronic obstructive pulmonary disease patients at their first hospitalisation. BMC Pulm Med. 2015;15:4.
33. Anthonisen NR, Skeans MA, Wise RA, Manfreda J, Kanner RE, Connett JE. The effects of a smoking cessation intervention on 14.5-year mortality: a randomized clinical trial. Ann Intern Med. 2005;142:233–9.
34. Shibata Y, Inoue S, Igarashi A, Yamauchi K, Abe S, Aida Y, Nunomiya K, Sato M, Nakano H, Sato K, Nemoto T, Kimura T, Watanabe T, Konta T, Daimon M, Ueno Y, Kato T, Kayama T, Kubota I. A lower level of forced expiratory volume in 1 second is a risk factor for all-cause and cardiovascular mortality in a Japanese population: the Takahata study. PLoS One. 2013;8, e83725.

Part II
Genetic Predisposition and Pathogenic Mechanisms

Chapter 3
Genetic Predisposition to COPD: Are There Any Relevant Genes Determining the Susceptibility to Smoking?

Takeo Ishii and Koichi Hagiwara

Abstract Chronic obstructive pulmonary disease (COPD) is a complex disease with both genetic and environmental determinants, and case–control association studies on candidate genes and also genomic approaches such as genome-wide association studies (GWASs) have been used to discover genes involved in COPD pathogenesis. Though the 15q25 locus which encodes a family of nicotinic cholinergic receptors including *CHRNA3* and *CHRNA5* and also the other novel loci were reported to be associated with COPD susceptibility, it is uncertain through which molecular pathways the genetic variants of these genes affect the pathogenesis in a concrete manner and whether the genetic effects are on susceptibility to smoking behavior and/or to lung destruction as emphysematous change of the lungs induced by smoking. Recent studies showed the functional genetic variations related to COPD pathogenesis by using two different types of omics data, such as GWAS and gene expression profiling in the lungs. A recent study with more than 50,000 individuals of European ancestry in the United Kingdom investigated the genes associated with COPD and reported the genes related to nicotine addiction, impaired lung development, and accelerated lung function decline, respectively. The genetic variations associated with COPD exacerbations and the ethnic difference of COPD pathogenesis also should be elucidated.

Keywords Chronic obstructive pulmonary disease [COPD] • Exacerbations • Genome-wide association study (GWAS) • Omics • Smoking

T. Ishii, M.D., Ph.D. (✉)
Department of Pulmonary Medicine and Oncology, Graduate School of Medicine, Nippon Medical School, 4-7-15-8 F Kudan-Minami, Chiyoda, Tokyo 102-0074, Japan
e-mail: tishii@nms.ac.jp

K. Hagiwara
Comprehensive Medicine 1, Saitama Medical Center, Jichi Medical University, Saitama, Japan

H. Nakamura, K. Aoshiba (eds.), *Chronic Obstructive Pulmonary Disease*, Respiratory Disease Series: Diagnostic Tools and Disease Managements, DOI 10.1007/978-981-10-0839-9_3

3.1 Introduction

Chronic obstructive pulmonary disease (COPD) is a complex disease with both genetic and environmental determinants, the latter of which includes smoking as a main and critical one. First, the case–control genetic association studies on candidate genes possibly related to COPD were performed, and for these 10 years, genome-wide association studies (GWASs) have been used to discover genes involved in COPD pathogenesis. However, many problems remain to be resolved, including whether they affect COPD through smoking-related behaviors, lung development, and structural change of the lungs including emphysema and airway thickening and the way how these genetic variations found in GWAS affect COPD pathogenesis through molecular pathways. Since GWASs were performed on common genetic variations only, minor alleles related to COPD should be investigated with exome analyses or next-generation sequencing. In this chapter, we would like to describe the investigation on the genes related to COPD pathogenesis before and after GWAS and the future of this research field.

3.2 Investigation of the Genes Related to COPD Pathogenesis: The Era Before GWAS

Though tobacco smoking is the most important risk factor for COPD, only 15–20 % of heavy smokers develop symptomatic COPD, which suggests that susceptibility to COPD for each individual is, at least in part, genetically determined [1]. Epidemiological studies on familial aggregation of COPD demonstrate that there is a genetic component to COPD [2–4]. Severe alpha1-antitrypsin (AAT) deficiency, which is the result of mutations in the *SERPINA1* gene, is only known as a definite genetic risk factor of COPD and is mainly found in Caucasians. Since AAT deficiency accounts for approximately 1 % of COPD cases [5], genes other than *SERPINA1*, which are related to COPD pathogenesis, have been investigated so far.

However, it was (and is) uncertain whether chronic diseases including COPD have a few or many genetic factors related to susceptibility and whether common and/or rare genetic variants mainly affect the pathogenesis. Two main approaches to search for susceptibility genes of the diseases were linkage analysis and association analysis, and both of them utilize the fact that the genetic variation close to a disease gene is coinherited with the disease. In linkage analysis, usually highly polymorphic short tandem repeats (STRs), which are more informative than single-nucleotide polymorphisms (SNPs), are genotyped in families to identify the chromosomal region related to the disease or phenotype. In the association analysis, SNPs are genotyped in case and control groups, and the frequencies of genotypes and/or allele of the genes are compared. Genetic linkage analyses would be relatively useful for the study of the disorders related to single or a few genes. Generally, linkage analyses relatively have low statistical power for detecting genes with low to modest risk (RR < 1.5), and rare alleles with high penetrance and high risk as is typical for monogenetic diseases are more likely to be identified by the analyses [6]. Though COPD could be a syndrome with several diseases with symptom like cough, sputum, and dyspnea on exercise and also airflow obstruction and a part of COPD could be a monogenic disease like AAT deficiency, COPD mostly seems to be one of the multigenic diseases as similar to other common chronic diseases (e.g., hypertension, diabetes, osteoporosis, etc.) [7]. It is thought to be better to perform case–control association studies to investigate the susceptibility genes in polygenic diseases like COPD. Thus, linkage analyses were used to investigate the genes related to early-onset and severe COPD which is similar to AAT deficiency, and case–control association studies including GWAS were performed to find susceptibility genes of typical COPD, i.e., gradually progressing and/or relatively mild one.

The Boston Early-Onset COPD Study has reported linkage results identifying genomic regions that may harbor susceptibility genes for the development of COPD in 1998 or later [2, 8]. It could be speculated that early-onset COPD with extreme phenotype (i.e., severe airflow limitation) would be monogenic or oligogenic and that linkage analyses would be useful to find susceptibility genes of COPD with this kind of subjects as families. In this study, probands were ascertained on the basis of a physician diagnosis of severe COPD with forced expiratory volume in one second (FEV1) less than 40 % predicted at age younger than 53 without severe AAT deficiency. Linkage analyses for qualitative and quantitative COPD-related phenotypes including post-bronchodilator values for FEV1 and FEV1/forced vital capacity (FVC) have been performed with an autosomal 10 cM genome-wide scan of short tandem repeat for 585 members of 72 families [9, 10]. The genome-wide linkage analysis showed significant and suggestive linkage to mild-to-severe airflow obstruction as the logarithm of odds (LOD) score on chromosomes 1, 12, and 19 and linkage to FEV1/FVC on chromosome 2q. The approximate regions described above were also reported to be associated with lung function in the other groups with genome scans [11–13]. *SERPINE2* was reported as a positional candidate gene on chromosome 2q, which has been associated with COPD-related phenotypes in the Boston Early-Onset COPD Study and case–control studies [14–16]. However, the investigation of the molecular mechanism with *SERPINE2* on COPD pathogenesis has not progressed yet with in vitro or in vivo study with transgenic mice. *TGFB1* is also a positional candidate gene on chromosome 19, and the genetic variations of *TGFB1* were associated with COPD in several multiethnic populations [17–22]. It was reported that loss of integrin alpha(v)beta6-mediated TGF-beta activation causes Mmp12-dependent emphysema in mice model [23] and that the progression of emphysema could be overcome by simultaneous transgenic expression of active TGF-beta1.

In the common disease/common variant (CD/CV) hypothesis, proposed in the end of the 1990s, the genetic risk for common diseases will often be due to disease-predisposing alleles with relatively high frequencies, which was supported by several groups including Reich DE [24, 25]. COPD is one of the common chronic diseases, and its pathogenesis was thought to be under this hypothesis in that era

[26]. Thus, on genes speculated to be related to COPD pathogenesis with hypotheses, common (and mainly functional) genetic variations were searched through literature or by sequencing with samples of a small population, and the associations between these genetic variants and COPD were investigated as case–control association studies. A series of candidate genes were investigated under the several hypotheses speculated to be related to COPD pathogenesis, e.g., the protease-antiprotease hypothesis, the oxidant-antioxidant hypothesis, and the hypotheses on persistence of airway inflammation, aging, apoptosis, and autophagy (details of each hypothesis are described in Chaps. 4, 5, 6, and 7). The knowledge on emphysema formation in the cases with AAT deficiency lead to the protease-antiprotease hypothesis, and the oxidant-antioxidant hypothesis was proposed because oxidant stress is induced in the lungs by smoking, one of the main causes of COPD, and leads to destruction of the lung structure including emphysema formation. Case–control association studies were performed on the genes which were selected as candidate genes related to COPD pathogenesis under the hypotheses described above. In parallel, transgenic and knockout mice were produced on these genes to investigate whether these genes have critical roles in COPD pathogenesis and how they do if so. Many COPD-related genes were reported according to the results of these studies, and they include *SERPINA1* and matrix metalloproteinase 9 (*MMP9*) which is also related to severe COPD, reported based on GWAS [27, 28]. We also reported the association between genetic variations and emphysema by a case–control association study on a gene surfactant protein D (*SFTPD*) which is a candidate as a COPD-related gene [29]. Surfactant protein D belongs to a group of carbohydrate-binding proteins called collectins and is expressed primarily in type II alveolar cells [30]. It antagonizes inflammation by inhibiting oxidative stress [31, 32] and stimulating innate immunity [33]. *Sftpd* knockout mice develop emphysema, and alveolar macrophages from these *sftpd* knockout mice produced more H2O2 and matrix metalloproteinases 2, 9, and 12 compared with wild-type mice [34]. Thus, *SFTPD* is a good candidate gene related to COPD pathogenesis based on protease-antiprotease hypothesis and oxidant-antioxidant hypothesis and also through modification of susceptibility to pulmonary infection and COPD exacerbation. The single-nucleotide polymorphism (SNP) rs721917 in a coding region of *SFTPD* affects the amino acid sequence of this gene; two protein isoforms with different functions are derived from this SNP [35, 36]. The association between this SNP and emphysema, a major characteristic of COPD, was reported by our group with two Japanese populations [29] and also by Evaluation of COPD Longitudinally to Identify Predictive Surrogate End points (ECLIPSE) study with Caucasian populations [37]. Since the results of the association between genetic variations and COPD were not so consistent among the reports in general, meta-analyses by using these data were also performed on several genes [38]. Case–control association studies were performed on so many candidate genes, which was reviewed by myself [39] and recently by Bosse Y [38]. The genes related to COPD in several studies and also in a meta-analysis, e.g., *GSTM1* [40–42], are good candidates to investigate further on its role in pathogenesis of COPD, by in vitro study and/or in vivo study with transgenic mice or other mouse models, which could lead to innovative drug development.

3.3 Genome-Wide Association Studies (GWASs) for Susceptibility Genes of COPD

As written above, since COPD mostly seems to be one of the multigenic diseases as similar to other common chronic diseases (e.g., hypertension, diabetes, osteoporosis, etc.) [6], it is thought to be better to perform case–control association studies to investigate the susceptibility genes on COPD pathogenesis. However, it would be difficult to find novel genes related to susceptibility of the diseases if we perform case–control association studies under the proposed hypotheses. According to the common disease/common variant hypothesis [24], it was thought to be possible to find genes that are truly novel on relationship to the disease susceptibility by performing case–control association study with genotyping SNPs in a genome-wide manner. Genome-wide association studies (GWASs) were performed for more than 10 years to investigate the genes related to chronic common diseases including COPD. GWASs are the studies to see the association between quantitative or qualitative traits mainly of the diseases and SNPs in a genome-wide manner, and GWAS could be performed in a practical manner after human HapMap Project showed the allele frequency of the SNPs in a whole genome (not all SNPs but more than one million SNPs (approximately one tenth of the SNPs) with relatively high frequency) [43]. According to the HapMap data, the SNPs with allele frequency more than 5 % are selected (usually, approximately 200–500 thousand SNPs) in a genome-wide manner, and the association between all of these SNPs and disease phenotypes was investigated to find a novel disease susceptibility genotype. Usually, after this kind of GWAS, the results of the GWAS would be verified by the replicated genetic association between the same genotypes or alleles and the disease phenotypes in a different population, which leads the results of the study easy to confident.

The firstly reported group conducted a GWAS in a homogenous case–control cohort from Bergen, Norway [GenKOLS] (823 COPD cases and 810 smoking controls) and evaluated the top 100 SNPs in the family-based International COPD Genetics Network (ICGN, 1891 Caucasian individuals from 606 pedigrees) study [44]. The polymorphisms that showed replication were further evaluated in 389 subjects from the US National Emphysema Treatment Trial (NETT) and 472 controls from the Normative Aging Study (NAS) and then in a fourth cohort of 949 individuals from 127 extended pedigrees from the Boston Early-Onset COPD population. Two SNPs at the alpha-nicotinic acetylcholine receptor (*CHRNA3*/*CHRNA5*) locus were identified. They showed unambiguous replication in the ICGN family-based analysis and in the NETT case–control analysis with combined p-values of $1.48 \times 10(-10)$ (rs8034191) and $5.74 \times 10(-10)$ (rs1051730). Furthermore, these SNPs were significantly associated with lung function in both the ICGN and Boston Early-Onset COPD populations. The C allele of the rs8034191 SNP was estimated to have a population attributable risk for COPD of 12.2 %. The association of hedgehog-interacting protein (*HHIP*) locus on chromosome 4 was also consistently replicated, but did not reach genome-wide significance levels. Genome-wide significant association of the *HHIP* locus with lung function was identified in the

Framingham Heart Study [45]. Thus, they concluded that the *CHRNA3/CHRNA5* and the *HHIP* loci make a significant contribution to the risk of COPD.

Next, another genome-wide association study for chronic obstructive pulmonary disease (COPD) was performed. They hypothesized that a larger genome-wide association study would reveal additional common variants that contribute to COPD susceptibility. Their study included white subjects from three populations: (1) the case–control population from GenKOLS, (2) NETT cases and NAS controls, and (3) cases and controls from the ECLIPSE study, including 2940 cases and 1380 controls who were current or former smokers with normal lung function. They replicated the association with *CHRNA3/CHRNA5/IREB2* and *HHIP* loci and also identified a new susceptibility locus at 4q22.1 in *FAM13A* and replicated this association in one case–control group (n = 1006) and two family-based cohorts (n = 3808) (rs7671167, combined P = 1.2 × 10(−11), combined odds ratio in case–control studies 0.76, 95 % confidence interval 0.69–0.83) [46]. Further, they performed a GWAS again using a total of 3499 cases and 1922 control subjects from four cohorts: ECLIPSE, NAS and NETT, GenKOLS, and the COPDGene studies. Genotyping was performed with additional markers imputed using 1000 Genomes data [the 1000 Genomes Project reconstructed the genomes of 2504 individuals from 26 populations using a combination of low-coverage whole-genome sequencing, deep exome sequencing, and dense microarray genotyping and collected more data of SNP in a dense manner] [47]. This time they identified a new genome-wide significant locus on chromosome 19q13 (rs7937, OR = 0.74, P = 2.9 × 10(−9)) [48]. Genotyping this SNP and another nearby SNP in linkage disequilibrium in 2859 subjects from ICGN demonstrated supportive evidence for association for pre-bronchodilator FEV1 (P = 0.08 and 0.04) and severe (GOLD 3&4) COPD (P = 0.09 and 0.017). This region includes *RAB4B, EGLN2, MIA*, and *CYP2A6*, which has previously been identified in association with cigarette smoking behavior [49, 50]. In addition, they sought to identify risk loci for moderate to severe and severe COPD with data from these cohort studies described above. Analysis of 6633 individuals with moderate to severe COPD and 5704 control individuals confirmed association at three known loci, namely, C*HRNA3*, *FAM13A*, and *HHIP*. They also showed significant evidence of association at a novel locus near *RIN3* and also identified associations at two additional loci: *MMP12* and *TGFB2* [28].

The other group also performed meta-analyses of GWAS for airflow obstruction in population-based cohorts examining all participants, ever smokers, never smokers, and asthma-free participants, and the subset of more severe airflow obstruction with FEV1 less than 65% predicted [51]. For discovery phase, 3368 affected and 29,507 unaffected were studied, and the data on 3837 cases and 4479 control subjects were used for replication. These populations were different from those described above, but are also European descent. This study replicated the association between airflow obstruction and one region on chromosome 15q25.1 meeting genome-wide significance in ever smokers that includes *AGPHD1*, *IREB2*, and *CHRNA5/CHRNA3* genes. An SNP in *HTR4*, a gene previously related to FEV1/FVC [52, 53], achieved genome-wide statistical significance on airflow obstruction in ever smokers.

In summary, by performing several GWASs on COPD with populations of NETT, NAS, ECLIPSE study, Genetic Epidemiology of COPDGene Study, GenKOLS study, and others, each of which has several to 10 thousand subjects (mainly Caucasian), novel genes or chromosomal regions related to COPD pathogenesis reported were as follows [28, 44, 46, 48, 51] (Table 3.1 [54]): chromosomes 4q22 (*FAM13A*), 4q31 (*HHIP*), 15q25 (*CHRNA3/CHRNA5/IREB2*), 14q32 (*RIN3*), and 19q13. Chromosomal regions 11q22 (*MMP12*) and 1q41 (*TGFB2*) were also found to be associated with severe COPD by GWASs.

Though the genes or genotypes related to the susceptibility of COPD could have a critical role in COPD pathogenesis, the mechanism whether and how these genes or genetic variations affect the pathogenesis should be differently investigated. Current evidence in this research field is concisely reviewed in a recent article [56]. *CHRNA3* and *CHRNA5* are subunits of the nicotinic cholinergic receptor, and the proteins are responsive to nicotine. The association between nicotine addiction and genetic variants of these genes was also reported including GWAS (Fig. 3.1a) [49, 57, 58]. It was also reported by using *chrna5* knockout mice that nicotine activates the habenulo-interpeduncular pathway through alpha5-containing nAChRs, triggering an inhibitory motivational signal that acts to limit nicotine intake [59]. Thus, it is speculated that genetic variations of this gene affect COPD susceptibility through modifying the extent of nicotine dependence. Though this idea was supported also by the mediation analysis on previous GWAS, *CHRNA3* and *CHRNA5* possibly affect COPD pathogenesis through direct and indirect manner, as shown in Fig. 3.1b [60]. The SNPs of these genes are related to the expression level of *CHRNA3* and *IREB2* in blood and sputum samples [61]. *IREB2*

Table 3.1 Summary of the COPD GWASs

First authors of the studies and references	Number of cases	Number of controls	Novel genes or genomic regions related to COPD	Replicate genes or regions
Pillai [44]	823	810	*CHRNA3/CHRNA5/IREB, HHIP*	
Cho [46]	2940	1380	*FAM13A*	*CHRNA3/CHRNA5/IREB2, HHIP*
Cho [48]	3499	1922	Chromosome 19q13	*CHRNA3/CHRNA5/IREB2, HHIP, FAM13A*
Wilk [51]	3368	29,507	*HTR4*	*CHRNA3/CHRNA5/IREB2, HHIP*
Cho [28]	6633	5704	*RIN3*	*CHRNA3/CHRNA5/IREB2, HHIP, FAM13A*
Cho (on severe COPD) [28]	3125	1468	*MMP12, TGFB2*	*CHRNA3/CHRNA5/IREB2, HHIP, FAM13A*
Hobbs [100]	6161	6004	*IL27*	*CHRNA5, etc*

Modified the table in the Ref. [54], with permission

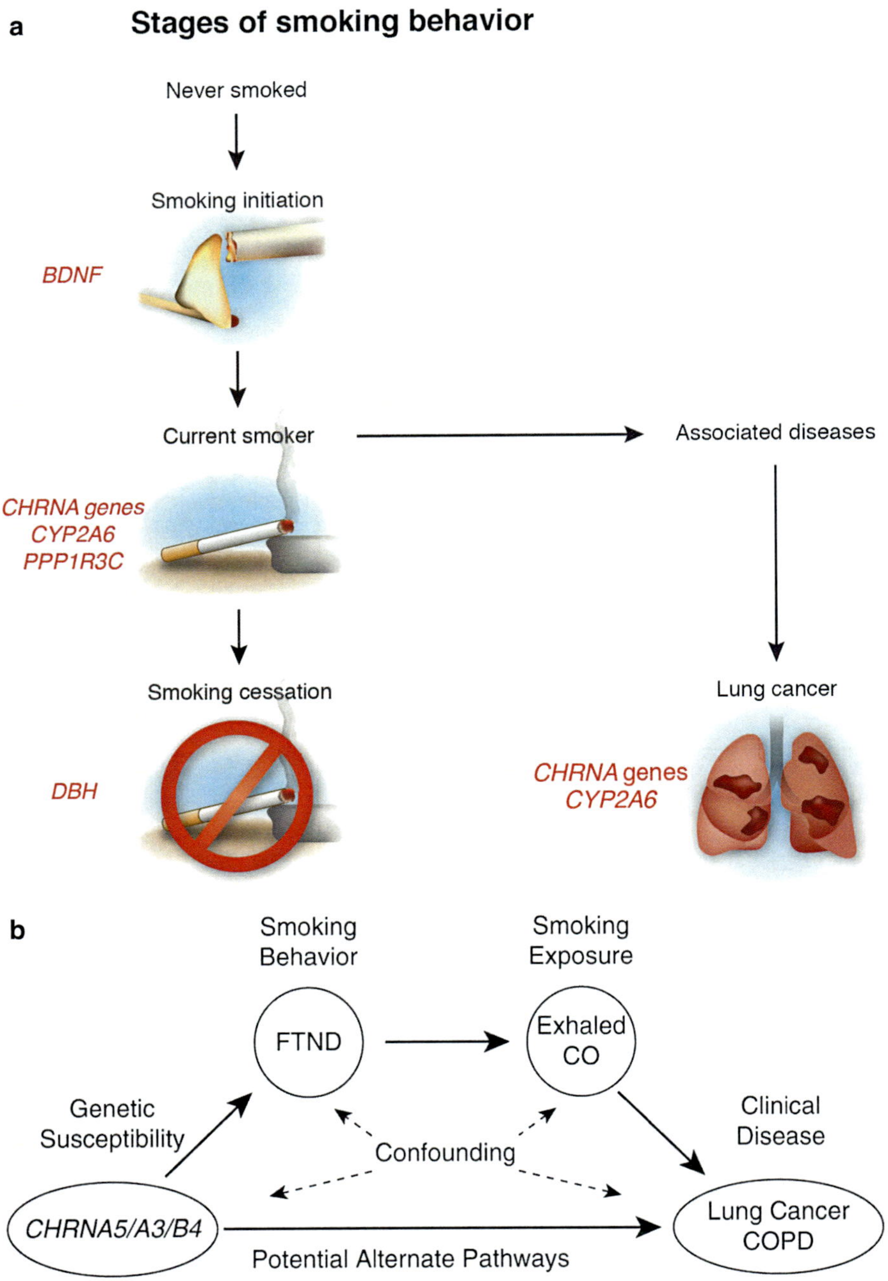

Fig. 3.1 Susceptibility genes on smoking and COPD. (**a**) The various phenotypes of smoking and the genes (*BDNF*, *CHRNA* genes, *CYP2A6*, and *PPP1R3C*) whose variations are related to these phenotypes (Reproduced with permission from Ref. [58]). (**b**) The model on the association between the genes related to smoking behavior (e.g., *CHRNA3*) and their direct and indirect effects on smoking-related diseases [60] (Reproduced with permission from the American Thoracic Society. Copyright © 2016 American Thoracic Society. Ann Am Thorac Soc. 2014 Sep;11(7):1082–3. Official Journal of the American Thoracic Society). FTND means Fagerstroem Test of Nicotine Dependence.

is a protein that binds iron-responsive elements which maintains cellular iron metabolism. Though mice with a targeted disruption of this gene *Ireb2* have been already generated, it was only reported that misregulation of iron metabolism leads to neurodegenerative disease and that there were no reports on COPD pathogenesis with these mice [62].

HHIP encodes a membrane glycoprotein that is an endogenous antagonist for the hedgehog pathway, which is critical for the morphogenesis of the lung and other organs. One of the COPD-related SNPs, rs1828591, is located in the enhancer region of *HHIP* and the expression of these protein non-tumor lung specimens reduced with the risk allele of this SNP [63]. Gene expression microarray analysis in a human bronchial epithelial cell line (Beas-2B) stably infected with *HHIP* shRNAs revealed that differential expression of the genes related to extracellular matrix and cell growth genes and these genes were also differentially expressed in lung tissues of COPD [64]. In mice with *hhip* haploinsufficiency exposed to cigarette smoking, severe airspace enlargement and enhanced lymphocyte activation pathways in lung tissues were observed [65].

The function of *FAM13A* is still largely unknown. However, it was reported that this protein is related to the activation of Wnt signaling pathway [66]. *FAM13A* was associated with pulmonary function in healthy and also asthmatic populations with GWAS [67], was associated with chronic bronchitis but not with emphysema [68], and was associated with idiopathic pulmonary fibrosis also with GWAS [69]. Thus, possibly this gene has a critical role in pathogenesis of various lung diseases, but in a complicated manner. Since knockout mice of *fam13a was recently generated* [66], the role of *FAM13A* on COPD pathogenesis could be further elucidated with this mice model in the near future. On the other genes, including *TGFB2* and *RIN3*, molecular mechanisms through which these genes affect COPD pathogenesis are still largely unknown.

3.4 Recent Progress of Studies of COPD Genetics in GWAS Era (I): Relevant Genes Determining the Susceptibility to Smoking

Since genes of nicotinic acetylcholine receptors, thought to be one of the critical factors affecting smoking behavior, were reported to be associated with COPD by GWASs with validation by using several populations [28, 44] as described above, it is speculated that relevant genes determining the susceptibility to smoking are also involved in COPD pathogenesis and progression in general. In addition, when we observed the association between genes related to smoking behavior like *CHRNA3*, it is a little unclear whether these genes affect COPD in a direct manner (e.g., by modifying the inflammation process in the local regions of the lungs) or in an indirect manner (e.g., by modifying susceptibility to smoking behavior). In fact, COPDGene and ECLIPSE investigators showed that the effects of two linked variants (rs1051730 and rs8034191) in the *AGPHD1/CHRNA3* cluster on COPD development were significantly, yet not entirely, mediated by the smoking-related phenotypes, and they confirmed the existence of direct effects of the *AGPHD1/CHRNA3*, *IREB2*, *FAM13A*, and *HHIP* loci on COPD development [70], as shown in Fig. 3.1b [60]. They also reported that the association of the *AGPHD1/CHRNA3* locus with COPD is significantly mediated by smoking-related phenotypes though *IREB2* appears to affect COPD independently of smoking [70]. Very recently, UK Biobank data were used to study the genetic causes of smoking behavior and lung health in UK Biobank Lung Exome Variant Evaluation (UK BiLEVE) study, and the study selected 50,008 unique samples which composed of 10 002 individuals with low FEV1, 10 000 with average FEV1, and 5002 with high FEV1 from each of the heavy-smoker and never-smoker groups [71] (Fig. 3.2 [72]). First, they showed a substantial sharing of genetic causes of low FEV1 between heavy smokers and never smokers and between individuals with and without doctor-diagnosed asthma. They also discovered six novel genome-wide significant signals of association with extremes of FEV1, including signals at four novel loci (*KANSL1*, *TSEN54*, *TET2*, and *RBM19/TBX5*) and independent signals at two previously reported loci (*NPNT* and *HLA-DQB1/HLA-DQA2*), and these variants also showed association with COPD, including in individuals with no history of smoking. In addition, they also discovered five new genome-wide significant signals for smoking behavior, including a variant in *NCAM1* and a variant on chromosome 2 (between *TEX41* and *PABPC1P2*) that has a trans effect on expression of *NCAM1* in brain tissue. This study is so unique especially on its design, namely, by sampling from the extremes of the lung function distribution in UK Biobank with a so large population. In summary, this study showed that *CHRNA3/CHRNA5* is associated with COPD pathogenesis through nicotine dependence, that *HHIP* is through disturbance of lung development, and that *GSTCD* and several other genes are through modification of oxidant stress and/or inflammation (Fig. 3.2) [72]. This study not only showed susceptibility genes of COPD but also successfully revealed how these genes affect COPD pathogenesis and suggests a new strategy on COPD genetics study with GWAS. Smoking behaviors include various phenotypes, including smoking initiation, increment of tobacco consumption, nicotine addiction, and smoking cessation, and these behaviors could be associated with different genes (Fig. 3.1a) [58]. Meta-analyses of genome-wide association studies for the number of cigarettes smoked per day (CPD) in smokers ($n = 31{,}266$) and smoking initiation ($n = 46{,}481$) using samples mainly from the ENGAGE Consortium and replication study with the Tobacco and Genetics (TAG) and Oxford-GlaxoSmithKline (Ox-GSK) consortium cohorts ($n = 45{,}691$ smokers) and also with a third sample of European ancestry ($n = 9040$) revealed the variants in three genomic regions associated with CPD, including previously identified SNPs at 15q25 represented by rs1051730[A] and SNPs at 19q13 and 8p11, where genes encoding nicotine-metabolizing enzymes (*CYP2A6* and *CYP2B6*) and nicotinic acetylcholine receptor subunits (*CHRNB3* and *CHRNA6*) are located [49]. Since *CHRNA3/CHRNA5* is only a gene related to both smoking behavior and COPD with GWAS, the other genes related to smoking behaviors, e.g., *CYP2A6*, could also have a critical role in

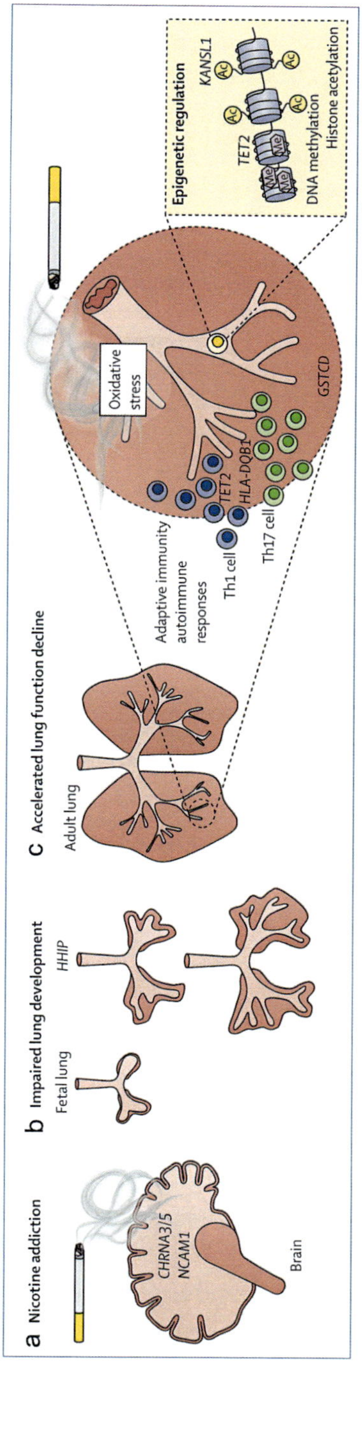

Fig. 3.2 The several processes of COPD pathogenesis and the results of a GWAS by UK BiLEVE (Reproduced with permission from Ref. [72])

COPD pathogenesis. Finding novel genes related to both smoking and COPD could be a supportive evidence that shows that therapeutics for nicotine addiction will also prevent from COPD and its progression, which leads to development of novel therapeutics for both smoking and COPD.

3.5 Recent Progress of Studies of COPD Genetics in GWAS Era (II): Gene Related to Critical Subtypes or Phenotypes of COPD

Though COPD is thought to result mostly from an accelerated decline in FEV1 over time (namely, the phenotype of "rapid decliner") which is possibly caused by smoking and also by frequent exacerbations of COPD, it is also possible that a normal decline in FEV1 could also lead to COPD in persons whose maximally attained FEV1 is less than population norms. This idea was proposed by Burrows long time ago [73] (Fig. 3.3), and it was actually shown in real world that low FEV1 in early adulthood is important in the genesis of COPD and that accelerated decline in FEV1 is not an obligate feature of COPD [74]. Thus, genes related to COPD pathogenesis also could affect COPD and its progression through these two models (namely, the pattern of rapid decliners and another one). On rapid decliners, case–control association studies on candidate genes with a population of Lung Health Study (283 rapid decliners (deltaFEV1 = −154 +/− 3 ml/year) and 308 nondecliners (deltaFEV1 = +15 +/− 2 ml/year) among smokers followed for 5 years) were performed, and the associations between the phenotype of rapid declining of FEV1 and MZ genotype of the alpha1-antitrypsin gene and haplotype of the microsomal epoxide hydrolase were suggested [75]. A recent GWAS to assess genetic contributions to lung function decline over a 5 year period in 4048

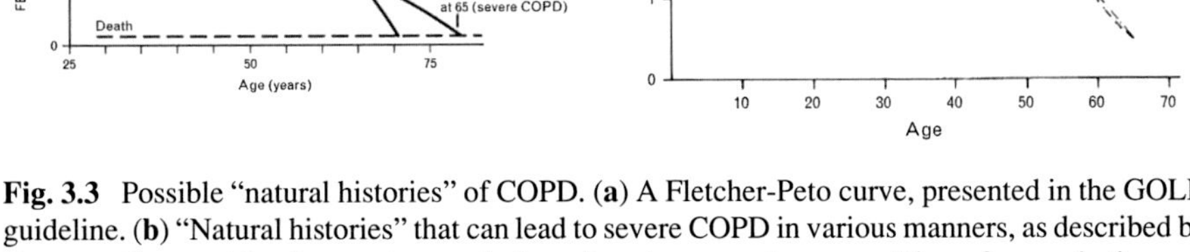

Fig. 3.3 Possible "natural histories" of COPD. (**a**) A Fletcher-Peto curve, presented in the GOLD guideline. (**b**) "Natural histories" that can lead to severe COPD in various manners, as described by Burrows. Some with a frequent exacerbation phenotype may have repetition of exacerbation and remission leading to progression of COPD, shown as "*B*." *COPD* chronic obstructive pulmonary disease (Reproduced with permission from Ref. [84])

European American Lung Health Study participants with largely mild COPD showed that two novel regions were associated with lung function decline in mild COPD and that genes within these regions (*TMEM26*, *FOXA1*, and *ANK3*) were expressed in relevant lung cells and their expression was related to airflow limitation [76]. However, the genes related to the subjects whose maximally attained FEV1 is less than population norms are less elucidated so far partly because this phenotype was not thought to be associated with COPD. *HHIP* could be one of the possible candidates of the genes related to this phenotype or subgroup of COPD (Fig. 3.2 [72]). *HHIP* was reported to be associated with COPD by GWASs as described above [44], and according to the results of UK BiLEVE study, *HHIP* is thought to affect COPD pathogenesis especially through modifying lung development [71]. The genes related to airflow obstruction were investigated as GWASs with larger populations than COPD studies [52, 53, 77] and include not only *HHIP* but also the other several genes. Thus, these genes except for *HHIP*, namely, *TNS1*, *GSTCD*, *AGER*, *HTR4*, *THSD4*, and others, are good candidates as COPD-related genes, and their possible roles on COPD pathogenesis should be investigated, including on their effect size.

Emphysema is one of the most important phenotypes in COPD, and the pathogenesis of emphysema should be investigated and clarified in a fine manner, partly in order to develop new therapeutic strategy of this phenotype. Airway wall thickening and emphysema phenotypes showed independent aggregation within families of individuals with COPD, suggesting that different genetic factors influence these disease processes [78]. Further, it is relatively easy to assess the extent of emphysema pathologically or by computed tomography (CT) in mice compared to assessing the airway disease; we can realistically proceed the research on molecular mechanism of emphysema formation with mice with knockdown of the gene related to emphysema. By GWASs with ECLIPSE, NETT, GenKOLS, and COPDGene populations, *BICD1*, *SNRPF*, and *PPT2* were associated with emphysema [79, 80] and *SERPINA10* and *DLC1* also, as reported recently [81]. One of the COPD phenotype comorbidities with interstitial lung diseases, combined pulmonary fibrosis and emphysema (CPFE) (reviewed in Chap. 18), is also a critical and definite category. The susceptibility genes of CPFE are speculated to the genes related to both emphysema and interstitial pulmonary fibrosis (e.g., *FAM13A* [82]), which remained to be elucidated. Though the research on the genes related to airway disease in COPD is also ongoing, the results are a little unclear, and these should be investigated further [81].

Frequent exacerbators are also one of the critical subgroups of COPD. Although exacerbations become more frequent and more severe as COPD progresses, the rate at which they occur appears to reflect an independent phenotype [83]. Exacerbation is a leading cause of mortality, decrement of pulmonary function and quality of life, and also is a major cost driver of COPD especially through hospitalization [84]. Fletcher and Peto [85] demonstrated the natural course of COPD, the "Fletcher-Peto curve," and they showed that the expiratory airflow limitation, defined as FEV1, declines with age throughout adulthood and that smoking, not the effect of mucus hypersecretion, accelerates its decline (Fig. 3.3a). In addition,

Burrows [73] indicated that some COPD individuals might have exacerbation and remission periods with each episode leading to a progressive loss of function (Fig. 3.3b). Thus, the susceptibility genes of COPD exacerbations should be also elucidated. Several reports exist regarding the association between exacerbation susceptibility and some gene variations, including surfactant protein B [86], mannose-binding lectin [87], and chemokine ligand 1 [88]; the proteins coded by these genes are a surfactant protein, a lectin that acts as a pattern recognition receptor in serum, and a chemokine, respectively, and they mainly have the capacity to protect against bacteria or viruses. The genetic variations that increase this capacity are thought to reduce susceptibility to infection and thus COPD exacerbations. Loss of Siglec-14, a lectin likely involved in host defense, was also associated with a reduced COPD exacerbation risk in a Japanese population [89]. However, minor allele frequency of this deletion polymorphism of *SIGLEC14* is rare in Caucasians; it is uncertain whether this gene has a critical role in the pathogenesis of COPD exacerbations in various ethnics. Since a protein involved in strengthening host defense such as Siglec-14, that could also trigger exaggerated response, might also generate unwanted local and systemic inflammation, which could be detrimental to a host and could generate COPD with a frequent exacerbation phenotype, its progression, and its comorbidities (Fig. 3.4) [84]. Thus, the genes related to signal transduction on inflammation and immunity like *SIGLEC*s, and components of gap junction, are thought to be good candidates for case–control association studies of COPD exacerbation genetics. However, to find truly "novel" genes related to COPD exacerbations, GWASs should be performed with multiethnic population with clear definition of exacerbations.

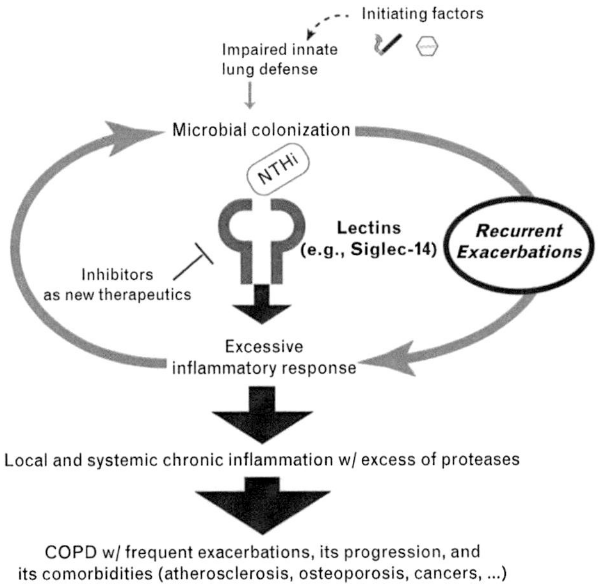

Fig. 3.4 The hypothesized role of an antibacterial but also proinflammatory molecules (e.g., Siglec-14) in the pathogenesis of COPD as a systemic disease (Reproduced with permission from Ref. [84])

Comorbidities are frequent in COPD and some of them negatively influence survival [90]. It was reported by cluster analysis that multimorbidity is common in patients with COPD and that different comorbidity clusters ((1) less comorbidity, (2) cardiovascular, (3) cachectic, (4) metabolic, and (5) psychological) were identified [91]. If we consider that COPD is a syndrome composed of these subgroups, each subgroup could have a different susceptibility gene to be investigated. COPD with asthma is called as asthma-COPD overlap syndrome (ACOS) and is thought to be relevant as a clinical entity. The non-Hispanic white GWAS identified single-nucleotide polymorphisms in the genes *CSMD1* and *SOX5*, and the meta-analysis identified single-nucleotide polymorphisms in the gene *GPR65* associated with ACOS [92].

3.6 Recent Progress of Studies of COPD Genetics in GWAS Era (III): Novel Strategy for Research on COPD Genetics with Multi-omics

Though a number of genes were reported to be associated with COPD so far, the functional relevance of these genetic variations is not so clear on most of or at least a part of them, similar to the results of the GWASs on other common chronic diseases. In this kind of situation, it is thought to be difficult to connect the results of GWASs and disease pathogenesis. Therefore, the associations between two different types of omics data, such as GWAS and gene expression profiling, were examined, which aim to correlate the results to the disease [54] (Fig. 3.5 [54]).

The genetic variants related to COPD were identified with GWASs as written above. In addition, the association between genetic variations and the mRNA expression in, first, lymphoblastoid cells [93] and then sputum and lung tissues was also reported [63, 94]. If these kinds of information are combined, we could find the disease-related genes and simultaneously the molecular mechanism of the genes to affect disease pathogenesis. Recently, the GWAS results on COPD with SpiroMeta-CHARGE, whose consortium undertook the largest GWAS so far (n = 48 201), were integrated with the lung expression quantitative trait loci (eQTLs) in lung tissue from 1111 individuals, and this group found that SNPs associated with lung function measures were more likely to be eQTLs, that the genes whose expression in lung tissues were regulated by these SNPs were enriched for developmental and inflammatory pathways, and that SNPs associated with lung function that were eQTLs in blood, but not in the lung, were only involved in inflammatory pathways [63, 94, 95].

Another group developed a systematic approach to identify key regulators of COPD that integrates genome-wide DNA methylation, gene expression, and phenotype data in lung tissue from COPD and control samples [96]. They identified 126 key regulators of COPD, including *EPAS1* as the only key regulator whose downstream genes significantly overlapped with multiple genes sets associated with

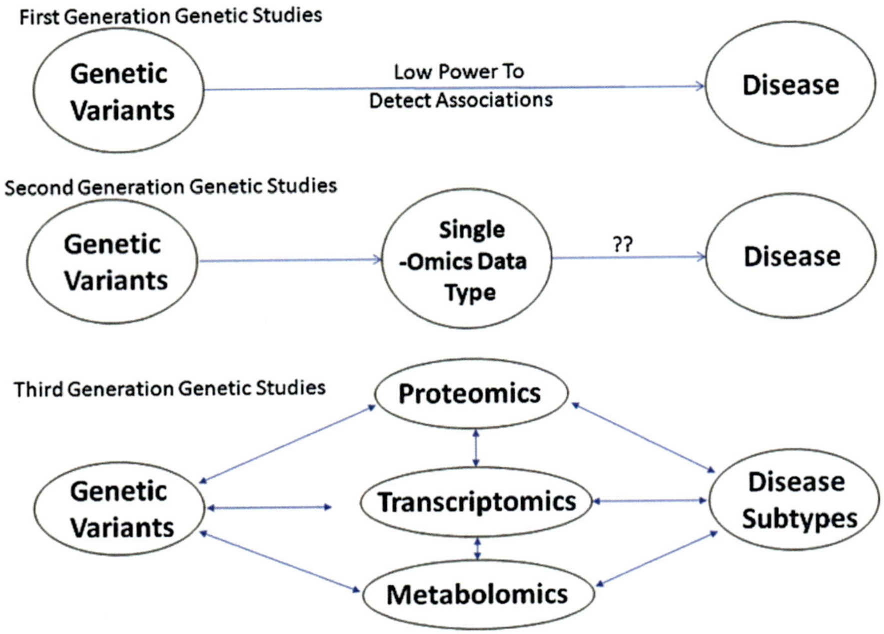

Fig. 3.5 Genetic and genomic studies on disease pathogenesis before and in GWAS era (Reproduced with permission from Ref. [54, 55])

COPD disease severity. *EPAS1* was distinct in comparison with other key regulators in terms of methylation profile and downstream target genes. They also confirmed that *EPAS1* protein levels are lower in human COPD lung tissue compared to non-disease controls and that Epas1 gene expression is reduced in mice chronically exposed to cigarette smoke. This kind of methodology could be leveraged to directly identify novel key mediators of this pathophysiology.

The other group hypothesized that by applying unbiased weights derived from unique populations, they could identify additional COPD susceptibility loci, and they performed a homozygosity haplotype analysis on a group of subjects with and without COPD to identify regions of conserved homozygosity haplotype (RCHHs), and weights were constructed based on the frequency of these RCHHs in case versus controls and used to adjust the p-values from a large collaborative GWAS of COPD. They identified two SNPs in a novel gene (fibroblast growth factor-7 (*FGF7*)) that gained genome-wide significance, and also the association with COPD was validated in an independent population. They also observed that increased lung tissue *FGF7* expression was associated with worse measures of lung function [97].

3.7 Recent Progress of Studies of COPD Genetics in GWAS Era (IV): Next-Generation Sequencing and Arrays

The technology to detect genetic variations rapidly progresses in these 10 years, which includes next-generation sequencing and GWAS with genotyping of more SNPs and imputation of genotypes. Parts of the reasons why genotypes of common variants (approximately 500,000 SNPs) were assessed in initial GWASs are the fact that CD/CV hypothesis was widely believed and also the fact at that time that it would be technically and economically difficult to genotype much more SNPs including not only common variants but also rare variants. The initial generation of GWAS was based on the data of HapMap Project which showed the allele frequency of the SNPs in a whole genome (not all SNPs but more than one million SNPs (approximately one tenth of the SNPs) with relatively high frequency) [43]. According to these data, the SNPs with allele frequency more than 5 % are selected in a genome-wide manner, and the association between these SNPs and disease phenotypes was investigated to find a novel disease susceptibility genotype. Thereafter, the 1000 Genomes Project was launched in January 2008 as an international research effort to establish the most detailed catalogue of human genetic variation including rare variations, and it planned to sequence the genomes of at least one thousand anonymous participants from a number of different ethnic groups within the following 3 years, using newly developed technologies which were faster and less expensive, including next-generation sequencing. The project finished its pilot phase in 2010 [98] and completed in 2015 [47]. In parallel, though genome-wide association studies have identified hundreds of genetic variants associated with complex human diseases and traits and have provided valuable insights into their genetic architecture, most variants identified so far confer relatively small increments in risk and explain only a small proportion of familial clustering, leading many to question how the remaining, "missing" heritability can be explained. Many explanations for this missing heritability have been suggested, including much larger numbers of variants of smaller effect yet to be found, rarer variants (possibly with larger effects) that are poorly detected by available genotyping arrays that focus on variants present in 5 % or more of the population, and structural variants poorly captured by existing arrays [99]. Thus, new GWASs with genotyping of minor alleles on which the allele frequency is 0.5–5 % (approximately two million or more SNPs are genotyped) and next-generation sequencing in exome- or genome-wide were performed and also ongoing to see the genetic aspects of COPD further including the aspect of missing heritability. To identify coding variants associated with COPD, non-synonymous, splice, and stop variants with a minor allele frequency above 0.5 % were assessed for association with COPD in five study populations, mainly Caucasians, enriched for COPD including COPDGene Study, and novel single-variant associations were validated in three additional COPD cohorts in a very recent study. The 6004 controls and 6161 COPD cases across five analysis cohorts and the genes related to COPD were not only those reported previously (*CHRNA5*, *AGER*, *MMP3*, and *SERPINA1*) but also a non-synonymous variant, rs181206, in *IL27* [100]. We also reported that serum IL27 levels are a promising biomarker for COPD [101] by using in vitro model in which we modify gene expression of *SIGLEC14*, which was reported as a susceptibility gene of COPD exacerbations [89]. Thus, it is speculated that *IL27* (and *SIGLEC*s possibly) has a critical role in the pathogenesis of COPD and its exacerbations in various ethnics. Also in a recent study, it was hypothesized that exome sequencing in families identified through a proband with severe, early-onset COPD would identify additional rare genetic determinants of large effect, and potential causal variants for COPD in whole exomes from 347 subjects in 49 extended pedigrees from the Boston Early-Onset COPD Study were investigated. However, novel susceptible or causal genes of COPD could not be found with this study, and they also demonstrated the limitations of the power of this approach under genetic heterogeneity through simulation [102]. The missing heritability on COPD could be explained by much larger numbers of variants of smaller effect yet to be found, similar to the case of the heritability of height, for example [103]. The other type of genetic variations, e.g., copy number variants (CNVs), could be also associated with COPD. The effects of polymorphic CNVs on quantitative measures of pulmonary function and chest computed tomography phenotypes among subjects enrolled in COPDGene were investigated, and they identified a polymorphic CNV on chromosome 5q35.2 located between two genes (*FAM153B* and *SIMK1*, but also harboring several pseudo-genes) giving genome-wide significance in tests of association with total lung capacity as measured by chest CT scans [104], but the associations between CNVs and COPD should be further elucidated in a near future.

3.8 Recent Progress of Studies of COPD Genetics in GWAS Era (V): Pharmacogenetics and Pharmacogenomics in COPD

Though pharmacogenetics is a clinically important research field also for COPD, few COPD pharmacogenetics studies have been completed, and most studies have focused on the role of variants in the beta(2)-adrenergic receptor gene on bronchodilator response, but the findings have been inconclusive. The use of pharmacogenetics to determine initial smoking cessation therapy may be closer to clinical application [105]. In the research of COPD pharmacogenomics, GWAS should be also applied. The in silico drug repurposing approach by using the data of GWAS, expression quantitative trait loci, and the Connectivity Map database [106] suggested several compounds that reverse the COPD gene expression signature, including a nicotine receptor antagonist, and the findings represent novel therapeutic pathways for COPD [95].

3.9 Conclusions

Several novel genes related to COPD were found by having performed GWASs for these 8 years. However, it is sometimes still not clear how these genes affect COPD pathogenesis on molecular mechanism and which phenotypes of COPD they affect, which could lead to development of novel therapies and thus should be elucidated.

Combination of omics and novel technologies like next-generation sequencing and recently improved GWASs also worked to find more on novel susceptibility genes. However, there are still problems to be solved to assess genetic variations and COPD in a more precise and fine manner. Though SNPs were widely assessed on the relationship with COPD, other types of genetic variations, e.g., deletion, insertion, and CNVs, which are thought to be functionally relevant, have not been assessed on the association with COPD enough. The Structural Variation Analysis Group of the 1000 Genomes Project reported recently an integrated structural variation map based on discovery and genotyping of eight major structural variation classes in genomes for 2504 unrelated individuals from across 26 populations, and they characterized structural variation within and between populations and quantify its functional effect and also created a phased reference panel that will be valuable for population genetic and disease association studies [107]. Thus, possibly, the association studies as genome-wide association studies on these kinds of genetic variations will be also performed, and novel COPD-related genes (like *SIGLEC14*, which is a kind of CNV [89]) will be found in the near future. On omics data, the data on gene expression, for example, are usually collected from "lung tissues," but not from some definite types of cells in the lung tissues. Therefore, definite types of cells which are thought to have critical roles in COPD pathogenesis, e.g., alveolar macrophages, should be selected and collected as samples (this was already collected in some studies [108] but the data were not combined with GWAS), and the expression data on these samples also should be combined with GWAS. Several models of interconnection between genotypes, gene expression, and disease phenotypes are suggested [109], and it is uncertain whether the model presently used in which the genotype affects disease by modifying the expression level of the gene suits to understand the relationship between the disease and the susceptibility gene. As written above, the missing heritability on COPD could be explained by much larger numbers of variants of smaller effect yet to be found, similar to the case of the heritability of height [98].

Studies on disease susceptibility genes by combining the data of omics progress with the Biobank data mainly of Caucasian populations [110]. Also on COPD, research on genomics will mainly proceed with Caucasian populations by SPIROMICS (http://www.cscc.unc.edu/spir/) [111], Lung Genomics Research Consortium (www.lung-genomics.org), and others. However, the GWAS data on COPD with Asian populations are scarce, and studies with multiethnic populations should be performed. The susceptibility genes of COPD exacerbations should be also elucidated.

References

1. Snider GL. Chronic obstructive pulmonary disease: risk factors, pathophysiology and pathogenesis. Annu Rev Med. 1989;40:411–29.
2. Silverman EK, Chapman HA, Drazen JM, Weiss ST, Rosner B, Campbell EJ, et al. Genetic epidemiology of severe, early-onset chronic obstructive pulmonary disease. Risk to relatives for airflow obstruction and chronic bronchitis. Am J Respir Crit Care Med. 1998;157(6 Pt 1):1770–8.
3. Khoury MJ, Beaty TH, Tockman MS, Self SG, Cohen BH. Familial aggregation in chronic obstructive pulmonary disease: use of the loglinear model to analyze intermediate environmental and genetic risk factors. Genet Epidemiol. 1985;2(2):155–66.
4. McCloskey SC, Patel BD, Hinchliffe SJ, Reid ED, Wareham NJ, Lomas DA. Siblings of patients with severe chronic obstructive pulmonary disease have a significant risk of airflow obstruction. Am J Respir Crit Care Med. 2001;164(8 Pt 1):1419–24.
5. Silverman EK, Sandhaus RA. Clinical practice. Alpha1-antitrypsin deficiency. N Engl J Med. 2009;360(26):2749–57.
6. Halapi E, Hakonarson H. 1. Introduction to genetics. In: Postma DS, Weiss ST, editors. Genetics of asthma and chronic obstructive pulmonary disease. New York: Informa Healthcare; 2006. p. 1–16.
7. Molfino NA. Genetic predisposition to accelerated decline of lung function in COPD. Int J Chron Obstruct Pulmon Dis. 2007;2(2):117–9.
8. Demeo DL, HC, Silverman EK. 11. Linkage analysis of spirometric phenotypes and chronic obstructive pulmonary disease. In: Postma DS, Weiss ST, editors. Genetics of asthma and chronic obstructive pulmonary disease. New York: Informa Healthcare; 2006. p. 211–22.
9. Silverman EK, Palmer LJ, Mosley JD, Barth M, Senter JM, Brown A, et al. Genomewide linkage analysis of quantitative spirometric phenotypes in severe early-onset chronic obstructive pulmonary disease. Am J Hum Genet. 2002;70(5):1229–39.
10. Silverman EK, Mosley JD, Palmer LJ, Barth M, Senter JM, Brown A, et al. Genome-wide linkage analysis of severe, early-onset chronic obstructive pulmonary disease: airflow obstruction and chronic bronchitis phenotypes. Hum Mol Genet. 2002;11(6):623–32.
11. Joost O, Wilk JB, Cupples LA, Harmon M, Shearman AM, Baldwin CT, et al. Genetic loci influencing lung function: a genome-wide scan in the Framingham Study. Am J Respir Crit Care Med. 2002;165(6):795–9.
12. Malhotra A, Peiffer AP, Ryujin DT, Elsner T, Kanner RE, Leppert MF, et al. Further evidence for the role of genes on chromosome 2 and chromosome 5 in the inheritance of pulmonary function. Am J Respir Crit Care Med. 2003;168(5):556–61.
13. Wilk JB, DeStefano AL, Arnett DK, Rich SS, Djousse L, Crapo RO, et al. A genome-wide scan of pulmonary function measures in the National Heart, Lung, and Blood Institute Family Heart Study. Am J Respir Crit Care Med. 2003;167(11):1528–33.
14. Demeo DL, Mariani TJ, Lange C, Srisuma S, Litonjua AA, Celedon JC, et al. The SERPINE2 gene is associated with chronic obstructive pulmonary disease. Am J Hum Genet. 2006;78 (2):253–64.
15. Zhu G, Warren L, Aponte J, Gulsvik A, Bakke P, Anderson WH, et al. The SERPINE2 gene is associated with chronic obstructive pulmonary disease in two large populations. Am J Respir Crit Care Med. 2007;176(2):167–73.
16. Fujimoto K, Ikeda S, Arai T, Tanaka N, Kumasaka T, Ishii T, et al. Polymorphism of SERPINE2 gene is associated with pulmonary emphysema in consecutive autopsy cases. BMC Med Genet. 2010;11:159.
17. Celedon JC, Lange C, Raby BA, Litonjua AA, Palmer LJ, DeMeo DL, et al. The transforming growth factor-beta1 (TGFB1) gene is associated with chronic obstructive pulmonary disease (COPD). Hum Mol Genet. 2004;13(15):1649–56.

18. Ito M, Hanaoka M, Droma Y, Hatayama O, Sato E, Katsuyama Y, et al. The association of transforming growth factor beta 1 gene polymorphisms with the emphysema phenotype of COPD in Japanese. Intern Med. 2008;47(15):1387–94.
19. Kim WJ, Hoffman E, Reilly J, Hersh C, Demeo D, Washko G, et al. Association of COPD candidate genes with computed tomography emphysema and airway phenotypes in severe COPD. Eur Respir J. 2011;37(1):39–43.
20. Kukkonen MK, Tiili E, Vehmas T, Oksa P, Piirila P, Hirvonen A. Association of genes of protease-antiprotease balance pathway to lung function and emphysema subtypes. BMC Pulm Med. 2013;13:36.
21. Wu L, Chau J, Young RP, Pokorny V, Mills GD, Hopkins R, et al. Transforming growth factor-beta1 genotype and susceptibility to chronic obstructive pulmonary disease. Thorax. 2004;59(2):126–9.
22. Su ZG, Wen FQ, Feng YL, Xiao M, Wu XL. Transforming growth factor-beta1 gene polymorphisms associated with chronic obstructive pulmonary disease in Chinese population. Acta Pharmacol Sin. 2005;26(6):714–20.
23. Morris DG, Huang X, Kaminski N, Wang Y, Shapiro SD, Dolganov G, et al. Loss of integrin alpha(v)beta6-mediated TGF-beta activation causes Mmp12-dependent emphysema. Nature. 2003;422(6928):169–73.
24. Reich DE, Lander ES. On the allelic spectrum of human disease. Trends Genet. 2001;17 (9):502–10.
25. Schork NJ, Murray SS, Frazer KA, Topol EJ. Common vs. rare allele hypotheses for complex diseases. Curr Opin Genet Dev. 2009;19(3):212–9.
26. Hoidal JR. Genetics of COPD: present and future. Eur Respir J. 2001;18(5):741–3.
27. Hunninghake GM, Cho MH, Tesfaigzi Y, Soto-Quiros ME, Avila L, Lasky-Su J, et al. MMP12, lung function, and COPD in high-risk populations. N Engl J Med. 2009;361 (27):2599–608.
28. Cho MH, McDonald ML, Zhou X, Mattheisen M, Castaldi PJ, Hersh CP, et al. Risk loci for chronic obstructive pulmonary disease: a genome-wide association study and meta-analysis. Lancet Respir Med. 2014;2(3):214–25.
29. Ishii T, Hagiwara K, Kamio K, Ikeda S, Arai T, Mieno MN, et al. Involvement of surfactant protein D in emphysema revealed by genetic association study. Eur J Hum Genet. 2012;20 (2):230–5.
30. Hartl D, Griese M. Surfactant protein D in human lung diseases. Eur J Clin Invest. 2006;36 (6):423–35.
31. Bridges JP, Davis HW, Damodarasamy M, Kuroki Y, Howles G, Hui DY, et al. Pulmonary surfactant proteins A and D are potent endogenous inhibitors of lipid peroxidation and oxidative cellular injury. J Biol Chem. 2000;275(49):38848–55.
32. Yoshida T, Tuder RM. Pathobiology of cigarette smoke-induced chronic obstructive pulmonary disease. Physiol Rev. 2007;87(3):1047–82.
33. McCormack FX, Whitsett JA. The pulmonary collectins, SP-A and SP-D, orchestrate innate immunity in the lung. J Clin Invest. 2002;109(6):707–12.
34. Wert SE, Yoshida M, LeVine AM, Ikegami M, Jones T, Ross GF, et al. Increased metalloproteinase activity, oxidant production, and emphysema in surfactant protein D gene-inactivated mice. Proc Natl Acad Sci U S A. 2000;97(11):5972–7.
35. Sorensen GL, Hjelmborg J, Kyvik KO, Fenger M, Hoj A, Bendixen C, et al. Genetic and environmental influences of surfactant protein D serum levels. Am J Physiol Lung Cell Mol Physiol. 2006;290(5):L1010–7.
36. Leth-Larsen R, Garred P, Jensenius H, Meschi J, Hartshorn K, Madsen J, et al. A common polymorphism in the SFTPD gene influences assembly, function, and concentration of surfactant protein D. J Immunol. 2005;174(3):1532–8.
37. Foreman MG, Kong X, DeMeo DL, Pillai SG, Hersh CP, Bakke P, et al. Polymorphisms in surfactant protein-D are associated with chronic obstructive pulmonary disease. Am J Respir Cell Mol Biol. 2011;44(3):316–22.

38. Bosse Y. Updates on the COPD gene list. Int J Chron Obstruct Pulmon Dis. 2012;7:607–31.
39. Ishii T, Sandford AJ. 14. Association studies in chronic obstructive pulmonary disease. In: Postma DS, Weiss ST, editors. Genetics of asthma and chronic obstructive pulmonary disease. New York: Informa Healthcare; 2006. p. 273–97.
40. Castaldi PJ, Cho MH, Cohn M, Langerman F, Moran S, Tarragona N, et al. The COPD genetic association compendium: a comprehensive online database of COPD genetic associations. Hum Mol Genet. 2010;19(3):526–34.
41. Hu G, Yao W, Zhou Y, Hu J, Shi Z, Li B, et al. Meta- and pooled analyses of the effect of glutathione S-transferase M1 and T1 deficiency on chronic obstructive pulmonary disease. Int J Tuberc Lung Dis. 2008;12(12):1474–81.
42. Smolonska J, Wijmenga C, Postma DS, Boezen HM. Meta-analyses on suspected chronic obstructive pulmonary disease genes: a summary of 20 years' research. Am J Respir Crit Care Med. 2009;180(7):618–31.
43. A haplotype map of the human genome. Nature. 2005;437(7063):1299–320.
44. Pillai SG, Ge D, Zhu G, Kong X, Shianna KV, Need AC, et al. A genome-wide association study in chronic obstructive pulmonary disease (COPD): identification of two major susceptibility loci. PLoS Genet. 2009;5(3), e1000421.
45. Wilk JB, Chen TH, Gottlieb DJ, Walter RE, Nagle MW, Brandler BJ, et al. A genome-wide association study of pulmonary function measures in the Framingham Heart Study. PLoS Genet. 2009;5(3), e1000429.
46. Cho MH, Boutaoui N, Klanderman BJ, Sylvia JS, Ziniti JP, Hersh CP, et al. Variants in *FAM13A* are associated with chronic obstructive pulmonary disease. Nat Genet. 2010;42 (3):200–2.
47. Auton A, Brooks LD, Durbin RM, Garrison EP, Kang HM, Korbel JO, et al. A global reference for human genetic variation. Nature. 2015;526(7571):68–74.
48. Cho MH, Castaldi PJ, Wan ES, Siedlinski M, Hersh CP, Demeo DL, et al. A genome-wide association study of COPD identifies a susceptibility locus on chromosome 19q13. Hum Mol Genet. 2012;21(4):947–57.
49. Thorgeirsson TE, Gudbjartsson DF, Surakka I, Vink JM, Amin N, Geller F, et al. Sequence variants at *CHRNB3-CHRNA6* and *CYP2A6* affect smoking behavior. Nat Genet. 2010;42 (5):448–53.
50. Tobacco and Genetics Consortium. Genome-wide meta-analyses identify multiple loci associated with smoking behavior. Nat Genet. 2010;42(5):441–7.
51. Wilk JB, Shrine NR, Loehr LR, Zhao JH, Manichaikul A, Lopez LM, et al. Genome-wide association studies identify CHRNA5/3 and HTR4 in the development of airflow obstruction. Am J Respir Crit Care Med. 2012;186(7):622–32.
52. Hancock DB, Eijgelsheim M, Wilk JB, Gharib SA, Loehr LR, Marciante KD, et al. Meta-analyses of genome-wide association studies identify multiple loci associated with pulmonary function. Nat Genet. 2010;42(1):45–52.
53. Repapi E, Sayers I, Wain LV, Burton PR, Johnson T, Obeidat M, et al. Genome-wide association study identifies five loci associated with lung function. Nat Genet. 2010;42 (1):36–44.
54. Hobbs BD, Hersh CP. Integrative genomics of chronic obstructive pulmonary disease. Biochem Biophys Res Commun. 2014;452(2):276–86.
55. Silverman EK, Loscalzo J. Network medicine approaches to the genetics of complex diseases. Discov Med. 2012;14(75):143–52.
56. Kim WJ, Lee SD. Candidate genes for COPD: current evidence and research. Int J Chron Obstruct Pulmon Dis. 2015;10:2249–55.
57. Thorgeirsson TE, Geller F, Sulem P, Rafnar T, Wiste A, Magnusson KP, et al. A variant associated with nicotine dependence, lung cancer and peripheral arterial disease. Nature. 2008;452(7187):638–42.
58. Amos CI, Spitz MR, Cinciripini P. Chipping away at the genetics of smoking behavior. Nat Genet. 2010;42(5):366–8.

59. Fowler CD, Lu Q, Johnson PM, Marks MJ, Kenny PJ. Habenular alpha5 nicotinic receptor subunit signalling controls nicotine intake. Nature. 2011;471(7340):597–601.
60. Lutz SM, Hokanson JE. Genetic influences on smoking and clinical disease. Understanding behavioral and biological pathways with mediation analysis. Ann Am Thorac Soc. 2014;11 (7):1082–3.
61. Castaldi PJ, Cho MH, Zhou X, Qiu W, McGeachie M, Celli B, et al. Genetic control of gene expression at novel and established chronic obstructive pulmonary disease loci. Hum Mol Genet. 2015;24(4):1200–10.
62. LaVaute T, Smith S, Cooperman S, Iwai K, Land W, Meyron-Holtz E, et al. Targeted deletion of the gene encoding iron regulatory protein-2 causes misregulation of iron metabolism and neurodegenerative disease in mice. Nat Genet. 2001;27(2):209–14.
63. Lamontagne M, Couture C, Postma DS, Timens W, Sin DD, Pare PD, et al. Refining susceptibility loci of chronic obstructive pulmonary disease with lung eQTLs. PLoS One. 2013;8(7), e70220.
64. Zhou X, Qiu W, Sathirapongsasuti JF, Cho MH, Mancini JD, Lao T, et al. Gene expression analysis uncovers novel hedgehog interacting protein (HHIP) effects in human bronchial epithelial cells. Genomics. 2013;101(5):263–72.
65. Lao T, Glass K, Qiu W, Polverino F, Gupta K, Morrow J, et al. Haploinsufficiency of Hedgehog interacting protein causes increased emphysema induced by cigarette smoke through network rewiring. Genome Med. 2015;7(1):12.
66. Jin Z, Chung JW, Mei W, Strack S, He C, Lau GW, et al. Regulation of nuclear-cytoplasmic shuttling and function of Family with sequence similarity 13, member A (Fam13a), by B56-containing PP2As and Akt. Mol Biol Cell. 2015;26(6):1160–73.
67. Li X, Hawkins GA, Ampleford EJ, Moore WC, Li H, Hastie AT, et al. Genome-wide association study identifies TH1 pathway genes associated with lung function in asthmatic patients. J Allergy Clin Immunol. 2013;132(2):313–20 e15.
68. Lee JH, Cho MH, Hersh CP, McDonald ML, Crapo JD, Bakke PS, et al. Genetic susceptibility for chronic bronchitis in chronic obstructive pulmonary disease. Respir Res. 2014;15:113.
69. Fingerlin TE, Murphy E, Zhang W, Peljto AL, Brown KK, Steele MP, et al. Genome-wide association study identifies multiple susceptibility loci for pulmonary fibrosis. Nat Genet. 2013;45(6):613–20.
70. Siedlinski M, Tingley D, Lipman PJ, Cho MH, Litonjua AA, Sparrow D, et al. Dissecting direct and indirect genetic effects on chronic obstructive pulmonary disease (COPD) susceptibility. Hum Genet. 2013;132(4):431–41.
71. Wain LV, Shrine N, Miller S, Jackson VE, Ntalla I, Artigas MS, et al. Novel insights into the genetics of smoking behaviour, lung function, and chronic obstructive pulmonary disease (UK BiLEVE): a genetic association study in UK Biobank. Lancet Respir Med. 2015;25.
72. Brusselle GG, Bracke KR. Elucidating COPD pathogenesis by large-scale genetic analyses. Lancet Respir Med. 2015;3(10):737–9.
73. Burrows B. An overview of obstructive lung diseases. Med Clin North Am. 1981;65 (3):455–71.
74. Lange P, Celli B, Agusti A, Boje Jensen G, Divo M, Faner R, et al. Lung-function trajectories leading to chronic obstructive pulmonary disease. N Engl J Med. 2015;373(2):111–22.
75. Sandford AJ, Chagani T, Weir TD, Connett JE, Anthonisen NR, Pare PD. Susceptibility genes for rapid decline of lung function in the lung health study. Am J Respir Crit Care Med. 2001;163(2):469–73.
76. Hansel NN, Ruczinski I, Rafaels N, Sin DD, Daley D, Malinina A, et al. Genome-wide study identifies two loci associated with lung function decline in mild to moderate COPD. Hum Genet. 2013;132(1):79–90.
77. Soler Artigas M, Loth DW, Wain LV, Gharib SA, Obeidat M, Tang W, et al. Genome-wide association and large-scale follow up identifies 16 new loci influencing lung function. Nat Genet. 2011;43(11):1082–90.

78. Patel BD, Coxson HO, Pillai SG, Agusti AG, Calverley PM, Donner CF, et al. Airway wall thickening and emphysema show independent familial aggregation in chronic obstructive pulmonary disease. Am J Respir Crit Care Med. 2008;178(5):500–5.
79. Kong X, Cho MH, Anderson W, Coxson HO, Muller N, Washko G, et al. Genome-wide association study identifies *BICD1* as a susceptibility gene for emphysema. Am J Respir Crit Care Med. 2011;183(1):43–9.
80. Manichaikul A, Hoffman EA, Smolonska J, Gao W, Cho MH, Baumhauer H, et al. Genome-wide study of percent emphysema on computed tomography in the general population. The Multi-Ethnic Study of Atherosclerosis Lung/SNP Health Association Resource Study. Am J Respir Crit Care Med. 2014;189(4):408–18.
81. Cho MH, Castaldi PJ, Hersh CP, Hobbs BD, Barr RG, Tal-Singer R, et al. A genome-wide association study of emphysema and airway quantitative imaging phenotypes. Am J Respir Crit Care Med. 2015;192(5):559–69.
82. Corvol H, Hodges CA, Drumm ML, Guillot L. Moving beyond genetics: is FAM13A a major biological contributor in lung physiology and chronic lung diseases? J Med Genet. 2014;51 (10):646–9.
83. Hurst JR, Vestbo J, Anzueto A, Locantore N, Mullerova H, Tal-Singer R, et al. Susceptibility to exacerbation in chronic obstructive pulmonary disease. N Engl J Med. 2010;363 (12):1128–38.
84. Ishii T, Kida K. Predictors of chronic obstructive pulmonary disease exacerbations. Curr Opin Pulm Med. 2014;20(2):138–45.
85. Fletcher CM. Causes and development of chronic airways obstruction and its further investigation. Bull Physiopathol Respir (Nancy). 1973;9(4):1131–48.
86. Foreman MG, DeMeo DL, Hersh CP, Carey VJ, Fan VS, Reilly JJ, et al. Polymorphic variation in surfactant protein B is associated with COPD exacerbations. Eur Respir J. 2008;32(4):938–44.
87. Lin CL, Siu LK, Lin JC, Liu CY, Chian CF, Lee CN, et al. Mannose-binding lectin gene polymorphism contributes to recurrence of infective exacerbation in patients with COPD. Chest. 2011;139(1):43–51.
88. Takabatake N, Shibata Y, Abe S, Wada T, Machiya J, Igarashi A, et al. A single nucleotide polymorphism in the CCL1 gene predicts acute exacerbations in chronic obstructive pulmonary disease. Am J Respir Crit Care Med. 2006;174(8):875–85.
89. Angata T, Ishii T, Motegi T, Oka R, Taylor RE, Soto PC, et al. Loss of Siglec-14 reduces the risk of chronic obstructive pulmonary disease exacerbation. Cell Mol Life Sci. 2013;70 (17):3199–210.
90. Divo M, Cote C, de Torres JP, Casanova C, Marin JM, Pinto-Plata V, et al. Comorbidities and risk of mortality in patients with chronic obstructive pulmonary disease. Am J Respir Crit Care Med. 2012;186(2):155–61.
91. Vanfleteren LE, Spruit MA, Groenen M, Gaffron S, van Empel VP, Bruijnzeel PL, et al. Clusters of comorbidities based on validated objective measurements and systemic inflammation in patients with chronic obstructive pulmonary disease. Am J Respir Crit Care Med. 2013;187(7):728–35.
92. Hardin M, Cho M, McDonald ML, Beaty T, Ramsdell J, Bhatt S, et al. The clinical and genetic features of COPD-asthma overlap syndrome. Eur Respir J. 2014;44(2):341–50.
93. Stranger BE, Nica AC, Forrest MS, Dimas A, Bird CP, Beazley C, et al. Population genomics of human gene expression. Nat Genet. 2007;39(10):1217–24.
94. Qiu W, Cho MH, Riley JH, Anderson WH, Singh D, Bakke P, et al. Genetics of sputum gene expression in chronic obstructive pulmonary disease. PLoS One. 2011;6(9), e24395.
95. Obeidat M, Hao K, Bosse Y, Nickle DC, Nie Y, Postma DS, et al. Molecular mechanisms underlying variations in lung function: a systems genetics analysis. Lancet Respir Med. 2015;21.

96. Yoo S, Takikawa S, Geraghty P, Argmann C, Campbell J, Lin L, et al. Integrative analysis of DNA methylation and gene expression data identifies *EPAS1* as a key regulator of COPD. PLoS Genet. 2015;11(1), e1004898.
97. Brehm JM, Hagiwara K, Tesfaigzi Y, Bruse S, Mariani TJ, Bhattacharya S, et al. Identification of FGF7 as a novel susceptibility locus for chronic obstructive pulmonary disease. Thorax. 2011;66(12):1085–90.
98. Abecasis GR, Altshuler D, Auton A, Brooks LD, Durbin RM, Gibbs RA, et al. A map of human genome variation from population-scale sequencing. Nature. 2010;467 (7319):1061–73.
99. Manolio TA, Collins FS, Cox NJ, Goldstein DB, Hindorff LA, Hunter DJ, et al. Finding the missing heritability of complex diseases. Nature. 2009;461(7265):747–53.
100. Hobbs BD, Parker MM, Chen H, Lao T, Hardin M, Qiao D, et al. Exome array analysis identifies a common variant in *IL27* associated with chronic obstructive pulmonary disease. Am J Respir Crit Care Med. 2016;15.
101. Angata T, Ishii T, Gao C, Ohtsubo K, Kitazume S, Gemma A, et al. Association of serum interleukin-27 with the exacerbation of chronic obstructive pulmonary disease. Physiol Rep. 2014;2(7).
102. Qiao D, Lange C, Beaty TH, Crapo JD, Barnes KC, Bamshad M, et al. Exome sequencing analysis in severe, early-onset chronic obstructive pulmonary disease. Am J Respir Crit Care Med. 2016;193(12):1353–63.
103. Wood AR, Esko T, Yang J, Vedantam S, Pers TH, Gustafsson S, et al. Defining the role of common variation in the genomic and biological architecture of adult human height. Nat Genet. 2014;46(11):1173–86.
104. Begum F, Ruczinski I, Li S, Silverman EK, Cho MH, Lynch DA, et al. Identifying a deletion affecting total lung capacity among subjects in the COPDGene study cohort. Genet Epidemiol. 2016;40(1):81–8.
105. Hersh CP. Pharmacogenetics of chronic obstructive pulmonary disease: challenges and opportunities. Pharmacogenomics. 2010;11(2):237–47.
106. Lamb J, Crawford ED, Peck D, Modell JW, Blat IC, Wrobel MJ, et al. The Connectivity Map: using gene-expression signatures to connect small molecules, genes, and disease. Science. 2006;313(5795):1929–35.
107. Sudmant PH, Rausch T, Gardner EJ, Handsaker RE, Abyzov A, Huddleston J, et al. An integrated map of structural variation in 2,504 human genomes. Nature. 2015;526 (7571):75–81.
108. Ishii T, Abboud RT, Wallace AM, English JC, Coxson HO, Finley RJ, et al. Alveolar macrophage proteinase/antiproteinase expression in lung function and emphysema. Eur Respir J. 2014;43(1):82–91.
109. Lamontagne M, Timens W, Hao K, Bosse Y, Laviolette M, Steiling K, et al. Genetic regulation of gene expression in the lung identifies *CST3* and *CD22* as potential causal genes for airflow obstruction. Thorax. 2014;69(11):997–1004.
110. Kaiser J. Who has your DNA–or wants it. Science. 2015;349(6255):1475.
111. Couper D, LaVange LM, Han M, Barr RG, Bleecker E, Hoffman EA, et al. Design of the Subpopulations and Intermediate Outcomes in COPD Study (SPIROMICS). Thorax. 2014;69 (5):491–4.

Chapter 4
Pathogenesis of COPD (Persistence of Airway Inflammation): Why Does Airway Inflammation Persist After Cessation of Smoking?

Akane Kato and Masayuki Hanaoka

Abstract The structural features of airways in patients with COPD are airway wall inflammation, fibrosis, muscle hypertrophy, and goblet cell metaplasia. These structural cellular changes contribute to mucus hypersecretion and destruction of the alveolar walls and a decline in forced expiratory volume in one second (FEV_1). At the cellular level, macrophages, T lymphocytes, and neutrophils, driven by cytokines including interleukin-8 (IL-8), gather on the airways. The main cause of COPD inflammation is cigarette smoke. Smoke causes an increase in the secretion of matrix metalloproteinase (MMPs) and neutrophilic elastase from epithelial cells and neutrophils, which are responsible for mucin production and destruction of the lung. Initially, cigarette smoke influences the expression of pattern recognition receptors (PRRs) including Toll-like receptors (TLRs), the intracellularly located nucleotide-binding oligomerization domain (NOD)-like receptors (NLRs), retinoic acid-inducible gene I (RIG-I)-like receptors (RLRs), and receptors for advanced glycation end products (RAGE) on lung epithelial cells, endothelial cells, and leukocytes in the lung. These actions bring about the production of cytokines and activation of inflammatory cells, leading to production of MMPs and neutrophilic elastase. The inflammatory changes persist for several months and years after smoking cessation and are sometimes irreversible. Damage-associated molecular patterns (DAMPs) released from dying cells after cigarette smoking increase the number of apoptotic cells, suppress efferocytosis, induce hypoxia and oxidative stress, and prolong the inflammatory changes, even after smoking cessation. Viral and bacterial infections of the respiratory tract then fortify these inflammatory responses. Exacerbations of COPD then worsen the deterioration of COPD.

A. Kato • M. Hanaoka (✉)
The First Department of Internal Medicine, Shinshu University of Medicine, 3-1-1 Asahi, Matsumoto City 390-8621, Japan
e-mail: masayuki@shinshu-u.ac.jp

H. Nakamura, K. Aoshiba (eds.), *Chronic Obstructive Pulmonary Disease*, Respiratory Disease Series: Diagnostic Tools and Disease Managements,
DOI 10.1007/978-981-10-0839-9_4

Keywords Matrix metalloproteinase (MMPs) • Interleukin-8 (IL-8) • Neutrophils • CD4 T cells • COPD exacerbations

4.1 Introduction

Global Initiative for Chronic Obstructive Lung Disease 2006 (GOLD 2006) states that "Smoking cessation is the single most effective and cost-effective intervention in most people to reduce the risk of developing COPD and stop its progression (Evidence A)." However, once a patient smokes and develops COPD, the inflammatory changes persist through the innate and adaptive immune systems, which are commonly activated during infection. In this chapter, we will explain why the pathogenesis of COPD progresses, even after smoking cessation, from the point of view of inflammation. The airway inflammation is related not only to the cigarette smoke itself but also viral and bacterial infections occurring before and after smoking cessation. First, the structural and cellular aspects of the inflammatory changes that are also seen with respiratory infection and that occur during COPD formation will be described in general. Then, the progression of COPD after smoking cessation will be discussed. Finally, the relationships between latent respiratory infections, COPD exacerbations, and COPD progressions will be reviewed.

4.2 Airway Inflammation and Changes in COPD

Clinically, most COPD patients are current or former smokers. In this chapter, we will first explain what happens in the airways of patients with COPD.

4.2.1 Airway Structure and Mucus Production in Patients with COPD

At the end of the peripheral airways are the alveoli, which are composed of type 1 and type 2 pneumocytes. Bronchiolar patency is stabilized by surfactant secreted from alveoli. Small airways adjacent to alveoli are lined by the epithelium. The epithelial cells are composed of two principal cell types—ciliated and secretory cells. Secretory cells are further divided into goblet and Clara cells [1]. Beneath the epithelium is the basal membrane, and further down the smooth muscle layer (Fig. 4.1) [2]. The secretory cells release mucus, which contains mucins or large glycoproteins [1]. Mucins form polymers. Two of the polymers, mucin 5 AC (MUC5AC) and MUC5B, are highly expressed in the airways [1].

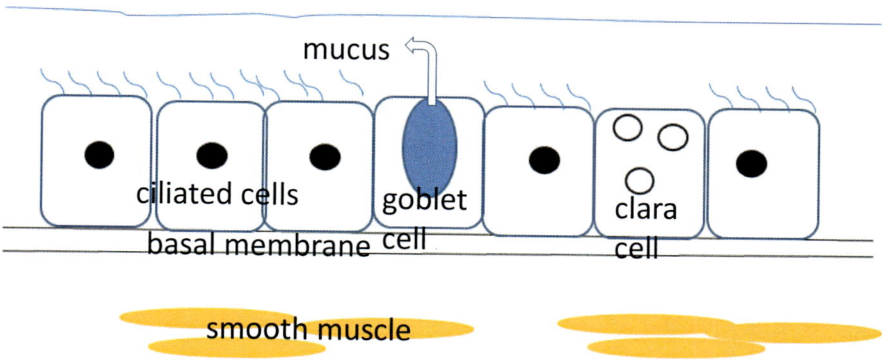

Fig. 4.1 Airway structure and mucus production. The epithelial cells are composed of ciliated and secretory cells. Goblet and Clara cells are secretory cells. Secretory cells release mucus, which contains mucins MUC5AC and MUC5B

In patients with COPD, the development of airflow obstruction is associated with structural and cellular changes in both the peripheral and central airways. The structural level of peripheral changes involves airway wall inflammation, fibrosis, smooth muscle hypertrophy, goblet cell metaplasia, and lumen occlusion by mucus plugging [3]. These are all possible causes of airflow limitation (Fig. 4.2). However, despite that airway wall fibrosis can be a major contributor to the irreversible component of airflow obstruction in smokers with COPD, the presence of a precise characterization of the fibrotic tissue in peripheral airways has never been reported [4]. Goblet cell metaplasia produces an excess of mucus, which can obstruct the lumen and alter the surface tension of the fluid lining the airway, rendering the peripheral airways unstable and facilitating their closure [4]. Mucus hypersecretion from hyperplastic airway goblet cells is a hallmark of COPD [5]. A recent study showed that chronic sputum production was significantly associated with both excess of FEV_1 decline and increased risk of subsequent hospitalization [4].

4.2.2 *Lung Destruction in COPD*

Airway wall inflammatory reaction contributes not only to the mucus hypersecretion described above but also to the destruction of the alveolar walls, allowing the airway wall to deform and narrowing the airway lumen [4]. Activated inflammatory cells are thought to release elastases, which destroy the lung tissue [4]. The major sources of elastases in the lung are granulocytes and macrophages, and their products include leukocyte elastase, proteinase 3, MMPs, cysteine proteinases, and plasminogen activators [4]. Because anti-elastin antibodies are found in patients with COPD, it is thought that COPD is also an autoimmune disease of elastin [6]. MMP9 gene expression is regulated by numerous stimulatory and suppressive factors, including several cytokines and growth factors such as

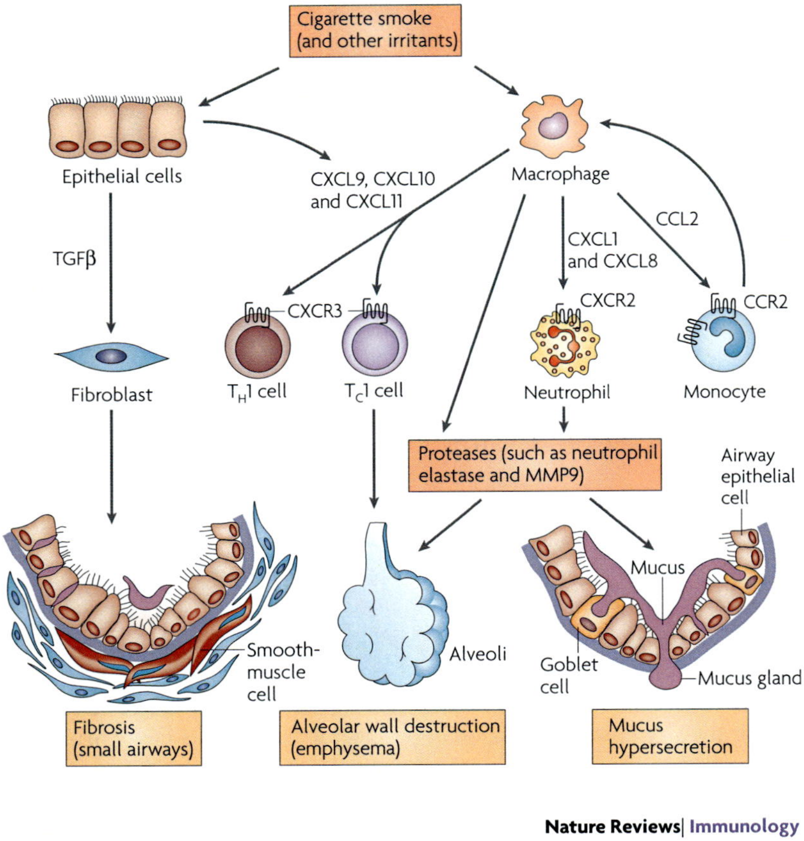

Fig. 4.2 Inflammatory and immune cells involved in COPD. Structural level of peripheral changes involved in airway wall inflammation, fibrosis, smooth muscle hypertrophy, goblet cell metaplasia, and destruction of the alveolar walls. Inflammatory cells include macrophages, T lymphocytes, and neutrophils in the airway lumen (From "Peter J. Barns. Nature. 2008;8:183-92"). *CCL2* CC-chemokine ligand 2, *CCR2* CC-chemokine receptor 2, *CXCL1* CXC-chemokine ligand 1, *MMP9* matrix metalloproteinase-9, *Tc1 cell* type 1 cytotoxic T cell, *TGF-β* transforming growth factor-β, *T_H1 cell* T helper 1 cell

interleukin-1α (IL-1α), IL-2, IL-8, and interferon-γ (IFN-γ) [7]. MMPs bring about not only MUC5AC accumulation but also the destruction of the lung that leads to emphysema. MMPs probably participate in a proteolytic attack on the alveolar wall matrix [8]. MMP9 is known as gelatinase B. It has multiple potential substrates including collagens, gelatin, elastin, and pro-MMP9 and 13. It is secreted by bronchial epithelial cells, neutrophils, eosinophils, mast cells, and alveolar macrophages.

4.2.3 Inflammatory Cells and Cytokines in the Airway in COPD

The development of airflow obstruction is associated with an increase of macrophages and T lymphocytes in the airway wall and of neutrophils in the airway lumen [4]. Although the mechanism of neutrophil accumulation in the airway lumen of smokers with COPD is not entirely clear, it is possible that an imbalance between pro- and anti-inflammatory cytokines may play a role. For example, IL-8 is a cytokine that promotes neutrophil chemotaxis, and tumor necrosis factor (TNF-α) is a cytokine that activates an increase in adhesion molecules [4]. There is a shift in the balance of the CD4-/CD8-positive T lymphocyte ratio in favor of CD8-positive ones [4]. Indeed, the CD8-positive cytotoxic T lymphocytes infiltrate the central airways [4], peripheral airways [4], and lung parenchyma [4] suggesting a consistent inflammatory process along the entire tracheobronchial tree in smokers with COPD.

4.3 Airway Inflammation After Smoking Cessation

Inflammatory changes persist for several months after smoking cessation and are sometimes irreversible [3]. The association observed between smoking and the incidence of COPD is more likely to reflect an early interaction between tobacco exposure and genetic or immunologic host characteristics rather than the effect of the cumulative exposure to cigarette smoke [3].

During cessation of smoking, the number of blood leukocytes immediately falls, goblet cell hyperplasia in the airway declines remarkably, and the number of macrophages and neutrophils in bronchoalveolar lavage fluid (BALF) decreases. However, IL-8, and consequently neutrophils in the airways of ex-smokers, still remains higher than those in nonsmokers [3]. A recent cross-sectional study in which bronchial inflammation was compared between smokers and ex-smokers in patients with COPD [9] showed that the CD3+, CD4+, and plasma cell numbers were significantly higher in the ex-smokers with COPD than current smokers with COPD. Furthermore, compared with current smokers, the short-term ex-smokers showed significantly higher CD4+ and CD8+ cell numbers, whereas the long-term ex-smokers showed significantly lower CD8+ cell numbers and CD8/CD3 ratios and higher plasma cell numbers [9]. These results indicate that the inflammation persists in the airways of patients with COPD even after smoking cessation [10], though the progression of inflammation might attenuate gradually.

Unfortunately, once mild COPD occurs, smoking cessation is not always effective in terminating the progression of COPD. The alterations in squamous metaplasia, gland size, smooth muscle mass, and fibrosis after exposure to smoking do not always recover after smoking cessation [3], though the situation is much better than not quitting smoking [11]. The hypersecretion of mucus, formation of emphysema, and fibrosis in COPD begin with the inhalation of cigarette smoke, which acts on epithelial cells, macrophages, and T lymphocytes in the airway lumen. Activation of epithelial growth factor receptor (EGFR) is responsible for mucin production after inhalation of cigarette smoke in the airways [1, 5, 7]. Meanwhile, acrolein is one of the main cigarette smoke constituents, which increases MUC5AC-positive cells, lung MMP9 transcripts, and EGFR/mitogen-activated protein kinase (MAPK) signaling. These, in turn, contribute to MUC5AC accumulation in the airways [12]. Systemic administration of acrolein causes the stress response in the endoplasmic reticulum and lung cell apoptosis, and chronic administration leads to an enlargement of the alveolar air spaces and emphysema in rats [13].

4.3.1 Innate Immune System

Both the innate and adaptive immune systems are involved during the progression of the pulmonary inflammation that occurs in COPD [14]. Lung epithelium is always exposed to external microbes in the air such that the innate and adaptive immune responses play important roles in reacting to those external pathogens [15]. Innate immunity is the first line of defense against foreign pathogens. Contrary to adaptive immune responses by which we can obtain protective immunity throughout our lifetime against the same pathogens once we are infected, the innate immune response occurs only once, though it can react to diverse pathogens, including the varied constituents in cigarette smoke. The role of innate immunity in the airways involves detection of pathogen-associated molecular patterns (PAMPs) or DAMPs by PRRs including TLRs and NLRs (Fig. 4.3) [14].

4.3.1.1 The Role of TLRs

Cells that are associated with innate immunity in the lung include macrophages, dendritic cells, monocytes, and neutrophils [15]. The recognition of microbes is first done by PRRs expressed in alveolar macrophages, dendritic cells, and epithelial cells. TLRs are a major family of PRRs, and humans have ten kinds of TLRs to recognize pathogens. The TLRs associated with COPD are TLR6 and TLR9 [16, 17]. They usually recognize bacteria or viruses, but cigarette smoke can also induce pulmonary inflammation via TLRs [17–19]. Additionally, the interaction between TLRs and EGFR increases IL-8 and vascular endothelial growth factor (VEGF) [20]. Through TLR stimulation, reactive oxygen species (ROS) activate the latent form of TNF-α-converting enzyme (TACE), which cleaves the transforming growth factor (TGF)-α proligand that activates EGFR. This results in signaling that leads to IL-8 and VEGF production [21, 22]. Indeed, it was reported that cigarette smoke augments TLR3, which stimulates IL-8 release and

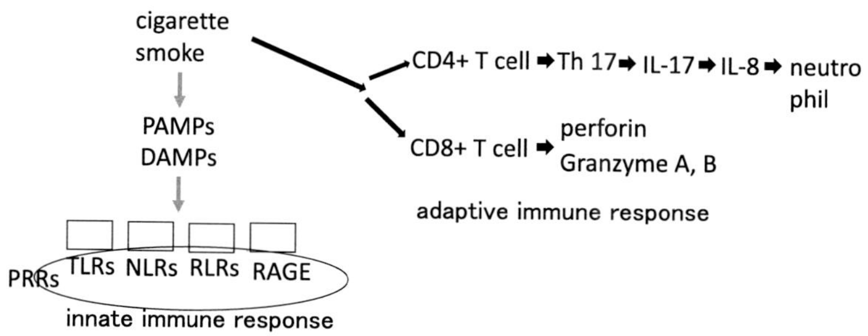

Fig. 4.3 Innate and adaptive immune responses in the airway after smoking cessation. Cigarette smoke brings about PAMPs and DAMPs, which stimulate PRRs on the inflammatory or epithelial cells in the innate immune system and finally cause COPD. In the adaptive immune system, T cells induce notable cytokines, neutrophils, and proteinase and are also causes of COPD formation. *DAMPs* damage-associated molecular patterns, *IL-17* interleukin-17, *NLRs* nucleotide-binding oligomerization domain (NOD)-like receptors, *PAMPs* pathogen-associated molecular patterns, *PRRs* pattern recognition receptors, *RAGE* receptors for advanced glycation end products, *RLRs* retinoic acid-inducible gene I (RIG-I)-like receptors, *Th17* T helper 17 cell, *TLRs* Toll-like receptors

increases total MMP9 activity in the airways [19]. IL-8 leads to the recruitment and activation of neutrophils in the airways (see Sect. 4.3.2.2).

4.3.1.2 The Role of NLRs

NLRs represent a group of key sensors of infections and tissue damage in the lung [23]. Activation of most known NLRs leads to the production and release of proinflammatory cytokines and induction of cell death [23]. Ligand recognition by NOD1 and NOD2 receptors leads to signal transduction through receptor-interacting protein 2 (RIP2) kinase, with downstream activation of MAPKs and transcription factor nuclear factor-kappa B (NF-kB). This then leads to the activation of genes encoding different cytokines and chemokines such as IL-8 [23]. Inflammasomes consisting of one or two NLR proteins serve as platforms for autocatalytic caspase-1 activation, which in turn critically regulates IL-1β and IL-18 production, inducing an inflammatory form of cell death called pyroptosis. Importantly, the NLR protein 3 (NLRP3) inflammasome responds to a vast range of sterile stimuli particularly DAMPs released by dying cells such as adenosine triphosphate (ATP), uric acid metabolites, and biglycan as well as hyaluronan [23]. Experimental studies in mice suggest that activation of NLRPs by some of those DAMPs might have important functions in the pathogenesis of acute lung injury/acute respiratory distress syndrome (ALI/ARDS), COPD/emphysema, and lung fibrosis [23].

4.3.1.3 The Role of RLRs

Unlike other PRRs, there are almost no reports about the relationship between the components in cigarette smoke and RLRs. However, RLRs are indispensable in viral infection, and they are intimately associated with COPD progression after smoking cessation.

RLRs, including RIG-1 and melanoma differentiation-associated gene 5 (MDA-5), are important pattern recognition receptors for viral elimination [14]. When viral RNA binds to the C-terminal regulatory domain of RIG-1 or MDA-5, it can initiate a signaling cascade. This cascade leads to activation and nuclear translocation of the transcription factors NF-kB and interferon regulatory transcription 3 (IRF-3), which are needed to turn on transcription of interferons (IFNs) [14]. Viral infection is a significant cause of COPD and acute exacerbations of COPD [14]. Up to half of COPD exacerbation cases are associated with viral infections [14]. The top four causes are rhinovirus (RV), coronavirus, influenza virus, and respiratory syncytial virus [14]. Recent studies provide evidence that MDA-5 is responsible for recognizing RV and subsequently activating signaling pathways, causing an exaggerated inflammatory response in patients with COPD. These responses include increased levels of IL-8, IL-6, CXC-chemokine ligand 1 (CXCL1), TNF-α, IL-1β, and monocyte chemotactic protein 1 (MCP-1) [14].

4.3.1.4 The Role of RAGE

RAGE are members of an immunoglobulin superfamily of cell surface receptors that function as pattern recognition receptors capable of signal transduction after interaction with diverse ligands [24]. RAGE is upregulated wherever its ligands accumulate in chronic conditions such as inflammation, cardiovascular disease, diabetes, cancer, and neurodegeneration [25]. RAGE expression increases in the pulmonary epithelium when tobacco smoke is present [24]. RAGE engagement activates an inflammatory signaling pathway. Smoke-induced RAGE expression mediates cytokine secretions via Ras, a GTPase that influences Raf/MAP kinase, phosphoinositide 3-kinase (PI3K), c-Jun N-terminal kinase (JNK)/p38, NF-kB [25], and the Rho proinflammatory pathway [24]. At minimum, RAGE signaling orchestrates polymorphonucleocyte recruitment and reservoirs of elastolytic enzymes including MMP9 and other mediators of emphysema regulated by RAGE signaling [24]. Recently, both soluble and circulating forms of RAGE were said to be the useful biomarkers for the presence or progression of emphysema because RAGE is generated via cleavage of full-length RAGE from the cell surface by metalloproteinases such as disintegrin, metalloproteinase domain-containing protein 10 (ADAM10), and MMP9 [25].

4.3.2 Adaptive Immune System

Similar to the importance of the innate immune reaction, the adaptive immune system is also a necessary element in the mechanism of COPD formation. Animal models of autoimmune emphysema not related to cigarette smoke are known [26, 27]. In this model, anti-endothelial cell antibodies (AECA) have been shown to trigger emphysema because of the reduction of the endothelium in the lung.

4.3.2.1 The Role of B Cells

Little is known about the role of B cells in the development of COPD [28]. The presence of B cells in lymphoid follicles has been reported in the airways and parenchyma of patients with COPD and of mice exposed to cigarette smoke [29]. In mice, the development of lymphoid follicles was progressive over time and correlated with the increase in airspace enlargement [28]. The B-cell follicles are surrounded by T cells, with the majority being CD4+ [28]. The B cells are interspaced by follicular dendritic cells that are necessary for antigen presentation and affinity maturation [28]. Follicle formation is associated with increased levels of cytokines including IL-4, IL-6, IL-8, and IL-13 [28]. These cytokines are essential for the formation and differentiation of germinal centers [28]. Overexpression of IL-13 in mice results in severe emphysema [28]. The absence of bacterial and viral products in the follicles suggests that oligoclonal B cells arise in response to lung antigens [30]. Nevertheless, viral and bacterial infections could be important in perpetuating the inflammatory process and are regarded as the main cause of the exacerbations in COPD. Barry et al. [28] hypothesized that cigarette smoke-induced breakdown products of the extracellular matrix might also be immunogenic and trigger a specific B-cell reaction [28].

4.3.2.2 The Role of T Cells

It is likely that antigens from necrotic and apoptotic cells in the lungs of smokers are taken up by dendritic cells and presented as antigens to CD8+ T lymphocytes [29]. Activated T cells leave the blood vessels and enter the lung parenchyma. In the lungs of smokers with COPD, CD8+ and CD4+ T cells express the tissue-specific chemokine receptors CXCR3, CXCR5, and CXCR6 [30]. These receptors correlate with the severity of the disease [29]. In both the airway and alveolar compartments, the CD8+ cytotoxic T cell is the predominant T cell in patients with COPD and causes tissue injury [29]. Any cell that displays MHC class I can be a target of CD8+ cytolytic T cells. After a cytolytic attack, target cells die of apoptosis or necrosis from the damage done by perforin, granulysin, or granzyme A or B (Fig. 4.3), all of which are proteolytic enzymes released by CD8+ T cells [15] in the lungs of patients with COPD.

CD4+ T cells also play an important role in COPD. The cytokine IL-17 is a 17-kDa molecule that is produced in vitro by CD4+ and CD8+ subsets of T lymphocytes from humans and mice [31]. IL-17A signaling appears to be crucial for the formation of cigarette smoking-induced emphysema [16]. The frequencies of Th17 (CD4 + IL-17+) and Tc17 (CD8 + IL-17+) cells in the lungs of smoke-exposed mice and smoke-ceased mice are positively correlated with emphysematous lesions [30].

IL-17A plays several important roles in COPD formation. First, it causes lung destruction. IL-17 induces IL-8, which is a chemoattractant for neutrophilic migration (Fig. 4.3). Activated neutrophils and macrophages cause lung destruction through the release of oxygen radicals and proteolytic enzymes such as neutrophil elastase and MMPs including MMP8, MMP9, and MMP12 (macrophage elastase) [15]. As mentioned above for "the innate immune system," proteolytic enzymes cause cleavage of TGF-α proligands, which bind to EGFR and lead to hypersecretion of MUC5AC [20]. This results in the destruction of the extracellular matrix, tissue damage, and formation of emphysema. Second, IL-17A leads to mucus hypersecretion. In addition to recruitment and activation of the epithelial cells in the lungs, IL-17A also induces MUC5AC expression together with IL-1β, TNF-α, CXCL1, granulocyte colony-stimulating factor (G-CSF), and intracellular adhesion molecule-1 (ICAM-1) in the lungs, resulting in hypersecretion of mucus [16]. Moreover, there is evidence that both IL-6 and IL-17 mediate MUC5B expression through the extracellular signal-regulated kinase (ERK) signaling pathway [16].

Though the definition of emphysema is "non-fibrotic lesions," fibrosis is said to play an important role in COPD, for example, pulmonary hypertension. In a recent study, IL-1β caused fibrosis in the lung. SMAD4 and NF-kB cooperate to mediate IL-1β and integrin $\alpha_v\beta_8$-dependent dendritic cell chemokine CCL20 expression [32]. Driving CCL20 expression involves integrin $\alpha_v\beta_8$-mediated activation of TGF-β [33]. Dendritic cell depletion or deficiency in the crucial dendritic cell chemokine receptor CCR6 protects cells from adenoviral IL-1β-induced adaptive T cell immune responses and fibrosis in the airways of mice [33].

4.3.3 COPD Deterioration After Smoking Cessation

The average duration of smoking cessation before lung volume reduction surgery is 9.2 years [10], proving that COPD deteriorates for several years after smoking cessation. The immunological changes in the lungs of COPD patients during this period are key to understanding the mechanisms involved in this pathologic progression.

4.3.3.1 COPD Deterioration by COPD Itself

Needless to say, cigarette smoking is not a significant cause of the progression of COPD after smoking cessation. Before explaining the relationship between COPD and infection after smoking cessation, we will first take a look at the mechanism of COPD deterioration caused by COPD itself.

First, DAMPs arise from the direct stimulation of acute exposure to cigarette smoke, but COPD itself is a cause of DAMPs. In COPD, apoptotic cells are increased because of enhanced induction of apoptosis and deficient phagocytosis of the apoptotic cells by alveolar macrophages. The increased apoptosis of lung parenchyma leads to impaired resolution of inflammation. On the other hand, apoptosis of neutrophils followed by efferocytosis (the process by which dying or dead cells are removed by phagocytic cells) not only prevents damage but also induces an anti-inflammatory macrophage phenotype (M2 or alternatively activated macrophages). In a murine model of COPD, acute cigarette exposure suppresses efferocytosis by alveolar macrophages (Fig. 4.4) [15]. Failed efferocytosis of apoptotic neutrophils leads to secondary necrosis, resulting in the release of DAMPs, neutrophil elastase, and other toxic components into the extracellular space [15]. All of these might be recognized by PRRs initially mediating the inflammatory response, eventually leading to worsening of COPD.

Second, hypoxia is another factor involved in COPD deterioration. Recently, a close relationship between hypoxia and inflammation was identified [34]. Hypoxia could perpetuate inflammatory changes in COPD [15]. Hypoxia seen in COPD also promotes prolonged COPD deterioration. Under hypoxic conditions, hypoxia-inducible factor 1α (HIF1α) translocates from the cytoplasm to the nucleus, inducing transcription of multiple genes, including those of TLRs and nuclear factor-kB, which are the influential factors in COPD progression. HIF1α also prolongs the life span of neutrophils by inhibiting apoptosis and promoting COPD progression [34]. On the other hand, the decrease of HIF1α is reported to bring about emphysema or COPD by reducing VEGF [35]. More research is necessary to clarify the impact of HIF1α on COPD or emphysema.

Other factors include oxidative stress, which is discussed in another chapter.

4.3.3.2 COPD Deterioration by Latent Respiratory Infection

While smoking is a very important determinant for adult lung function and COPD, there is a wide variation in adult lung function that is not related to smoking [36]. An association between lower respiratory infections and adult lung function impairment is reasonably well documented (Fig. 4.5) [36]. Viral infection plays an important role. Recently, the subject of viral infection and COPD was taken up mainly in the topic of COPD exacerbation (mainly rhinovirus), but the groundwork of COPD could already be set by respiratory viral infections during childhood, and adult lung function could be determined early in life [36]. The estimates for

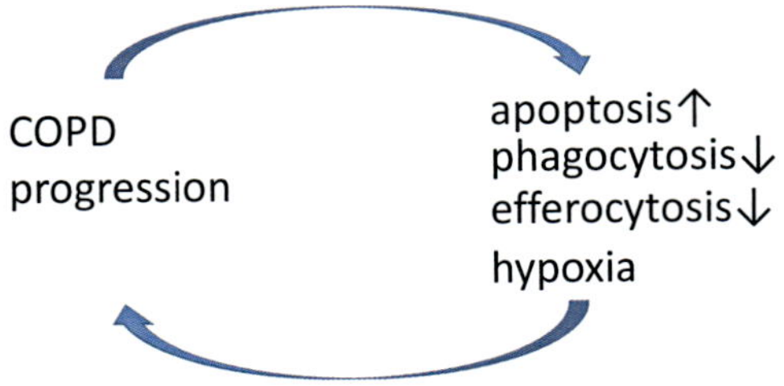

Fig. 4.4 COPD deterioration by COPD itself. In COPD, apoptotic cells are increased, while phagocytosis and efferocytosis are deficient. This condition is thought to cause activation of pattern recognition receptors (PRRs) and makes COPD even worse

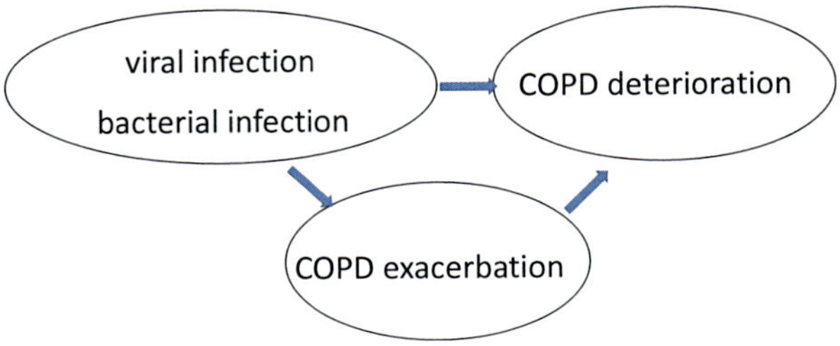

Fig. 4.5 COPD deterioration by respiratory infection and COPD exacerbation. Viral and bacterial infections of the airways bring about COPD exacerbation and accelerate COPD progression

individual childhood disadvantage factors such as maternal asthma, paternal asthma, childhood asthma, and severe respiratory infection were comparable to or larger than the estimate for smoking 10–19 cigarettes daily [36]. One of the most well-known viruses in relation with COPD is adenovirus. Latent adenoviral infection may amplify inflammation and predispose to COPD [10]. Double-stranded DNA viruses have the ability to persist in the airway epithelial cells long after the acute infection has cleared. The expression of the adenoviral trans-activating protein has been demonstrated in the airway epithelium and is associated with an amplification of the cigarette smoke-induced inflammatory response and emphysema. In vitro, human airway epithelial cells with viral genes upregulate the expression of intercellular adhesion molecule 1 (ICAM-1) and IL-8 in these cells [37]. Human rhinovirus (HRV) is also a main virus of respiratory infection and closely related with COPD. IL-17A synergistically enhances HRV type 16 (HRV-16)-induced epithelial production of neutrophil chemoattractant of IL-8 [38].

Bacterial infection is also reported to be the cause of COPD. Tuberculosis is an important matter. The results of a nationwide survey of adults in South Africa suggested that the strongest predictor of COPD was a history of pulmonary tuberculosis [36], but other pathogenic bacteria are, of course, important. Viral infections yield a negative chain of succeeding bacterial infections. Preceding rhinovirus infections precipitate secondary bacterial infections in 60 % of COPD patients by the production of rhinovirus-induced neutrophil elastase and reductions in antimicrobial molecules [39]. In COPD, impaired innate lung defenses predispose patients to microbial colonization and infection of the lower respiratory tract, which causes additional airway epithelial injury. This cyclical sequence of events amplifies chronic inflammation and perpetuates microbial infections. The frequency of chronic bacterial colonization and infection increases progressively with disease severity [15]. In a study of bacterial colonization of the lower respiratory tract, potentially pathogenic bacteria were recovered in 34.6 % of patients with COPD compared with 6.7 % in ex-smokers without COPD and nonsmokers by means of BAL culture. Neutrophilia and decreases in macrophages were seen among subjects with COPD after smoking cessation. Additionally, patients with COPD demonstrated increased levels of IL-8 in the BAL. COPD patients also had increased levels of proteinase and proteinase inhibitors, including neutrophil elastase/antineutrophil elastase (NE-A1AT) complex, MMP9, and tissue inhibitor of matrix metalloproteinase-1 (TIMP-1) [40]. In short, bacterial colonization in the lower respiratory tract is related to IL-8 and neutrophils and could contribute to airway inflammation and progressive airway destruction and obstruction in COPD [40].

On the contrary, COPD prolongs bacterial infections. The alveolar macrophage is a key defense against inhaled particulate matter and pathogens. Indeed, the phagocytosis of bacteria such as *Haemophilus influenzae* and *Streptococcus pneumoniae* by alveolar macrophages is impaired in COPD [15, 41]. Histone deacetylase (HDAC) is a key molecule in the repression of proinflammatory cytokine production in alveolar macrophages, and its expression is diminished in COPD patients [42]. The decreased TLR2 expression on alveolar macrophages has also been observed in patients with COPD, and the decrements in TLR4 expression in nasal and tracheal epithelium have been noted in severe COPD [41]. Additional important factors of attacking infections in COPD include the impairment of mucociliary clearance because the airway surface liquid is rich in endogenous antimicrobial polypeptides, including cationic polypeptides and collectins. Several of these molecules also have important immunoregulatory functions [41].

4.3.3.3 COPD Deterioration by Exacerbation

Lastly, we look at the relationship between acute exacerbations and subsequent COPD progression (Fig. 4.5). There is a considerable new evidence that infection is the predominant cause of exacerbations and likely contributes to the pathogenesis of COPD [41]. Viruses can be detected in 10–15 % of sputum samples from patients with COPD and 30–60 % of those with COPD exacerbations, depending on the sensitivity of the detection method [15]. Exacerbations of COPD result in elevated levels of circulating fragments of structural proteins. This suggests that patients with COPD have accelerated extracellular matrix turnover during exacerbations that is related to disease severity [43]. The worsening of airway obstruction is also caused by viral infection in COPD exacerbation. The CD4+ T cells of BALF from patients with COPD showed a mixed Th1 and Th2 cell cytokine phenotype during acute rhinovirus infection [15]. Though Th1-biased immunity has previously been linked to the immunopathology of COPD and emphysema, Th2 as well as Th1 bias is seen in acute exacerbations of COPD [44]. HRV-encoded proteinase 2A induces strong Th1 and Th2 immune responses from CD4+ T cells, implicating this microbial proteinase as an adjuvant factor during respiratory tract infections in patients with COPD. Th2 induces the production of cytokines such as IL-13, IL-4, IFN-γ, and IL-2, which causes an asthma-like attack [44]. This mechanism of the worsening obstruction in acute exacerbations of COPD triggered by viral infection could accumulate the inflammatory microbes and particles, such as the bacteria themselves and the related DAMPs and PAMPs, in the respiratory airways, eventually accelerating COPD deterioration.

4.4 Conclusion

COPD deterioration is not just the result of exposure to substances in cigarette smoke. The progression of COPD is associated with delayed immunological reactions caused by neutrophils, macrophages, and lymphatic cells and the cytokines secreted by these cells. The viral and bacterial infections accelerate pathological processes in the respiratory tract, even several years after smoking cessation. In view of these, airway inflammation persists after smoking cessation.

References

1. Fahy JV, Dickey BF. Airway mucus function and dysfunction. N Engl J Med. 2010;363(23):2233–47.
2. Hogg JC, Chu F, Utokaparch S, et al. The nature of small-airway obstruction in chronic obstructive pulmonary disease. N Engl J Med. 2004;350(26):2645–53.
3. Willemse BW, Postma DS, Timens W, et al. The impact of smoking cessation on respiratory symptoms, lung function, airway hyperresponsiveness and inflammation. Eur Respir J. 2004;23(3):464–76.
4. Saetta M, Turato G, Maestrelli P, et al. Cellular and structural bases of chronic obstructive pulmonary disease. Am J Respir Crit Care Med. 2001;163(6):1304–9.
5. Takeyama K, Jung B, Shim JJ, et al. Activation of epidermal growth factor receptors is responsible for mucin synthesis induced by cigarette smoke. Am J Physiol Lung Cell Mol Physiol. 2001;280(1):L165–72.
6. Kasahara Y, Tuder RM, Taraseviciene-Stewart L, et al. Inhibition of VEGF receptors causes lung cell apoptosis and emphysema. J Clin Invest. 2000;106(11):1311–9.
7. Deshmukh HS, Shaver C, et al. Acrolein-activated matrix metalloproteinase 9 contributes to persistent mucin production. Am J Respir Cell Mol Biol. 2008;38(4):446–54.
8. Churg A, Zhou S, Wright JL. Series "matrix metalloproteinases in lung health and disease": matrix metalloproteinases in COPD. Eur Respir J. 2012;39(1):197–209.
9. Gamble E, Grootendorst DC, Hattotuwa K, O'Shaughnessy T, Ram FS, Qiu Y, Zhu J, Vignola AM, Kroegel C, Morell F, Pavord ID, Rabe KF, Jeffery PK, Barnes NC. Airway mucosal inflammation in COPD is similar in smokers and ex-smokers: a pooled analysis. Eur Respir J. 2007;30(3):467–71. Epub 2007 May 15.
10. Shapiro SD. End-stage chronic obstructive pulmonary disease: the cigarette is burned out but inflammation rages on. Am J Respir Crit Care Med. 2001;164(3):339–40.

11. Vlies BH, Walker PP. Improving the diagnosis and management of COPD. Practitioner. 2015;259(1787):15–9, 2.
12. Haswell LE, Hewitt K, Thorne D, et al. Cigarette smoke total particulate matter increases mucous secreting cell numbers in vitro: a potential model of goblet cell hyperplasia. Toxicol In Vitro. 2010;24(3):981–7.
13. Kitaguchi Y, Taraseviciene-Stewart L, Hanaoka M, et al. Acrolein induces endoplasmic reticulum stress and causes airspace enlargement. PLoS One. 2012;7(5), e38038.
14. Zhang Q, Wan H, Huang S, et al. Critical role of RIG-I-like receptors in inflammation in chronic obstructive pulmonary disease. Clin Respir J. 2014;3:22–31.
15. Brusselle GG, Joos GF, Bracke KR. New insights into the immunology of chronic obstructive pulmonary disease. Lancet. 2011;378(9795):1015–26.
16. Nyunoya T, Mebratu Y, Contreras A, et al. Molecular processes that drive cigarette smoke-induced epithelial cell fate of the lung. Am J Respir Cell Mol Biol. 2014;50(3):471–82.
17. Doz E, Noulin N, Boichot E, et al. Cigarette smoke-induced pulmonary inflammation is TLR4/MyD88 and IL-1R1/MyD88 signaling dependent. J Immunol. 2008;180(2):1169–78.
18. Todt JC, Freeman CM, Brown JP, et al. Smoking decreases the response of human lung macrophages to double-stranded RNA by reducing TLR3 expression. Respir Res. 2013;14:33.
19. Koarai A, Yanagisawa S, Sugiura H, Ichikawa T, Akamatsu K, Hirano T, Nakanishi M, Matsunaga K, Minakata Y, Ichinose M. Cigarette smoke augments the expression and responses of toll-like receptor 3 in human macrophages. Respirology. 2012;17(6):1018–25.
20. Koff JL, Shao MX, Ueki IF, Nadel JA. Multiple TLRs activate EGFR via a signaling cascade to produce innate immune responses in airway epithelium. Am J Physiol Lung Cell Mol Physiol. 2008;294(6):L1068–75.
21. Nakanaga T, Nadel JA, Ueki IF, Koff JL, Shao MX. Regulation of interleukin-8 via an airway epithelial signaling cascade. Am J Physiol Lung Cell Mol Physiol. 2007;292(5):L1289–96.
22. Richter A, O'Donnell RA, Powell RM, Sanders MW, Holgate ST, Djukanović R, Davies DE. Autocrine ligands for the epidermal growth factor receptor mediate interleukin-8 release from bronchial epithelial cells in response to cigarette smoke. Am J Respir Cell Mol Biol. 2002;27(1):85–90.
23. Chaput C, Sander LE, Suttorp N, Opitz B. NOD-like receptors in lung diseases. Front Immunol. 2013;4:393.
24. Stogsdill MP, Stogsdill JA, Bodine BG, et al. Conditional overexpression of receptors for advanced glycation end-products in the adult murine lung causes airspace enlargement and induces inflammation. Am J Respir Cell Mol Biol. 2013;49(1):128–34.
25. Yonchuk JG, Silverman EK, Bowler RP, Agustí A, Lomas DA, Miller BE, Tal-Singer R, Mayer RJ. Circulating soluble receptor for advanced glycation end products(sRAGE) as a biomarker of emphysema and the RAGE axis in the lung. Am J Respir Crit Care Med. 2015;192(7):785–92.
26. Taraseviciene-Stewart L, Scerbavicius R, Voelkel NF. An animal model of autoimmune emphysema. Am J Respir Crit Care Med. 2005;171(7):734–42.
27. Hanaoka M, Nicolls MR, Taraseviciene-Stewart L, et al. Immunomodulatory strategies prevent the development of autoimmune emphysema. Respir Res. 2010;11:179.
28. van der Strate BW, Postma DS, Brandsma CA, Melgert BN, et al. Cigarette smoke-induced emphysema: a role for the B cell? Am J Respir Crit Care Med. 2006;173(7):751–8.
29. Cosio MG, Saetta M, Agusti A. Immunologic aspects of chronic obstructive pulmonary disease. N Engl J Med. 2009;360(23):2445–54.
30. Duan MC, Tang HJ, Zhong XN, et al. Persistence of Th17/Tc17 cell expression upon smoking cessation in mice with cigarette smoke-induced emphysema. Clin Dev Immunol. 2013;2013:350727.
31. Chen Y, Thai P, Zhao YH, Ho YS, DeSouza MM, Wu R. Stimulation of airway mucin gene expression by interleukin (IL)-17 through IL-6 paracrine/autocrine loop. J Biol Chem. 2003;278(19):17036–43.

32. Brand OJ, Somanath S, Moermans C, et al. Transforming growth factor-β and Interleukin-1β signaling pathways converge on the Chemokine CCL20 promoter. J Biol Chem. 2015;290(23):14717–28.
33. Hashimoto M, Yanagisawa H, Minagawa S, Sen D, Goodsell A, Ma R, Moermans C, McKnelly KJ, Baron JL, Krummel MF, Nishimura SL. A critical role for dendritic cells in the evolution of IL-1β-mediated murine airway disease. J Immunol. 2015;194(8):3962–9.
34. Eltzschig HK, Carmeliet P. Hypoxia and inflammation. N Engl J Med. 2011;364(7):656–65.
35. Yasuo M, Mizuno S, Kraskauskas D, et al. Hypoxia inducible factor-1α in human emphysema lung tissue. Eur Respir J. 2011;37(4):775–83.
36. Svanes C, Sunyer J, Plana E, et al. Early life origins of chronic obstructive pulmonary disease. Thorax. 2010;65(1):14–20.
37. Hogg JC. Role of latent viral infections in chronic obstructive pulmonary disease and asthma. Am J Respir Crit Care Med. 2001;164(10 Pt 2):S71–5.
38. Wiehler S, Proud D. Interleukin-17A modulates human airway epithelial responses to human rhinovirus infection. Am J Physiol Lung Cell Mol Physiol. 2007;293(2):L505–15.
39. Mallia P, Footitt J, Sotero R, et al. Rhinovirus infection induces degradation of antimicrobial peptides and secondary bacterial infection in chronic obstructive pulmonary disease. Am J Respir Crit Care Med. 2012;186(11):1117–24.
40. Sethi S, Maloney J, Grove L, Wrona C, Berenson CS. Airway inflammation and bronchial bacterial colonization in chronic obstructive pulmonary disease. Am J Respir Crit Care Med. 2006;173(9):991–8.
41. Sethi S, Murphy TF. Infection in the pathogenesis and course of chronic obstructive pulmonary disease. N Engl J Med. 2008;359(22):2355–65.
42. Ito K, Ito M, Elliott WM, Cosio B, et al. Decreased histone deacetylase activity in chronic obstructive pulmonary disease. N Engl J Med. 2005;352(19):1967–76.
43. Sand JM, Knox AJ, Lange P, et al. Accelerated extracellular matrix turnover during exacerbations of COPD. Respir Res. 2015;16:69.
44. Singh M, Lee SH, Porter P, et al. Human rhinovirus proteinase 2A induces TH1 and TH2 immunity in patients with chronic obstructive pulmonary disease. J Allergy Clin Immunol. 2010;125(6):1369–78.e2.

Chapter 5
Pathogenesis of COPD 3: Oxidative Stress – Is There a Possibility of Developing New Drugs from the Standpoint of This Pathogenetic Mechanism?

Tadashi Sato and Kuniaki Seyama

Abstract Growing evidence suggests that oxidative stress plays an important role in the pathogenesis of chronic obstructive pulmonary disease (COPD). However, the pathogenetic mechanisms underlying this disease are not fully understood. Although current therapies for COPD, which are mainly bronchodilators, can provide symptomatic relief, no available therapy can reverse or even slow the progression of COPD. A better understanding of the underlying mechanisms by which oxidative stress drives disease pathogenesis is critical for developing novel and more effective therapies. This chapter focuses first on the relationship between cigarette smoking and oxidative stress in COPD. Next, the role of antioxidants in the lung and the antioxidant capacity in COPD is explained. The latest information on genetic predisposition and epigenetic regulation of oxidative stress in COPD is then specifically reviewed, focusing on the role of microRNAs in this disease. Finally, the current state and the future direction of antioxidant therapeutics in COPD are presented. Certain classes of antioxidants are expected to be developed into promising treatments for COPD. However, their current therapeutic potential remains limited due to the complexity of this disease. Hence, multidisciplinary therapeutic approaches are necessary for developing novel strategies of COPD treatment.

Keywords Chronic obstructive pulmonary disease (COPD) • Oxidative stress • Reactive oxygen species (ROS) • Cigarette smoking • Antioxidant

---

T. Sato (✉) • K. Seyama
Department of Respiratory Medicine, Juntendo University Graduate School of Medicine, 3-1-3 Hongo, Bunkyo-ku, Tokyo 113-8431, Japan
e-mail: satotada@juntendo.ac.jp

H. Nakamura, K. Aoshiba (eds.), *Chronic Obstructive Pulmonary Disease*, Respiratory Disease Series: Diagnostic Tools and Disease Managements,
DOI 10.1007/978-981-10-0839-9_5

5.1 Introduction

Chronic obstructive pulmonary disease (COPD) is one of the leading causes of death worldwide and is the only major cause of death that is on the rise. It is characterized by the progressive development of expiratory airflow limitation that is not completely reversible. The airflow limitation is usually progressive and associated with an abnormal inflammatory response of the lungs. The pathogenesis of COPD is incompletely defined and can involve recurrent inflammation, oxidative stress (oxidant/antioxidant imbalance), protease/antiprotease imbalance, environmental insult, and host genetics. Cigarette smoking is the most important cause as it is the major source of oxidants/reactive oxygen species (ROS) in the lungs and throughout the body. Smoking cessation, early in the course of the disease, can slow the rate at which lung function is lost [1]. Cessation later in the course of the disease may be less effective. While current therapies can mitigate symptoms to some extent, no currently available therapy other than smoking cessation slows the rate at which lung function is lost, and no available therapy can restore lung function. The relentless progression of the disease, despite currently available therapies, portends COPD mortality that will rise among those who previously smoked for the next several decades, even if cigarette smoking were eliminated from the population.

5.2 Oxidative Stress in the Lung

Oxidative stress is the imbalance between the production of oxidants and the body's ability to detoxify the reactive intermediates or repair the resulting damage. Oxidant generation is part of normal cellular metabolism and is critical for cell homeostasis. Inflammatory cells, such as macrophages, neutrophils, and eosinophils, are the most important endogenous generators of oxidants. Cigarette smoking is the most common source of exogenous oxidants (Table 5.1).

5.2.1 Cigarette Smoking and COPD

Cigarette smoking is the most important cause of COPD and is among the leading causes of preventable morbidity and mortality. The most effective way to prevent disease due to cigarette smoking is to prevent smoking initiation. For those who have started smoking, cessation substantially reduces many adverse health consequences. Unfortunately, cessation does not eliminate health consequences of cigarette smoke exposure. Lung cancer risk, for example, remains high for the remainder of an ex-smoker's life. In COPD, cessation does not result in the restoration of lung function. If cessation occurs early in the course of disease, however, the rate at which lung function is lost with aging normalizes. In the face

Table 5.1 Exogenous and endogenous sources of oxidants

Exogenous source	Origin
Cigarette smoking	Cigarette smoke
Air pollution (ozone, SO_2, NO_2)	Polluted air
Infection	Bacteria/virus/fungus/protozoa
Endogenous source	Location
Electron transport chain of mitochondria	Endothelial cells
Xanthine oxidase system	Airway epithelial cells
Inflammatory cells	
1. NADPH oxidase (NOX)	Phagocytes (neutrophils, macrophages)
2. Oxidative bursts:	
Myeloperoxidase (MPO)	Neutrophils, macrophages
Eosinophil peroxidase	Eosinophils, macrophages
Heme peroxidase	Macrophages
3. Nitric oxide synthase (NOS)	

of more substantial disease, emphysema may progress despite cessation. Understanding the mechanisms that lead to progressive disease despite smoking cessation will be key in preventing smoke-induced diseases for former smokers.

5.2.2 *Cigarette Smoke and Oxidative Stress*

The most common source of exogenous oxidants is cigarette smoke. Cigarette smoke contains approximately 10^{15}–10^{17} oxidants and free radicals per puff in the gas phase. Numerous oxidant compounds are present among the 4000–7000 constituents in cigarette smoke. In the particular fraction, phenols and semiquinones are identified among these compounds, while superoxide (O_2^-), epoxides, peroxides, nitric oxide (NO), nitrogen dioxide, peroxynitrite, peroxynitrates, and acrolein are included in the gas phase. Cigarette smoke can induce increased oxidant burden and cause irreversible changes to endogenous antioxidant protection in the airways. In addition, the oxidants derived from cigarette smoke damage airway epithelial cells, inducing direct injury to membrane lipids, proteins, carbohydrates, and DNA, which leads to the persistent inflammation that characterizes COPD. The combination of oxidative stress and persistent inflammation accounts for the increased free radicals in the airways and further enhances pro-inflammatory gene expression, inflammatory protein release, and inactivation of antiproteases, leading to a vicious cycle of oxidative injury and inflammatory cell recruitment (Fig. 5.1) [2].

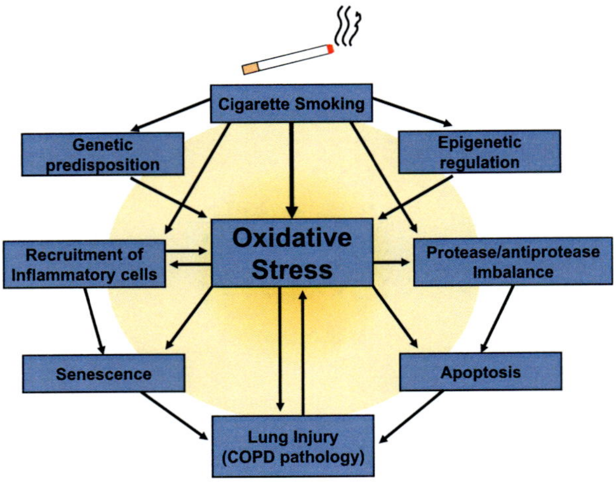

Fig. 5.1 Schema of oxidative stress in COPD pathogenesis

5.2.3 Endogenous Oxidant Generation

The ROS of endogenous origin are produced through enzymatic and nonenzymatic reactions of electron transfer. The principal cellular sites and processes that generate oxidants are the mitochondria, the microsomes, the xanthine/xanthine oxidase system, and the nicotinamide adenine dinucleotide phosphate hydrogen (NADPH) oxidase. The mitochondria are currently recognized to be the main source of endogenous intracellular oxidants through an electron leak from the mitochondrial respiratory chain. The important role of mitochondrial proteolytic enzymes was shown to provide resistance toward oxidative stress [3]. A recent study further highlighted the precious role of mitochondria in COPD pathogenesis: mitochondrial dysfunction in patients with COPD is associated with excessive mitochondrial ROS levels, which contributes to enhanced inflammation and cell hyperproliferation [4]. In the airways, the endogenous sources of oxidants are alveolar macrophages, epithelial cells, endothelial cells, and recruited inflammatory cells such as neutrophils, eosinophils, monocytes, and lymphocytes. The number of macrophages and neutrophils in cigarette smokers are increased, both in the lung and systemically, generating ROS. The activation of these cells results in the formation of O_2^-, which is converted into hydrogen peroxide (H_2O_2) by the enzyme superoxide dismutase (SOD). Phagocytes from cigarette smokers spontaneously release increased amounts of O_2^- and H_2O_2 compared to those from nonsmokers. H_2O_2 is also increased in bronchoalveolar lavage fluid (BALF) and exhaled breath condensate (EBC) collected from cigarette smokers [5]. In contrast, the enzymes catalase and glutathione (GSH) peroxidase, which breakdown H_2O_2, are downregulated in smokers.

5.2.4 *Measurement of Oxidative Stress*

Oxidative stress markers indicate the level of free oxidants and ROS-generating capacity. However, quantifying them remains difficult because oxidants and ROS are highly reactive. Multiple sample types, such as exhaled air, EBC, sputum, blood, endobronchial or surgical biopsy samples, and BALF, have been used to determine oxidative stress. These materials differ considerably in availability and significance.

H_2O_2 is a reactive oxygen species that can produce highly reactive oxidants and free radicals. It is also a product of many redox-active metal catalyzed reactions, leading to more oxidant-generating potential. There is some evidence that the concentration of H_2O_2 is elevated in the EBC and sputum from COPD patients. Determination of EBC pH is a reproducible method of sampling airway acidity; however, it is an indirect and nonspecific marker of oxidative stress. A study has shown that pH in EBC is inversely correlated with respiratory disease conditions such as asthma, COPD, and acute exacerbations [6]. Nitric oxide (NO) and reactive nitrogen species contribute to oxidative injury via their interactions with oxygen radicals. The levels of NO in exhaled air are known to be correlated with the disease activity of bronchial asthma; however, the involvement of NO and reactive nitrogen species in the development of COPD remains controversial. 8-Isoprostane, which is an end product of lipid peroxidation, is relatively stable at physiological temperature and significantly elevated in the EBC from patients with COPD [7]. F_2-α-Isoprostane, 4-hydroxy-2-nonenal (4-HNE), and malondialdehyde (MDA) are also highly reactive lipid peroxidation products and have been evaluated in samples from COPD subjects. In the case of MDA, it is not clear whether thiobarbituric acid reactive substances (TBARS) or specifically MDA have been measured. MDA/TBARS can be determined in EBC, serum, and biopsy samples. Additionally, 3-nitrotyrosine, 8-hydroxy-deoxyguanosine (8-OH-dG), and protein carbonyls have been investigated to assess oxidative stress in inflammatory lung diseases including COPD. Despite numerous studies aimed at identifying ideal oxidative stress markers, none have been found to be specific for COPD. Therefore, there are as yet no relevant standardized clinical methods or treatment guidelines toward oxidative stress in COPD.

5.3 Oxidative Stress in COPD

Oxidative stress resulting from oxidant and antioxidant imbalance is proposed as the mechanical basis of COPD. Alveolar macrophages and peripheral blood neutrophils from COPD patients are more activated and release increased amount of ROS in the form of the superoxide radical and H_2O_2. The significance of oxidative stress has been described by several studies that have identified the elevated markers of oxidative stress and free radicals in patients with COPD. The level of

8-OH-dG was increased in urine from COPD patients, and the level of 3-nitrotyrosine and $F_2\alpha$-isoprostane was elevated in the lungs of patients with COPD [8]. Furthermore, these markers demonstrated a strong correlation with COPD severity, defined by forced expiratory volume in the first second (FEV_1). The levels of lipid peroxidation products, such as 4-HNE and MDA, were also increased in the lungs and respiratory muscles, and this increase was negatively correlated with lung function [9].

5.3.1 Protein Carbonylation and COPD

Protein carbonylation is a type of protein oxidation that can be promoted by reactive oxygen species. It usually refers to a process that forms reactive ketones or aldehydes that can be reacted with 2,4-dinitrophenylhydrazine (DNPH) to form hydrazones. The development of the antibody against DNPH-derivatized proteins revolutionized the studies of carbonylated proteins by allowing for the use of immunological techniques and, more recently, mass spectrometry. Barreiro et al. reported that protein carbonyls are elevated in the respiratory muscle from severe COPD patients compared with control subjects and further showed that the increase of protein carbonyls was correlated negatively with FEV_1 [10]. The same group also reported that the intensity of creatine kinase carbonylation was significantly greater in the quadriceps femoris muscles of patients with COPD as compared with control subjects and correlated negatively with FEV_1 and maximal oxygen consumption (VO_2 max) [11]. Burcham et al. demonstrated that intermediate filament proteins are targets of acrolein-induced protein carbonylation in A549 cells, providing evidence for the involvement of carbonylation of these proteins during smoke-induced lung injury [12]. Sato et al. showed that protein carbonyls in the lungs of mice tended to increase with aging and were enhanced after chronic exposure of cigarette smoke [13]. Protein carbonylation can modify protein function, disrupting normal cell function and physiological mechanisms.

5.3.2 Oxidative Stress and COPD Pathogenesis

The pathogenesis of COPD involves several pathogenetic processes, such as oxidative stress, inflammation, protease/antiprotease imbalance, apoptosis, and cellular senescence, which are modified by genetic and epigenetic factors (Fig. 5.1). In particular, oxidative stress has several important consequences for the pathogenesis of COPD.

Oxidative stress activates the transcription factor nuclear factor-kB (NF-kB) pathway, leading to an increase in inflammation. NF-kB expression and activation are increased in the lungs from COPD subjects and correlate with airflow limitation. ROS are also intracellular second messengers, acting as inflammatory stimuli that induce micro-oxidative bursts, which are essential for cellular activation. The ability of corticosteroids to repress pro-inflammatory gene expression is impaired in COPD because of oxidative stress. Carbonylation and nitration reduce the activity and expression of histone deacetylase 2 (HDAC2), which is essential for the suppression of activated inflammatory genes and the anti-inflammatory effects of corticosteroids. HDAC2 is markedly reduced in COPD since there is another pathway activated by oxidative stress, phosphoinositide-3-kinase-δ, which is responsible for reducing HDAC2 activity and expression [14, 15]. Nuclear factor erythroid 2-related factor 2 (Nrf2) is a key transcriptional factor that regulates a number of antioxidant and cytoprotective genes. Loss of HDAC2 activity in COPD has also been demonstrated to lead to loss of Nrf2 activity through increased Nrf2 acetylation, thereby decreasing Nrf2 stability and expression [16]. Another transcriptional corepressor, sirtuin 1 (SIRT1), is similarly impacted by oxidative stress, reducing both its expression and activity leading to an accelerated aging process and the development of emphysema. Many studies have analyzed the relationship between aging and oxidative stress. Moderate oxidative stress may gradually develop with age because plasma levels of lipoperoxidation products and antioxidant enzyme activities in red blood cells increase with aging, whereas plasma levels of nutritional antioxidants decrease. Senescence marker protein-30 (SMP30), a gluconolactonase involved in L-ascorbic acid biosynthesis that is known to decrease with aging in rats and mice, has been shown to protect mouse lungs from oxidative stress associated with aging and smoking [13]. Oxidative stress can result in enhanced inflammatory gene expression, failure to resolve the inflammatory response, corticosteroid insensitivity, impaired antioxidant defenses, and accelerated aging, all of which are associated with the development of COPD pathology.

Oxidative stress can potentiate the effect of proteases on COPD through the activation of enzymes such as serine proteases, cysteine proteases, and matrix metalloproteinases. ROS increase the activity of matrix metalloproteinases by activating metalloproteinase precursors. The increase of epithelial and endothelial cell apoptosis in the lungs has been known to result in tissue destruction and in the development of emphysema. There are several reports that demonstrated the association between oxidative stress and apoptosis. Vascular endothelial growth factor (VEGF) is a pluripotent growth factor that has a broad impact on endothelial cell survival and its function and plays a critical role in the maintenance of lung structure. An experimental emphysema in rat lungs induced by VEGF blockade demonstrated that apoptosis predominates in the lungs under oxidative stress and that the blockade of apoptosis decreased the expression of oxidative stress markers [17]. The administration of the SOD mimetic can also prevent the development of alveolar cell apoptosis. Petrache et al. demonstrated that SOD overexpression protects against alveolar cell apoptosis and alveolar enlargement induced by ceramide, a second messenger lipid, which is upregulated in the lungs with smoking-induced emphysema [18, 19]. Koike et al. also reported that the administration of vitamin C to SMP30 knockout mice following chronic exposure of cigarette smoke attenuates oxidative stress and alveolar septal cell apoptosis, restoring the concentration of VEGF in the BALF and in the lungs [20].

5.4 Antioxidants in the Lung

Antioxidants are agents that decrease steady-state ROS and protect cellular macromolecules from oxidative modification. Antioxidants can be classified into two categories: enzymatic and nonenzymatic. The principal components of the enzymatic antioxidants are SOD, catalase, glutathione (GSH) peroxidases, GSH S-transferase, peroxiredoxin, and the heme oxygenase (HO). Nonenzymatic antioxidants include GSH, uric acid, bilirubin, ferritin, vitamin A (retinol), vitamin C (ascorbic acid), vitamin E (α-tocopherol), carotenoids, and polyphenols.

5.4.1 Superoxide Dismutases and COPD

SODs are a class of enzymatic antioxidants that catalyze the dismutation of superoxide into oxygen and hydrogen peroxide. There are three forms of superoxide dismutase in humans: Cu/Zn SOD, MnSOD, and extracellular SOD (EcSOD). Cu/Zn SOD is the most abundant in the lung tissue and is especially concentrated in ciliated epithelial cells. MnSOD is predominantly located in airway wall cells and mitochondria of the lungs. EcSOD is the major SOD in the extracellular fluid that exists in abundance in the lungs. The levels of EcSOD were increased in sputum from smokers, whereas the activity of EcSOD was reduced in COPD patients, and polymorphism in the EcSOD gene has been linked to both reduced lung function in COPD and susceptibility to emphysema [21].

5.4.2 Glutathione Redox System and COPD

GSH is a vital intracellular and extracellular protective antioxidant because of its strong electron-donor potential via the sulfhydryl groups of cysteine residues and its high concentration in cells. GSH is more concentrated in the epithelial lining fluids and plays an important role in the maintenance of the redox balance in the lungs. Glutathione peroxidases catalyze a variety of GSH reactions including the breakdown of H_2O_2. The levels of GSH are upregulated in the BALF from chronic smokers. However, this increase in GSH levels might not be enough to neutralize the excessive load of oxidants during acute exposure to cigarette smoke, since a depletion of GSH is observed after chronic cigarette smoke exposure in a time and dose-dependent manner.

5.4.3 *Catalase, Heme Oxygenase, and COPD*

Catalase is a common enzymatic antioxidant found in living organisms, which catalyzes the decomposition of H_2O_2 to water and oxygen. Betsuyaku et al. demonstrated that catalase is significantly downregulated in pulmonary macrophages from COPD patients compared with those that have never smoked and ex-smokers without COPD [22].

HO is an enzyme that catalyzes the degradation of heme and generates bilirubin, iron, and carbon monoxide. These downstream products of heme catabolism mediate the antioxidant properties of HO. HO-1 expression is upregulated in several respiratory diseases including COPD. Shinohara et al. demonstrated that overexpression of HO-1 in the lungs of mice attenuates elastase-induced pulmonary emphysema [23]. Bilirubin is one of the HO-1 downstream products and has been known to have potent antioxidant properties. A recent study showed that higher serum bilirubin concentration is associated with a higher FEV_1 and less annual decline of FEV_1 in patients with mild to moderate COPD. This suggested that bilirubin has a protective effect on COPD disease progression and a potential to be an easy access biomarker for this disease [24]. More recently, an in vivo study further indicated that the administration of bilirubin attenuated smoking-induced pulmonary injury by suppressing inflammatory cell recruitment and pro-inflammatory cytokine secretion, increasing anti-inflammatory cytokine levels and SOD activity [25].

5.4.4 *Dietary Antioxidants and COPD*

Dietary antioxidants include the micronutrients vitamins, carotenoids, and polyphenols. Vitamins A, C, and E and carotenoids (including lycopene which is a major carotenoid in tomatoes) have been well studied, possess strong antioxidant activities, and are well absorbed with relatively high bioavailability. As they are unable to be synthesized in humans, their concentration in serum/plasma, as well as a local milieu in the lungs, is reflected by dietary intake of vegetables and fruits as major sources. Several epidemiologic studies showed the association between lung function and dietary intake of vitamins and carotenoids, as well as manipulating antioxidant-rich diets, has led to altered clinical outcomes in chronic respiratory diseases including COPD [26]. Many studies have reported reduced levels of antioxidant nutrients, such as vitamins A, C, and E and carotenoids in serum or plasma from COPD patients. Recently, Kodama et al. showed that plasma vitamin C, lycopene, and total carotenoid levels were significantly lower in Japanese COPD patients than that of healthy elderly people [27]. Furthermore, Ford et al. demonstrated the prospective associations between concentrations of antioxidant nutrients and all causes of mortality among adults with obstructive lung function in the United States, showing that only the concentrations of vitamin C and lycopene were found to be significantly and inversely associated with all causes of mortality [28]. Interestingly, animal studies, which showed the benefits of both vitamin C and lycopene supplementation to COPD model mice, have already been reported. As noted above, vitamin C treatment successfully prevented cigarette smoke-induced pulmonary emphysema in SMP30 knockout mice, a strain that is genetically engineered to preclude vitamin C synthesis [20]. Similarly, lycopene also prevented cigarette smoke-induced emphysema in the senescence-accelerated mouse prone 1 by decreasing oxidative stress in the lungs [29]. Overall, the intake of these antioxidant nutrients could be beneficial for the treatment of COPD by modulating oxidative stress in this disease. However, it has so far failed to meet expectations in several clinical trials.

On the other hand, the polyphenols are a family of complex molecules that are ubiquitous in plants and include the flavonoids and phenolic acids. Dietary intake of polyphenols has been reported to improve the symptoms, FEV_1, and arterial oxygen tension in COPD patients. Resveratrol, a polyphenolic compound derived from red wine, was able to improve both corticosteroid efficacy and lung function in a general population. Resveratrol significantly reduced steroid-resistant cytokines from bacterial endotoxin-exposed alveolar macrophages from COPD patients [30]. Similarly, curcumin, a phenolic yellowish pigment and ingredient of turmeric, has been found to modulate cigarette smoke- or peroxide-induced steroid resistance by restoring HDAC2 activity and expression [31]. Suzuki et al. has also demonstrated that oral curcumin administration significantly attenuates elastase- and cigarette smoke-induced pulmonary emphysema in mice [32]. However, the efficacy of many polyphenols is limited either by low bioavailability or by transformation in the gastrointestinal tract.

Although there is not enough evidence to indicate the direct relationship between vitamin D and oxidative stress in COPD, vitamin D supplementation may be beneficial because the majority of COPD patients have vitamin D deficiency [33]. Many in vitro studies demonstrated important anti-inflammatory and immunomodulatory effects of vitamin D. A recent in vivo study showed that vitamin D deficiency both accelerates lung function decline and aggravates the development of emphysema following chronic exposure to cigarette smoke [34]. Moreover, a recent systematic review and meta-analysis reported that major deficiencies in 25-hydroxyvitamin D were associated with COPD severity [35]. Collectively, these studies indicate that vitamin D supplementation may be an important therapeutic strategy, in particular, for the prevention of COPD exacerbation, which is worthy of further investigation.

5.5 Genetic and Epigenetic Regulation of Oxidative Stress in COPD

Although cigarette smoking is clearly the most common risk factor in the development of COPD, only a small portion of smokers develop the disease, highlighting the important role of the individual's genetic predisposition to COPD. In addition, due to the heterogeneity of this disorder, epigenetic regulation of specific molecular and cellular pathways is also believed to be relevant to COPD pathogenesis. Epigenetics describes heritable changes in gene expression that do not involve changes to the underlying DNA sequence. Epigenetic change is a regular and natural occurrence but can also be influenced by several factors including age, environment, and disease state. DNA methylation, histone modification, and non-coding RNA-associated gene silencing are currently considered to initiate and sustain epigenetic changes.

5.5.1 Genetic Predisposition in COPD

The alpha 1-antitrypsin gene, *SERPINA1*, is the best described genetic risk factor for COPD; the most frequent mutation causing severe alpha 1-antitrypsin deficiency among Caucasians is called *PI**Z*. However, many genes are supposed to contribute to the individual predisposition to this multifactorial disorder. Major COPD susceptibility loci have recently been identified on chromosome 4 by genome-wide association studies [36]. The hedgehog-interacting protein (*HHIP*), a developmental transcription factor, was identified as a COPD susceptibility gene, while family with sequence similarity 13 member A (*FAM13A*) was associated with the regulation of oxidative stress and lung function. On chromosome 15, nicotinic acetylcholine receptor (*CHRNA*3/5) loci were associated with increased smoking intensity and emphysema in COPD patients. On chromosome 2q, *SERPINE2* and *XRCC5* have been linked to lung function and airflow obstruction in family-based genetics studies. Several genetic mutations in antioxidant genes are identified: polymorphisms in glutathione S-transferase (*GST*), superoxide dismutase 3 (*SOD3*), and microsomal epoxide hydrolase (*EPHX1*) are associated with the rapid decline of lung function characteristic of COPD [37]. Apart from the inherited genetic changes, the acquired somatic mutations constitute an important component in the pathogenesis of COPD. The oxidative stress in COPD can directly damage lung DNA. The distribution of oxidative damage in the genome depends on the varying susceptibilities of sequences to oxidative attack and preferential targeting of repair processes.

5.5.2 DNA Methylation and Histone Acetylation in COPD

DNA methylation is shown to regulate the expression of pro-inflammatory genes during the development of COPD. In patients with COPD, DNA methylation of the promoters of pro-inflammatory genes has been observed both in airway epithelial cells and in alveolar macrophages. Furthermore, methylation of the p16 gene promoter was frequently observed in the sputum of patients with COPD and positively correlated with heavy cigarette smoking. A recent analysis of methylation and gene expression indicated that DNA methylation is a genome-wide phenomenon in small airways of patients with COPD, and associated with altered expression of genes and pathways important to COPD, such as the Nrf2 oxidative response pathway [38].

The histone modifications include acetylation, methylation, ubiquitination, phosphorylation, and sumoylation. In particular, histone acetylation may play a role in airway diseases through the involvement of HDAC in inflammation. Indeed, HDAC2 is an important corepressor protein in inflammation. It is suggested that oxidants and free radicals could alter this sensitive protein, causing reduced expression level of these deacetylases in the lungs of smokers and COPD patients [14]. Furthermore, HDAC2 downregulation impairs Nrf2 activation in the lung by decreasing the half-life of Nrf2 [39]. SIRT1 is a class III HDAC with anti-inflammatory, anti-senescence, and anti-apoptotic activity mediated by the deacetylation of histone and nonhistone proteins, including transcription factors such as NF-kB and forkhead box O3 (FOXO3). It has been reported that SIRT1 is reduced in the lungs of cigarette smoke-exposed mice and patients with COPD and that SIRT1 attenuates cigarette smoke-induced lung inflammation and injury. A recent animal study showed that SIRT1 protects against cigarette smoke-induced oxidative stress, which is mediated by FOXO3 but is independent of Nrf2 [40].

5.5.3 MicroRNA Regulation upon Cigarette Smoking and in COPD

MicroRNAs (miRNAs) are noncoding endogenous RNAs, approximately 19–25 nucleotides in length, which play a role in the posttranscriptional regulation of gene expression. miRNA biogenesis begins with the cleavage of a pri-miRNA into a pre-miRNA, which is mediated by the Drosha enzyme (Fig. 5.2). The pre-miRNA is then actively transported from the nucleus into the cytoplasm by exportin-5. Next, the RNase III enzyme Dicer processes the pre-miRNA to generate a double-stranded RNA. One strand is degraded and the other is incorporated into the RNA-induced silencing complex (RISC), which then functions as a mature miRNA against its target mRNAs. The mature miRNAs, which are expressed during development in a tissue- or cell type-specific manner, mediate posttranscriptional repression of gene expression by increasing mRNA degradation or by

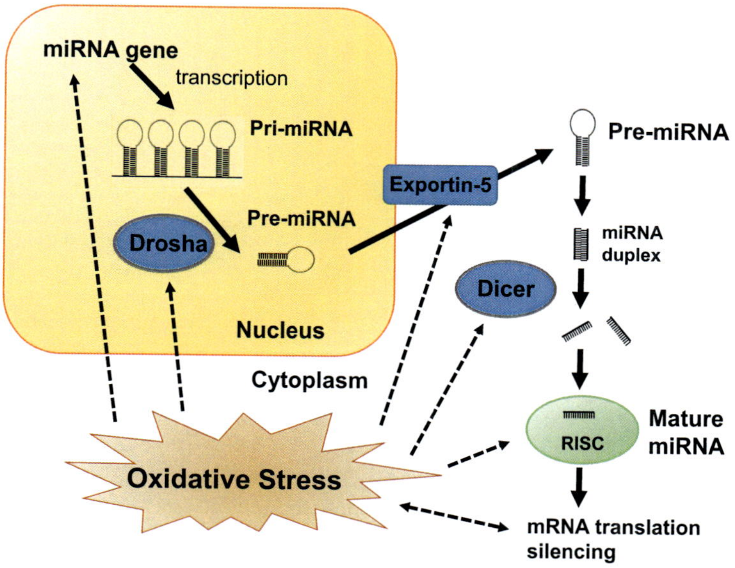

Fig. 5.2 MicroRNA biogenesis and oxidative stress

inhibiting translation. This is achieved by direct binding between the miRNA 5′ region and the 3′ untranslated region of the target mRNA. miRNAs may also indirectly alter gene expression by epigenetic mechanisms such as DNA methylation and histone acetylation. These processes enable a fine-tuning of gene expression as opposed to an on-off switch.

miRNAs have been associated with diverse biological processes such as the development, cellular differentiation, and pathogenesis of various diseases including COPD (Table 5.2). Graff et al. found that cigarette smoking downregulates global miRNA expression in human alveolar macrophages, possibly by modification of Dicer [41]. Similarly, Izzotti et al. reported a downregulation of miRNA expression in the lungs of cigarette smoke-exposed rats [42]. Schembri et al. examined whole-genome miRNA and mRNA expression in the bronchial airway epithelium in current smokers versus those who have never smoked and found that miR-218 levels modulate airway epithelial gene expression in response to exposure to cigarette smoke [43]. In contrast, Ezzie et al. compared the miRNA profile in the lung tissue from non-COPD smokers with that in the lung tissue from COPD subjects and found that 70 miRNAs are differentially expressed (57 miRNAs are upregulated and 13 miRNAs downregulated) and that miR-15b, in particular, is upregulated in COPD [44]. miR-15b was increased in COPD samples compared with controls and was differentially expressed in correlation with disease severity by the Global Initiative for Chronic Obstructive Lung Disease classification. The authors have further described that expression of Smad7, which is a validated target for miR-15b, is decreased in bronchial epithelial cells in COPD. More recently, Van Pottelberge et al. analyzed the miRNA profile from induced sputum samples and

Table 5.2 Representative microRNAs associated with smoking and COPD

Disease/condition	microRNA(s)	Expression	Source
Smoking related	Let-7, miR-10a, 34, 123, 145	↓	Lung (rat)
	miR-150, 222	↓	Sputum
	miR-199b, 218	↓	Bronchial epithelial cells
	miR-101, 144	↑	Bronchial epithelial cells
COPD	miR-15b, 223, 1274a	↑	Lung
	miR-146a	↓	Lung fibroblasts
	let-7c	↓	Sputum
	miR-638	↑	Lung
	miR-1, 133, 206, 499	↑	Plasma
	miR-1	↓	Quadriceps

showed that let-7c is significantly reduced in COPD subjects compared with smokers without COPD [45]. Hassan et al. examined the effect of cigarette smoke extract (CSE) on human bronchial epithelial cells and showed that miR-101 and miR-144 are upregulated by CSE and suppress the cystic fibrosis transmembrane conductance regulator protein, a chloride channel involved in the maintenance of fluid homeostasis in the lung [46].

miR-146a is known to downregulate NF-kB activity by repressing the NF-kB transducers interleukin (IL)-1 receptor-associated kinase and tumor necrosis factor (TNF) receptor-associated factor 6. Sato et al. reported reduced expression of miR-146a in lung fibroblasts from COPD patients compared with that observed in lung fibroblasts from non-COPD smokers following stimulation by the inflammatory cytokines IL-1β and TNF-α [47]. The authors further showed that miR-146a causes downregulation of prostaglandin E_2 production, an inflammatory mediator, by targeting cyclooxygenase-2. Interestingly, miR-146a was also identified to downregulate the expression of NADPH oxidase (NOX) 4 in human umbilical vein endothelial cells and to regulate cellular senescence in human umbilical vein endothelial cells [48]. miR-146a, therefore, may represent a promising therapeutic target for controlling abnormal inflammatory response and regulating oxidative stress in COPD. A recent analysis of the human lung tissue with regional emphysema revealed that miR-638 is positively correlated with emphysema severity and regulates gene expression networks associated with the oxidative stress response and aging in emphysematous lung tissue [49]. Additionally, Lewis et al. described that skeletal muscle-specific miRNAs (miR-1, 499, 133, and 206) are elevated in the plasma from patients with stable COPD compared with controls and showed that miR-1 is downregulated in the quadriceps of patients with COPD [50, 51]. One could speculate that these miRNAs may contribute to the development of skeletal muscle dysfunction in COPD, which may be associated with systemic oxidative stress in this condition.

5.5.4 Long Noncoding RNAs and Oxidative Stress in the Lung

Long noncoding RNAs (lncRNAs) are also receiving attention as regulators of gene expression. lncRNAs are nonprotein-coding transcripts longer than 200 nucleotides. The biological function of most lncRNAs remains unknown; however, growing evidence suggests that lncRNAs play complex roles in gene regulation and that some lncRNAs contribute to the development of neoplasms including lung cancer. Recently, Thai et al. have characterized a novel lncRNA, the smoke and cancer-associated lncRNA-1 (SCAL1), that is induced by cigarette smoke and elevated in lung cancer cell lines [52]. The authors also found that SCAL1 may act downstream of Nrf2 to regulate gene expression and protect against oxidative stress. SCAL1 may contribute to the pathogenesis of COPD by regulating cigarette smoke-induced oxidative stress.

5.6 Potential of Antioxidative Therapy in COPD

As noted earlier, smoking cessation is the best way to prevent development and progression of COPD. However, the progress of oxidant burden in the airways continues even after smoking cessation. Antioxidants and free radical scavenging compounds may provide directed therapeutics against persistent oxidative stress and subsequent tissue damage in COPD. Although several antioxidant agents have been evaluated as potential treatment candidates to date, none could be shown to protect against COPD and oxidative burden significantly (Table 5.3). For instance, N-acetyl-L-cysteine (NAC), a thiol antioxidant that serves as a precursor for GSH, is able to attenuate elastase-induced pulmonary emphysema in rats [53]. However, a large randomized placebo-controlled clinical trial (the BRONCUS) investigated the availability of NAC for the treatment of COPD and concluded that it failed to show any overall effect on slowing disease progression or exacerbation frequency [54]. In contrast, a recent randomized control trial (RCT), the PANTHEON study, showed that high-dose oral NAC therapy significantly decreases both exacerbation rate and duration of exacerbations [55]. Furthermore, carbocysteine, another thiol antioxidant, has also been evaluated for its impact on COPD exacerbation rate in a RCT [56].

A potential antioxidant therapeutic strategy has been focused on Nrf2, which has a central role in regulating antioxidant genes and is significantly reduced in COPD subjects [57]. Sulforaphane, derived from broccoli sprouts, is an Nrf2 activator that is being considered for potential clinical trials in COPD. Malhotra et al. demonstrated that sulforaphane has the ability to denitrosylate HDAC2, restoring glucocorticoid sensitivity in alveolar macrophages from patients with COPD [39]. As noted, EcSOD is an important extracellular antioxidant in the lungs. EcSOD mimetics are found to attenuate lung inflammation and emphysema

Table 5.3 Summary of antioxidants in COPD therapy

Class of antioxidants	Agent(s)	Current status for COPD therapy
Thiols	NAC	Decreased exacerbation rate (RCT)
	Carbocysteine	
Nrf2 activators	Sulforaphane	No RCTs, ex vivo study
SOD mimetics	EcSOD mimetics, PC-SOD	No RCTs, in vivo study
NOX inhibitors	Celestrol	No RCTs, in vivo study
MPO inhibitors	2-Thioxanthine	No RCTs, in vivo study
iNOS inhibitors	Manganese-metalloporphyrins	No RCTs, in vivo study
Polyphenols	Resveratrol, Curcumin	No RCTs, ex vivo/in vivo study
Vitamins	Vitamins C, E, A	No RCTs, in vivo study
	Vitamin D	Decreased exacerbation rate only in patients with severe deficiencies (RCT)
Carotenoids	Lycopene	No RCTs, in vivo study

NAC N-acetyl-L-cysteine, *Nrf2* nuclear factor erythroid 2-related factor 2, *SOD* superoxide dismutase, *EcSOD* extracellular superoxide dismutase, *PC-SOD* lecithinized superoxide dismutase, *NOX* nicotinamide adenine dinucleotide phosphate hydrogen oxidase, *MPO* myeloperoxidase, *iNOS* inducible nitric oxide synthase, *RCT* randomized control trial

in mice exposed to cigarette smoke by decreasing oxidative stress in the lungs [58]. Recently, lecithinized SOD (PC-SOD) has been shown to overcome clinical limitations of SOD, including low-tissue affinity and low stability in plasma. Tanaka et al. reported that the inhalation of PC-SOD suppresses elastase-induced pulmonary emphysema and cigarette smoke-induced lung inflammation in mice [59]. Therefore, PC-SOD has been suggested as a novel candidate for antioxidant therapy in COPD. Other promising antioxidant agents include NOX inhibitors, myeloperoxidase (MPO) inhibitors, and inducible nitric oxide synthase (iNOS) inhibitors. However, these candidates are currently still at the preclinical trial stage. Dietary antioxidants such as vitamins C, E, and D and polyphenols may also be beneficial for the treatment of COPD based on their antioxidative properties, previously discussed in Sect. 5.4.4. The current review of the clinical effectiveness of antioxidant therapy for COPD indicates that a combination of several antioxidants would be more beneficial than a single antioxidant treatment. Further clinical trials using more antioxidative combination regimens are needed to explore the clinical utility of antioxidant agents in the treatment of COPD.

5.7 Conclusion

There are currently no treatments that reverse or even slow progression of COPD. There is no doubt that oxidative stress plays a pivotal role in the development and progression of COPD. Moreover, systemic oxidative stress may also cause several comorbidities of COPD such as cardiovascular diseases and metabolic syndrome. Therefore, certain classes of antioxidants such as Nrf2 activators and EcSOD mimetics are expected to be promising for the treatment of COPD. However, the evidence of their therapeutic potentials remains limited, in part, due to the heterogeneity of this disease. Further investigations for understanding genetic susceptibility to cigarette smoke-induced COPD might be beneficial for establishing a novel strategy of COPD therapeutics. Multidisciplinary therapeutic approaches are necessary because of the complexity of the cellular and molecular mechanisms involved in the pathogenesis of COPD. Combining antioxidants with anti-inflammatory drugs, bronchodilators, and antimicrobials may provide future directions for research. Finally, emerging evidence suggests that epigenetic approaches including miRNAs provide a promising therapeutic strategy for lung diseases. Since miRNAs can target multiple genes leading to fine-tuned, coordinated regulation of complex biological processes, miRNA-based therapeutics are believed to have great potential for pathologically complex diseases including COPD.

References

1. Anthonisen NR, Connett JE, Murray RP. Smoking and lung function of Lung Health Study participants after 11 years. Am J Respir Crit Care Med. 2002;166(5):675–9. doi:10.1164/rccm.2112096.
2. Lee W, Thomas PS. Oxidative stress in COPD and its measurement through exhaled breath condensate. Clin Transl Sci. 2009;2(2):150–5. doi:10.1111/j.1752-8062.2009.00093.x.
3. Bota DA, Davies KJ. Protein degradation in mitochondria: implications for oxidative stress, aging and disease: a novel etiological classification of mitochondrial proteolytic disorders. Mitochondrion. 2001;1(1):33–49.
4. Wiegman CH, Michaeloudes C, Haji G, Narang P, Clarke CJ, Russell KE, et al. Oxidative stress-induced mitochondrial dysfunction drives inflammation and airway smooth muscle remodeling in patients with chronic obstructive pulmonary disease. J Allergy Clin Immunol. 2015;136(3):769–80. doi:10.1016/j.jaci.2015.01.046.
5. Dekhuijzen PN, Aben KK, Dekker I, Aarts LP, Wielders PL, van Herwaarden CL, et al. Increased exhalation of hydrogen peroxide in patients with stable and unstable chronic obstructive pulmonary disease. Am J Respir Crit Care Med. 1996;154(3 Pt 1):813–6. doi:10.1164/ajrccm.154.3.8810624.
6. Kostikas K, Papatheodorou G, Ganas K, Psathakis K, Panagou P, Loukides S. pH in expired breath condensate of patients with inflammatory airway diseases. Am J Respir Crit Care Med. 2002;165(10):1364–70. doi:10.1164/rccm.200111-068OC.
7. Makris D, Paraskakis E, Korakas P, Karagiannakis E, Sourvinos G, Siafakas NM, et al. Exhaled breath condensate 8-isoprostane, clinical parameters, radiological indices and airway inflammation in COPD. Respiration. 2008;75(2):138–44. doi:10.1159/000106377.

8. Ichinose M, Sugiura H, Yamagata S, Koarai A, Shirato K. Increase in reactive nitrogen species production in chronic obstructive pulmonary disease airways. Am J Respir Crit Care Med. 2000;162(2 Pt 1):701–6. doi:10.1164/ajrccm.162.2.9908132.
9. Rahman I, van Schadewijk AA, Crowther AJ, Hiemstra PS, Stolk J, MacNee W, et al. 4-Hydroxy-2-nonenal, a specific lipid peroxidation product, is elevated in lungs of patients with chronic obstructive pulmonary disease. Am J Respir Crit Care Med. 2002;166(4):490–5. doi:10.1164/rccm.2110101.
10. Barreiro E, de la Puente B, Minguella J, Corominas JM, Serrano S, Hussain SN, et al. Oxidative stress and respiratory muscle dysfunction in severe chronic obstructive pulmonary disease. Am J Respir Crit Care Med. 2005;171(10):1116–24. doi:10.1164/rccm.200407-887OC.
11. Barreiro E, Gea J, Matar G, Hussain SN. Expression and carbonylation of creatine kinase in the quadriceps femoris muscles of patients with chronic obstructive pulmonary disease. Am J Respir Cell Mol Biol. 2005;33(6):636–42. doi:10.1165/rcmb.2005-0114OC.
12. Burcham PC, Raso A, Thompson CA. Intermediate filament carbonylation during acute acrolein toxicity in A549 lung cells: functional consequences, chaperone redistribution, and protection by bisulfite. Antioxid Redox Signal. 2010;12(3):337–47. doi:10.1089/ars.2009.2817.
13. Sato T, Seyama K, Sato Y, Mori H, Souma S, Akiyoshi T, et al. Senescence marker protein-30 protects mice lungs from oxidative stress, aging, and smoking. Am J Respir Crit Care Med. 2006;174(5):530–7. doi:10.1164/rccm.200511-1816OC.
14. Ito K, Ito M, Elliott WM, Cosio B, Caramori G, Kon OM, et al. Decreased histone deacetylase activity in chronic obstructive pulmonary disease. N Engl J Med. 2005;352(19):1967–76. doi:10.1056/NEJMoa041892.
15. To Y, Ito K, Kizawa Y, Failla M, Ito M, Kusama T, et al. Targeting phosphoinositide-3-kinase-delta with theophylline reverses corticosteroid insensitivity in chronic obstructive pulmonary disease. Am J Respir Crit Care Med. 2010;182(7):897–904. doi:10.1164/rccm.200906-0937OC.
16. Mercado N, Thimmulappa R, Thomas CM, Fenwick PS, Chana KK, Donnelly LE, et al. Decreased histone deacetylase 2 impairs Nrf2 activation by oxidative stress. Biochem Biophys Res Commun. 2011;406(2):292–8. doi:10.1016/j.bbrc.2011.02.035.
17. Tuder RM, Zhen L, Cho CY, Taraseviciene-Stewart L, Kasahara Y, Salvemini D, et al. Oxidative stress and apoptosis interact and cause emphysema due to vascular endothelial growth factor receptor blockade. Am J Respir Cell Mol Biol. 2003;29(1):88–97. doi:10.1165/rcmb.2002-0228OC.
18. Petrache I, Natarajan V, Zhen L, Medler TR, Richter AT, Cho C, et al. Ceramide upregulation causes pulmonary cell apoptosis and emphysema-like disease in mice. Nat Med. 2005;11(5):491–8. doi:10.1038/nm1238.
19. Petrache I, Medler TR, Richter AT, Kamocki K, Chukwueke U, Zhen L, et al. Superoxide dismutase protects against apoptosis and alveolar enlargement induced by ceramide. Am J Physiol Lung Cell Mol Physiol. 2008;295(1):L44–53. doi:10.1152/ajplung.00448.2007.
20. Koike K, Ishigami A, Sato Y, Hirai T, Yuan Y, Kobayashi E, et al. Vitamin C prevents cigarette smoke-induced pulmonary emphysema in mice and provides pulmonary restoration. Am J Respir Cell Mol Biol. 2014;50(2):347–57. doi:10.1165/rcmb.2013-0121OC.
21. Dahl M, Bowler RP, Juul K, Crapo JD, Levy S, Nordestgaard BG. Superoxide dismutase 3 polymorphism associated with reduced lung function in two large populations. Am J Respir Crit Care Med. 2008;178(9):906–12. doi:10.1164/rccm.200804-549OC.
22. Betsuyaku T, Fuke S, Inomata T, Kaga K, Morikawa T, Odajima N, et al. Bronchiolar epithelial catalase is diminished in smokers with mild COPD. Eur Respir J. 2013;42(1):42–53. doi:10.1183/09031936.00058912.
23. Shinohara T, Kaneko T, Nagashima Y, Ueda A, Tagawa A, Ishigatsubo Y. Adenovirus-mediated transfer and overexpression of heme oxygenase 1 cDNA in lungs attenuates

elastase-induced pulmonary emphysema in mice. Hum Gene Ther. 2005;16(3):318–27. doi:10.1089/hum.2005.16.318.
24. Apperley S, Park HY, Holmes DT, Man SF, Tashkin D, Wise RA, et al. Serum bilirubin and disease progression in mild COPD. Chest. 2015;148(1):169–75. doi:10.1378/chest.14-2150.
25. Wei J, Zhao H, Fan G, Li J. Bilirubin treatment suppresses pulmonary inflammation in a rat model of smoke-induced emphysema. Biochem Biophys Res Commun. 2015;465(2):180–7. doi:10.1016/j.bbrc.2015.07.133.
26. Keranis E, Makris D, Rodopoulou P, Martinou H, Papamakarios G, Daniil Z, et al. Impact of dietary shift to higher-antioxidant foods in COPD: a randomised trial. Eur Respir J. 2010;36(4):774–80. doi:10.1183/09031936.00113809.
27. Kodama Y, Kishimoto Y, Muramatsu Y, Tatebe J, Yamamoto Y, Hirota N, et al. Antioxidant nutrients in plasma of Japanese patients with chronic obstructive pulmonary disease (COPD), asthma-COPD overlap syndrome, and bronchial asthma. Clin Respir J. 2015. doi:10.1111/crj.12436.
28. Ford ES, Li C, Cunningham TJ, Croft JB. Associations between antioxidants and all-cause mortality among US adults with obstructive lung function. Br J Nutr. 2014;112(10):1662–73. doi:10.1017/S0007114514002669.
29. Kasagi S, Seyama K, Mori H, Souma S, Sato T, Akiyoshi T, et al. Tomato juice prevents senescence-accelerated mouse P1 strain from developing emphysema induced by chronic exposure to tobacco smoke. Am J Physiol Lung Cell Mol Physiol. 2006;290(2):L396–404. doi:10.1152/ajplung.00483.2004.
30. Knobloch J, Hag H, Jungck D, Urban K, Koch A. Resveratrol impairs the release of steroid-resistant cytokines from bacterial endotoxin-exposed alveolar macrophages in chronic obstructive pulmonary disease. Basic Clin Pharmacol Toxicol. 2011;109(2):138–43. doi:10.1111/j.1742-7843.2011.00707.x.
31. Meja KK, Rajendrasozhan S, Adenuga D, Biswas SK, Sundar IK, Spooner G, et al. Curcumin restores corticosteroid function in monocytes exposed to oxidants by maintaining HDAC2. Am J Respir Cell Mol Biol. 2008;39(3):312–23. doi:10.1165/rcmb.2008-0012OC.
32. Suzuki M, Betsuyaku T, Ito Y, Nagai K, Odajima N, Moriyama C, et al. Curcumin attenuates elastase- and cigarette smoke-induced pulmonary emphysema in mice. Am J Physiol Lung Cell Mol Physiol. 2009;296(4):L614–23. doi:10.1152/ajplung.90443.2008.
33. Lehouck A, Mathieu C, Carremans C, Baeke F, Verhaegen J, Van Eldere J, et al. High doses of vitamin D to reduce exacerbations in chronic obstructive pulmonary disease: a randomized trial. Ann Intern Med. 2012;156(2):105–14. doi:10.7326/0003-4819-156-2-201201170-00004.
34. Heulens N, Korf H, Cielen N, De Smidt E, Maes K, Gysemans C, et al. Vitamin D deficiency exacerbates COPD-like characteristics in the lungs of cigarette smoke-exposed mice. Respir Res. 2015;16:110. doi:10.1186/s12931-015-0271-x.
35. Zhu B, Zhu B, Xiao C, Zheng Z. Vitamin D deficiency is associated with the severity of COPD: a systematic review and meta-analysis. Int J Chron Obstruct Pulmon Dis. 2015;10:1907–16. doi:10.2147/COPD.S89763.
36. Hobbs BD, Hersh CP. Integrative genomics of chronic obstructive pulmonary disease. Biochem Biophys Res Commun. 2014;452(2):276–86. doi:10.1016/j.bbrc.2014.07.086.
37. Postma DS, Kerkhof M, Boezen HM, Koppelman GH. Asthma and chronic obstructive pulmonary disease: common genes, common environments? Am J Respir Crit Care Med. 2011;183(12):1588–94. doi:10.1164/rccm.201011-1796PP.
38. Vucic EA, Chari R, Thu KL, Wilson IM, Cotton AM, Kennett JY, et al. DNA methylation is globally disrupted and associated with expression changes in chronic obstructive pulmonary disease small airways. Am J Respir Cell Mol Biol. 2014;50(5):912–22. doi:10.1165/rcmb.2013-0304OC.
39. Malhotra D, Thimmulappa RK, Mercado N, Ito K, Kombairaju P, Kumar S, et al. Denitrosylation of HDAC2 by targeting Nrf2 restores glucocorticosteroid sensitivity in macrophages from COPD patients. J Clin Invest. 2011;121(11):4289–302. doi:10.1172/JCI45144.

40. Yao H, Sundar IK, Ahmad T, Lerner C, Gerloff J, Friedman AE, et al. SIRT1 protects against cigarette smoke-induced lung oxidative stress via a FOXO3-dependent mechanism. Am J Physiol Lung Cell Mol Physiol. 2014;306(9):L816–28. doi:10.1152/ajplung.00323.2013.
41. Graff JW, Powers LS, Dickson AM, Kim J, Reisetter AC, Hassan IH, et al. Cigarette smoking decreases global microRNA expression in human alveolar macrophages. PLoS One. 2012;7 (8), e44066. doi:10.1371/journal.pone.0044066.
42. Izzotti A, Calin GA, Arrigo P, Steele VE, Croce CM, De Flora S. Downregulation of microRNA expression in the lungs of rats exposed to cigarette smoke. FASEB J. 2009;23 (3):806–12. doi:10.1096/fj.08-121384.
43. Schembri F, Sridhar S, Perdomo C, Gustafson AM, Zhang X, Ergun A, et al. MicroRNAs as modulators of smoking-induced gene expression changes in human airway epithelium. Proc Natl Acad Sci U S A. 2009;106(7):2319–24. doi:10.1073/pnas.0806383106.
44. Ezzie ME, Crawford M, Cho JH, Orellana R, Zhang S, Gelinas R, et al. Gene expression networks in COPD: microRNA and mRNA regulation. Thorax. 2012;67(2):122–31. doi:10.1136/thoraxjnl-2011-200089.
45. Van Pottelberge GR, Mestdagh P, Bracke KR, Thas O, van Durme YM, Joos GF, et al. MicroRNA expression in induced sputum of smokers and patients with chronic obstructive pulmonary disease. Am J Respir Crit Care Med. 2011;183(7):898–906. doi:10.1164/rccm.201002-0304OC.
46. Hassan F, Nuovo GJ, Crawford M, Boyaka PN, Kirkby S, Nana-Sinkam SP, et al. MiR-101 and miR-144 regulate the expression of the CFTR chloride channel in the lung. PLoS One. 2012;7(11), e50837. doi:10.1371/journal.pone.0050837.
47. Sato T, Liu X, Nelson A, Nakanishi M, Kanaji N, Wang X, et al. Reduced miR-146a increases prostaglandin E(2)in chronic obstructive pulmonary disease fibroblasts. Am J Respir Crit Care Med. 2010;182(8):1020–9. doi:10.1164/rccm.201001-0055OC.
48. Vasa-Nicotera M, Chen H, Tucci P, Yang AL, Saintigny G, Menghini R, et al. miR-146a is modulated in human endothelial cell with aging. Atherosclerosis. 2011;217(2):326–30. doi:10.1016/j.atherosclerosis.2011.03.034.
49. Christenson SA, Brandsma CA, Campbell JD, Knight DA, Pechkovsky DV, Hogg JC, et al. miR-638 regulates gene expression networks associated with emphysematous lung destruction. Genome Med. 2013;5(12):114. doi:10.1186/gm519.
50. Lewis A, Riddoch-Contreras J, Natanek SA, Donaldson A, Man WD, Moxham J, et al. Downregulation of the serum response factor/miR-1 axis in the quadriceps of patients with COPD. Thorax. 2012;67(1):26–34. doi:10.1136/thoraxjnl-2011-200309.
51. Donaldson A, Natanek SA, Lewis A, Man WD, Hopkinson NS, Polkey MI, et al. Increased skeletal muscle-specific microRNA in the blood of patients with COPD. Thorax. 2013;68 (12):1140–9. doi:10.1136/thoraxjnl-2012-203129.
52. Thai P, Statt S, Chen CH, Liang E, Campbell C, Wu R. Characterization of a novel long noncoding RNA, SCAL1, induced by cigarette smoke and elevated in lung cancer cell lines. Am J Respir Cell Mol Biol. 2013;49(2):204–11. doi:10.1165/rcmb.2013-0159RC.
53. Rubio ML, Martin-Mosquero MC, Ortega M, Peces-Barba G, Gonzalez-Mangado N. Oral N-acetylcysteine attenuates elastase-induced pulmonary emphysema in rats. Chest. 2004;125 (4):1500–6.
54. Decramer M, Rutten-van Molken M, Dekhuijzen PN, Troosters T, van Herwaarden C, Pellegrino R, et al. Effects of N-acetylcysteine on outcomes in chronic obstructive pulmonary disease (Bronchitis randomized on NAC cost-utility study, BRONCUS): a randomised placebo-controlled trial. Lancet. 2005;365(9470):1552–60. doi:10.1016/S0140-6736(05) 66456-2.
55. Zheng JP, Wen FQ, Bai CX, Wan HY, Kang J, Chen P, et al. Twice daily N-acetylcysteine 600 mg for exacerbations of chronic obstructive pulmonary disease (PANTHEON): a randomised, double-blind placebo-controlled trial. Lancet Respir Med. 2014;2(3):187–94. doi:10.1016/S2213-2600(13)70286-8.

56. Zheng JP, Kang J, Huang SG, Chen P, Yao WZ, Yang L, et al. Effect of carbocisteine on acute exacerbation of chronic obstructive pulmonary disease (PEACE Study): a randomised placebo-controlled study. Lancet. 2008;371(9629):2013–8. doi:10.1016/S0140-6736(08)60869-7.
57. Malhotra D, Thimmulappa R, Navas-Acien A, Sandford A, Elliott M, Singh A, et al. Decline in NRF2-regulated antioxidants in chronic obstructive pulmonary disease lungs due to loss of its positive regulator, DJ-1. Am J Respir Crit Care Med. 2008;178(6):592–604. doi:10.1164/rccm.200803-380OC.
58. Yao H, Arunachalam G, Hwang JW, Chung S, Sundar IK, Kinnula VL, et al. Extracellular superoxide dismutase protects against pulmonary emphysema by attenuating oxidative fragmentation of ECM. Proc Natl Acad Sci U S A. 2010;107(35):15571–6. doi:10.1073/pnas.1007625107.
59. Tanaka K, Sato K, Aoshiba K, Azuma A, Mizushima T. Superiority of PC-SOD to other anti-COPD drugs for elastase-induced emphysema and alteration in lung mechanics and respiratory function in mice. Am J Physiol Lung Cell Mol Physiol. 2012;302(12):L1250–61. doi:10.1152/ajplung.00019.2012.

Chapter 6
Pathogenesis of COPD 4 – Cell Death, Senescence, and Autophagy: Is There a Possibility of Developing New Drugs from the Standpoint of This Pathogenetic Mechanism?

Kazuyoshi Kuwano, Jun Araya, Hiromichi Hara, Shunsuke Minagawa, Naoki Takasaka, Saburo Ito, and Katsutoshi Nakayama

Abstract The balance of cell survival and death is essential feature of homeostasis. Apoptosis is a well-known form of cell death and involved in the pathogenesis of chronic obstructive pulmonary disease (COPD). The number of apoptotic epithelial and endothelial cells is increased in lung tissues from patients with COPD. Protease-antiprotease imbalance and oxidative stress amplify alveolar destruction. Cellular senescence is one of the cellular stress responses and considered to be one of the processes of aging. COPD has been assumed to be a disease of accelerated lung aging, and cellular senescence has been widely implicated in the pathogenesis of COPD, presumably by impairing cell repopulation and by the aberrant cytokine secretion seen in senescence-associated secretory phenotype, which may exert deleterious effects on the tissue microenvironment of neighboring cells. Autophagy is a process of lysosomal self-degradation that helps maintain homeostatic balance between the synthesis, degradation, and recycling of cellular proteins and organelles. Autophagy is closely related with aging, since autophagy diminishes with aging, and accelerated aging can be attributed to reduced autophagy. Insufficient autophagic clearance is reported to be involved in accelerated cellular senescence in COPD, while excessive autophagy might induce epithelial cell necroptosis in COPD. The detailed molecular mechanism for regulation of autophagy and cellular senescence is complex, and the role of autophagy and cellular senescence is overlapped significantly. We review molecular mechanisms of cell death, cellular

K. Kuwano, M.D., Ph.D. (✉) • J. Araya, M.D., Ph.D. • H. Hara, M.D., Ph.D. •
S. Minagawa, M.D., Ph.D. • N. Takasaka, M.D., Ph.D. • S. Ito, M.D., Ph.D. •
K. Nakayama, M.D., Ph.D.
Division of Respiratory Diseases, Department of Internal Medicine, The Jikei University School of Medicine, 3-25-8 Nishi-shinbashi, Minato-ku, Tokyo 105-8461, Japan
e-mail: kkuwano@jikei.ac.jp

H. Nakamura, K. Aoshiba (eds.), *Chronic Obstructive Pulmonary Disease*, Respiratory Disease Series: Diagnostic Tools and Disease Managements,
DOI 10.1007/978-981-10-0839-9_6

senescence, and autophagy and summarize the role of these stress responses in the pathogenesis of COPD.

Keywords Apoptosis • Aging • Senescence • Autophagy • Chronic obstructive pulmonary disease (COPD)

6.1 The Role of Cell Death in the Pathophysiology of COPD

6.1.1 Apoptosis

The balance of cell survival and death is an essential feature of homeostasis. Apoptosis and necrosis are a well-known form of cell death and involved in various human diseases. Recently, other forms of cell death, such as caspase-independent cell death, oncosis, and autophagy-associated cell death, have also been investigated in various diseases. Apoptosis is characterized by cell shrinkage, apoptotic bodies, and intact cellular membranes. Biochemical markers of apoptosis are caspase activation, DNA fragmentation, and externalization of phosphatidylserine. There are two principle-signaling pathways of apoptosis. One is a direct pathway, named the extrinsic pathway, from death receptor ligation to caspase cascade activation and cell death. Death receptor ligation triggers recruitment of the precursor form of caspase-8 to a death-inducing complex, through the adaptor protein Fas-associating protein with death domain (FADD), which leads to caspase-8 activation. The other pathway, named the intrinsic pathway, triggered by stimuli such as drugs, radiation, infectious agents, and reactive oxygen species (ROS), is initiated in mitochondria. Mitochondrial outer membrane permeability is regulated by Bcl-2 family proteins. After cytochrome c is released into the cytosol from the mitochondria triggered by various stimuli, it binds to Apaf1 and ATP, which then activate caspase-9 [1]. The activation of initiator caspase-8 and caspase-9 resulted in activation of effecter caspases such as caspase-3. Active executioner caspases mediate the cleavage of protein substrates, resulting in morphological features of apoptosis. Recently, endoplasmic reticulum has also been shown to be the organelle to execute apoptosis. Various stresses can impair protein folding and induce endoplasmic reticulum stress, and severe endoplasmic reticulum stress can transduce apoptotic signals [2].

6.1.2 Cell Death and COPD

Increased numbers of apoptotic alveolar, bronchiolar, and endothelial cells in lung tissues from patients with COPD were demonstrated in several reports. Particles, xenobiotics, and oxidants contained in cigarette smoke induce inflammation, oxidative stress, and protease activation. Protease-antiprotease imbalance and oxidative stress amplify alveolar destruction [3]. Since a large number of lymph follicles are found in lung tissues from patients with COPD, T-cell-mediated immune response is also considered to have a role in inducing apoptosis [4].

Pulmonary emphysema is characterized by the enlargement of distal air spaces due to the destruction and loss of alveolar structures. Recently, endothelial and epithelial cell apoptosis have been implicated as one of important mechanisms of pulmonary emphysema. Intratracheal injection of activated caspase-3 induces epithelial cell apoptosis, enhances elastolytic activity, and subsequently induces emphysematous changes in mice [5]. In addition, overexpression of α-1 antitrypsin attenuated endothelial cell death, alveolar wall destruction, and oxidative stress caused by caspase-3 instillation. In TNF-α and IL-1β receptor deficient mice, the degree of emphysematous changes and lung cell apoptosis are decreased after intratracheal instillation of elastase. Therefore, inflammation and protease activation accelerate epithelial, endothelial cell apoptosis and emphysema.

Cigarette smoke induces epithelial cell apoptosis, activated caspases, protease activation, and chemokines via IL-18Rα-dependent manner. Cigarette smoke induces mitochondrial dysfunction by blocking mitochondrial respiratory chain, loss of ATP generation, which leads to cellular necrosis rather than apoptosis [6]. The mitochondrial localization of HO-1 in bronchiolar epithelial cells was confirmed using electron microscopy. Overexpression of HO-1 inhibited cigarette smoke extract (CSE)-induced cell death. As well as cigarette smoke, air pollution contains high levels of nitrogen/oxygen species and reactive oxygen species, which activate different sphingomyelinases to induce apoptosis in airway epithelial cells.

Chronic treatment of rats with the vascular endothelial growth factor (VEGF) receptor blocker induces alveolar cell apoptosis, which subsequently leads to enlargement of the alveolar spaces without inflammatory cell infiltration or fibrosis [7]. VEGF and VEGF receptor type II expressions are also decreased in lung tissues from patients with pulmonary emphysema compared with controls. These results suggest that the defect of alveolar wall maintenance factors may lead to alveolar cell apoptosis.

Apoptotic cells should be removed rapidly by phagocytosis also called "efferocytosis" for the resolution of inflammation without damaging the tissues. Defective removal of apoptotic cells as well as more apoptosis is thought to be important as a contributor to COPD [8]. Surfactant protein (SP)-D deficient mice accumulate apoptotic macrophages in the lung, and exogenous SP-D binds to apoptotic macrophages. These results suggest that SP-D may have an important role in the clearance of apoptotic cells and have preventive effects on the development of emphysema.

In lung tissues from patients with emphysema, alveolar cell apoptosis and expression of PCNA in epithelium are increased, which suggests the activation of regenerative processes. However, cigarette smoke extract induces oxidative stress and apoptosis not only epithelium but also lung fibroblast and impairs repair processes [9]. Since apoptosis is likely to be involved in not only the destructive phase but also remodeling process, regulating apoptosis may become an effective treatment against COPD. Concerning regulating apoptosis in COPD, cellular senescence and autophagy are also involved, although its mechanisms are not well understood.

6.2 The Role of Cellular Senescence in the Pathophysiology of COPD

6.2.1 Aging and Cellular Senescence

Aging is associated with the impaired function of maintaining homeostasis in organs and bodies. The phenotypes of aging include genomic instability, telomere erosion, epigenetic changes, loss of proteostasis, deregulated nutrient sensing, mitochondrial dysfunction, cellular senescence, stem cell exhaustion, and altered cellular communication [10]. Hayflick et al. firstly used the term "replicative senescence" to describe phenomenon of irreversible growth arrest of normal human fibroblasts after extensive serial passaging in culture [11]. Replicative senescence was caused by telomere shortening. Senescent cells in tissues have usually been identified using histological staining for DNA damage markers such as p21, p16, or senescent-associated β-galactosidase (SA-βgal) activity. In the liver, skin, lung, and spleen, a total of ~8 % and ~17 % senescent cells in young and old mice were identified, respectively, although there was no change in the heart, skeletal muscle, and kidney. Therefore, cellular senescence is not a generalized property of aged tissues, and aging and senescence are not equal. As the first identification of cellular senescence in lung diseases, the positive staining for senescence-associated heterochromatin foci marker γH2AX in the alveolar epithelial cells of old mice was demonstrated. In human lung tissue, human lung fibroblasts obtained from lung tissues from patients with COPD showed reduced proliferation rate compared with those from healthy lung. Cellular senescence is induced by not only telomere shortening but various cellular stresses such as oxidative stress, oncogene activation, DNA damage, and chromatin abnormality [12]. In addition, it is noteworthy that cellular senescence also plays instructive roles in organ and tissue development [13].

The characteristics of senescent cells include irreversible growth arrest, enlarged morphology, expression of cyclin-dependent kinase inhibitor (CDKI), the formation of senescence-associated heterochromatin foci, and senescence-associated secretory phenotype (SASP). CDKIs, such as p21 and p16, control cell cycling. The increased expression of CDKIs results in cell cycle arrest in senescent cells. Senescent cells affect microenvironment through gene expression of growth factors, cytokines, and proteases, so-called SASP. SASP presents biological activities and plays a key role in diverse effects on carcinogenesis and the pathogenesis of degenerative diseases [14]. Senescent cells increase in size in vitro but not in vivo, enlarging sometimes as double as non-senescent cells. The markers of senescent cells include positive staining for SA-βgal which reflects the increase of lysosome contents; senescence-associated CDKIs p21, p16, p15, and p27 expression; and senescence-associated heterochromatin foci which inhibit gene expression of cell proliferation. These markers are not entirely specific to cellular senescence; therefore, cellular senescence has been defined by a collection of these markers. The

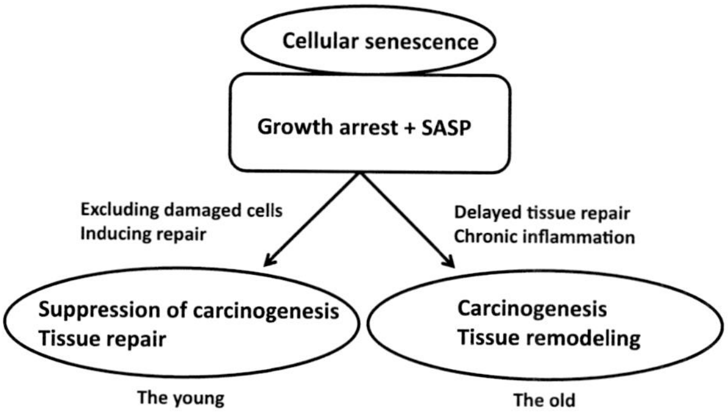

Fig. 6.1 The role of cellular senescence. Cellular senescence plays roles in tissue repair and carcinogenesis. SASP secreted from senescent cells stimulates the migration of phagocytic immune cells which play important roles in the clearance of senescent cells and the repair or resolution of damaged tissues. The tissue damage is prolonged when damaged tissue is not normally repaired. The prolongation of damaged tissues can lead to the accumulation of senescent cells. Senescent cells accumulate, secrete SASP, and induce remodeling of damaged tissues or proliferation of tumor cells in the old

phenotype of cellular senescence is various depending on the type of cell, senescent stimuli, and SASP [14].

Cellular senescence plays roles in tissue repair and regeneration [15]. SASP secreted from senescent cells stimulates the migration of phagocytic immune cells which play important roles in the clearance of senescent cells and the repair or resolution of damaged tissues. The tissue damage is prolonged when damaged tissue is not normally repaired or resolved. The prolongation of damaged tissues can lead to the accumulation of senescent cells. Therefore, senescent cells accumulate and secreted proteins, and other factors induce remodeling of damaged tissues or proliferation of tumor cells in the old [16] (Fig. 6.1). Recently, senescence has been reported to play important roles in the development processes and to compensate the role of apoptosis to remove unnecessary cells [13].

6.2.2 Cellular Senescence and COPD

COPD has been assumed to be a disease of accelerated lung aging, and cellular senescence has been widely implicated in the pathogenesis of COPD, presumably by impairing cell repopulation and by the aberrant cytokine secretion seen in SASP [17, 18]. Telomere length of neutrophils of COPD is shorter than that of healthy controls. Cellular senescence is found in lung epithelial cells, endothelial cells, and fibroblasts in patients with COPD [17, 19].

Sirtuin family belongs to class III histone deacetylases (HDAC), and one of sirtuin family SIRT1 has been extensively studied and well known as an antiaging molecule because of SIRT1-mediated longevity by calorie restriction [20]. SIRT1 expression is decreased in the lung tissues from patients with COPD by oxidative stress and smoking [21]. Decreased SIRT1 expression results in the increased expression of proinflammatory cytokines due to NF-kB activation and also results in the acceleration of cellular senescence mediated by the decrease of anti-senescent activity through FOXO3. Cellular senescence and emphysema were suppressed in SIRT1 transgenic mice by a FOXO3-mediated reduction of premature senescence in mice, while those are deteriorated in SITR1 knockout mice. SIRT1 activator SRT1720 suppressed emphysematous change in mice lung induced by elastase instillation and smoking inhalation [22].

6.3 The Role of Autophagy in the Pathophysiology of COPD

6.3.1 Autophagy

Autophagy is a process of lysosomal self-degradation that helps maintain homeostatic balance between the synthesis, degradation, and recycling of cellular proteins and organelles [23]. At the cellular level, autodigestion takes place within lysosomes and proteasomes. Proteasomes are involved in the clearance of ubiquitin-conjugated soluble proteins, whereas autophagy delivers diverse cytoplasmic components to the lysosome, including soluble proteins, aggregate-prone proteins, and organelles [24]. Autophagy is not simply machinery for amino acid supply in response to energy demand; it is an adaptive pathway of cytoprotection from cellular stresses, involving starvation, reactive oxygen species (ROS), endoplasmic reticulum (ER) stress, and microbe infection [24].

Three forms of distinct autophagy have been demonstrated: chaperon (Hsc70)-mediated autophagy (CMA), microautophagy, and macroautophagy. CMA degrades soluble proteins only, via direct translocation to the lysosome through Lamp2A, a lysosomal transmembrane protein. During microautophagy, small components of the cytoplasm are engulfed by direct invagination into lysosomes. Engulfment of cytoplasmic components by the isolation membrane (phagophore) is the initial step in autophagy and is followed by elongation and fusion, resulting in formation of double-membranous vesicles (autophagosome). Subsequent fusion of the autophagosome with the lysosome to form the autolysosome is absolutely required for proper degradation [25]. Recent advances in the molecular mechanisms of autophagy have mainly focused on macroautophagy, specifically on the detection of a series of autophagy-related (*Atg*) genes. Among 35 autophagy-related, (Atg), proteins identified in yeast, there are core Atg proteins required for autophagosome formation, which are well conserved in mammals. Hence, in general in the literature, macroautophagy is designated as autophagy [25].

Initially, autophagy was proposed to be a nonselective bulk degradation system, but recent advances demonstrate that a variety of ubiquitinated cargos, including protein aggregates, mitochondria, and microbes, are selective targets for autophagic degradation [25]. Accordingly, ubiquitination is an important tag for not only proteasomal degradation but also for selective autophagy. The p62 protein / sequestosome 1 (SQSTM1) has been shown to be an adaptor protein for selective autophagy based on its ability to bind both ubiquitin and microtubule-associated protein 1A/1B-light chain 3 (LC3), a crucial component for autophagosome formation [26]. Because of the dynamic nature of autophagy, in which autophagosome can be formed within several minutes, it is difficult to distinguish between increased autophagy flux and impaired subsequent clearance when using electron microscopic detection of autophagosomes or when examining Atg expression levels. Therefore, to detect the conversion of LC3-I to LC3-II (which is conjugated to phosphatidylethanolamine (PE) to ensure stable association to the autophagosomal membrane), the use of protease inhibitors is generally accepted to be standard methodology for evaluation of autophagy flux. In addition, based on the findings of selective autophagic degradation, concomitant accumulation of p62 and ubiquitinated protein is also recognized to at least partly reflect autophagy activity.

Due to the large number of physiological and aberrant intracellular components that are potential targets for autophagic degradation, autophagy status is linked to a diverse array of cellular processes and cell fates, including energy supply, homeostatic turnover of organelles, cell fate, cellular senescence, and immune responses [23]. In terms of the pathogenic role of autophagy, excessive activation may be associated with disease progression in extraphysiologic condition, whereas impairment of autophagy activity has been widely implicated in the pathogenic sequence of a variety of human disorders [26]. Indeed, recent in vitro and in vivo gene knockout studies revealed that insufficient autophagy is involved in the development of lung diseases [27–30].

Continuous ventilation of large amounts of air with high oxygen concentration, which may contain noxious particles and harmful microbes, is a fundamental function of the lungs and is required for sufficient gas exchange. Subsequently, indicating lung cells are serially exposed to a diverse array of cellular stresses, and it is reasonable to speculate that autophagy-mediated alleviation of cellular stress plays a key regulatory role in lung pathophysiology.

6.3.2 *Autophagy and Cell Death*

Apoptosis is necessary for the maintenance of homeostatic plasticity in the lung. However, the cell-type-specific imbalance of positive and negative regulation of apoptosis has been proposed to be a critical determination of lung disease progression [31]. Although autophagy had been postulated to be responsible for type II programmed cell death, current understanding is mainly that autophagic cell death is attributable simply to overwhelming autophagosome formation as a part of stress responses, in which cytosol and organelles are destroyed to an unrecoverable degree. Autophagy is an adaptation pathway for cellular stress, including starvation, ROS, endoplasmic reticulum (ER) stress, and microbe infection; hence autophagy is generally considered to be a mechanism for cell survival. However, *Atg*-gene-dependent cell death has been reported in the setting of dysfunction of apoptosis machinery. Indeed, double knockout of Bax/Bak, essential components of the mitochondrial apoptotic pathway, demonstrated a distinct type of cell death, marked by accumulation of autophagosomes [32]. *Atg5* knockdown ameliorated this cell death, indicating that autophagy may promote cell death in the setting of extraphysiologic apoptosis deficiency.

In addition, there is functional cross talk between apoptosis and autophagy. For instance, B-cell lymphoma-2 (Bcl-2), an anti-apoptotic protein, interferes with starvation-dependent autophagy by binding to Beclin1 (Atg6) [33], which is an important constituent of the class III phosphatidylinositol (Ptdlns) 3-kinase complex involved in nucleation and assembly of the initial phagophore membrane. During receptor-mediated apoptosis, cleavage of Atg3 protein by caspase-8-suppresses autophagy activation, resulting in increased cell death. Furthermore, irrespective of their known role in autophagy induction, several Atg proteins may exert diverse regulatory roles during both the apoptotic process and cell survival. Fragmented Atg5 cleaved by calpain promotes intrinsic mitochondrial apoptosis [34]. Atg5 on the autophagosomal membrane serves as a platform for an intracellular death-inducing signaling complex (iDISC) that recruits caspase-8 to initiate the apoptosis cascade [35]. LC3B has been demonstrated to regulate apoptosis through interaction with Fas and caveolin-1(Cav-1). Therefore, clarification of whether the autophagy process is involved in apoptosis regulation is a prerequisite for proper interpretation of experimental results in the setting of Atg manipulation.

6.3.3 Autophagy and Cellular Senescence

Cellular senescence has been widely implicated in disease pathogenesis in terms of not only impaired cell repopulation but also aberrant cytokine secretions of SASP. SASP may exert deleterious effects on the tissue microenvironment of neighboring cell [36]. Increased cellular senescence is one of major features of aging, and hence cellular senescence has been widely implicated in age-associated disorders. The detailed molecular mechanism for regulation of cellular senescence is complex and incompletely understood, but one of the typical manifestations is accumulation of damaged proteins and organelles, occasionally associated with ubiquitinated aggregations [37]. Therefore, it has been proposed that functional insufficiencies in the cellular cleaning and housekeeping mechanisms of autophagy play a pivotal role in the accumulation of deleterious cellular components and therefore in the regulation of cellular senescence [37].

Indeed, autophagy diminishes with aging, and accelerated aging can be attributed to reduced autophagy. Thus, autophagy activation appears to be associated with longevity [38]. Pathologic premature aging due to autophagy malfunction has been intensively examined using animal models of autophagy inhibition by tissue-specific knockout of *Atg* genes. Those animal models with insufficient autophagy demonstrated a cellular phenotype of progressive accumulation of ubiquitinated aggregates and disorganized mitochondria, suggesting the causal relationship between loss of autophagy and aging-associated disease phenotypes [38]. However, those phenotypic alterations were mainly evaluated in the central nervous system and liver, not in other organs. Among the variety of targets for autophagic degradation, selective autophagy of mitochondria (mitophagy) has been widely implicated in cellular senescence in terms of regulation of reactive oxygen species (ROS) of oxidative stress. Mitochondria are the main organelle responsible for intrinsic ROS release through respiratory chain reactions, and insufficient mitophagy results in accumulation of damaged mitochondria accompanied by increased ROS production [39].

The role of stress-induced autophagy activation in longevity has been mainly demonstrated in the case of caloric restriction (CR) [40]. CR induces autophagy through the inhibition of mammalian target of rapamycin (mTOR), an essential negative regulator of autophagy, and also through activation of adenosine monophosphate-activated protein kinase (AMPK) and sirtuin1 (SIRT1). In response to the rising AMP/ATP ratio during CR, AMPK induces autophagy via phosphorylation of ULK1, a mammalian orthologue of the yeast protein kinase Atg1. SIRT1 deacetylation of Atg proteins and transcription factors, including the FOXO family, is involved in autophagy induction [22]. The involvement of CR-induced autophagy in longevity was confirmed by inhibition of autophagy, and SIRT1-mediated longevity by CR is at least partly conferred by autophagy activation. Intriguingly, recent paper demonstrated that SIRT1 protects against emphysema by a FOXO3-mediated reduction of premature senescence in mice, but the involvement of autophagy was not examined.

Autophagy is getting more importance during the aging process, because proteasome pathway could not degrade protein aggregates in the presence of an enhanced prooxidant and aggregation-prone milieu characteristic of aging [41]. Pharmacological inhibition of autophagy prevented development of premature senescence but did lead to the enhanced rate of apoptosis in human umbilical vein endothelial cells. A subset of autophagy-related genes is upregulated during senescence [42]. Overexpression of one of those genes, ULK3, induces autophagy and senescence. Furthermore, inhibition of autophagy delays the senescence phenotype, including senescence-associated secretion [43]. Goehe et al. showed that autophagy and senescence tend to occur in parallel and furthermore that autophagy accelerates the development of the senescent phenotype [44]. Collectively, autophagy and cellular senescence are associated with each other in some situations, but these two important cellular processes may be interdependently involved in the pathophysiology of several diseases.

6.3.4 Autophagy and COPD

Chronic obstructive pulmonary disease (COPD) is one of the leading causes of death worldwide and is characterized by partially irreversible and progressive airflow limitation. Cigarette smoke, the major cause of COPD, is rich in toxic components including ROS, and a variety of biological responses to cigarette smoke exposure have been demonstrated. Although detailed molecular mechanisms for COPD development remain unclear, the possible participation of autophagy in the pathogenic sequence of COPD has been intensively explored (Fig. 6.2). It has been reported that autophagy in lung tissue from COPD patients is augmented by means of an increase in the LC3B-II/LC3B-I ratio, and Egr-1-induced LC3B expression is essential for autophagy activation [45]. LC3B−/− mouse experiments confirmed the pivotal role of LC3B in epithelial cell apoptosis induction by cigarette smoke exposure. The proposed mechanism of LC3B-induced apoptosis is attributed to the balance in a trimolecular interaction between LC3B with Fas and caveolin-1(Cav-1), a lipid raft protein. LC3B knockdown inhibits apoptosis by increasing Cav-1-dependent Fas sequestration, and dissociation of Fas and LC3B from Cav-1 in response to CSE exposure initiates apoptosis in epithelial cells. LC3B is a key component for autophagy machinery, and association between LC3B and Fas is an interesting observation; however it is still unclear whether autophagy activation by LC3B expression is crucial for apoptosis induction in these COPD models. Furthermore, in cases of hyperoxia-induced apoptosis in epithelial cells, LC3B interacts with Fas, resulting in prevention of apoptosis [46], suggesting that the role of association between LC3B and Fas in apoptosis regulation is dependent on the stimuli or experimental conditions. Intriguingly, decreased autophagy activity in alveolar macrophages derived from smokers has been reported in terms of impaired xenophagy. In spite of increased LC3B-II and autophagosomes in macrophages from smokers, impairment of autophagy flux was shown using protease inhibitors and also by detecting accumulation of p62 aggregates [47], indicating that autophagy activity in COPD lung may be regulated via cell-type-specific mechanisms.

Autophagy plays a pivotal regulatory role for cellular senescence; hence we have attempted to elucidate the involvement of autophagy in the regulation of cigarette smoke extract (CSE)-induced human bronchial epithelial cell (HBEC) senescence [27]. CSE transiently induces autophagy activation followed by accumulations of p62 and ubiquitinated proteins accompanied by an increase in HBEC senescence. Autophagy inhibition by 3MA, a specific inhibitor of autophagic sequestration, or by LC3B and Atg5 knockdown further enhanced HBEC senescence with concomitant accumulation of p62 and ubiquitinated proteins [27]. In contrast, autophagy activation by Torin1, a mammalian target of rapamycin (mTOR) inhibitor, suppressed p62 and ubiquitinated protein accumulations and also inhibited HBEC senescence. In line with the previous finding of increased autophagy activation in COPD epithelial cells, we observed an increase in baseline autophagy but also found significantly decreased autophagy induction in response to CSE exposure in

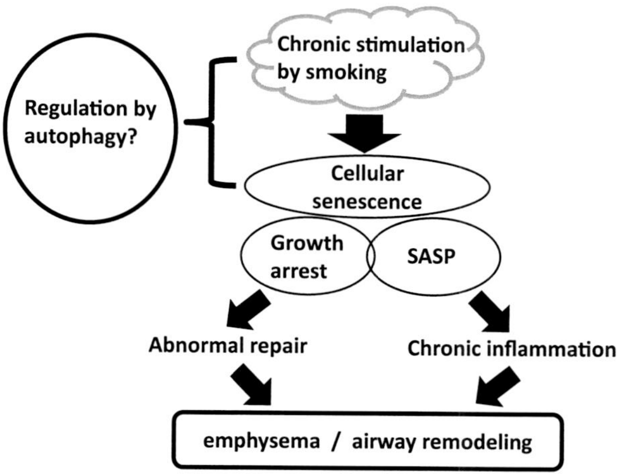

Fig. 6.2 The pathophysiology of COPD. Cigarette smoke, the major cause of COPD, is rich in toxic components including ROS, and a variety of biological responses to cigarette smoke exposure including cellular senescence has been demonstrated. Abnormal repair and SASP induce alveolar wall destruction and small airway remodeling. Although detailed molecular mechanisms for COPD development remain unclear, the possible participation of autophagy in the pathogenic sequence of COPD has been intensively explored

HBEC isolated from COPD patients compared to those from nonsmokers [27]. We speculated that the mechanism for enhanced baseline autophagy flux was attributed to increased oxidative stress, which was demonstrated by the accumulation of carbonylated proteins in HBEC from COPD patients [18]. Therefore, it is probable that the attenuation of autophagy flux in response to CSE exposure may reflect an insufficient reserve of autophagy activation in HBEC from COPD patients. Concomitant accumulation of p62 and ubiquitinated protein is also recognized to at least partly reflect autophagy activity. Increased accumulations of p62 and ubiquitinated proteins detected in lung homogenates support the notion that insufficient autophagic clearance is involved in accelerated cellular senescence in COPD [27] (Fig. 6.3).

SIRT6 has been demonstrated to regulate longevity by modulating insulin-like growth factor (IGF)-I signaling. IGF-I signaling activates mTOR, and a recent paper demonstrated that IGF-I exposure was sufficient to induce cellular senescence through inhibition of baseline autophagy [48]. Intriguingly, we demonstrated that CSE decreased the SIRT6 expression in HBEC and that CSE-induced HBEC senescence was inhibited by SIRT6 overexpression and that histone deacetylase (HDAC) activity of SIRT6 was indispensable for inhibition of CSE-induced HBEC senescence through autophagy activation, which was mainly attributed to attenuation of IGF-Akt-mTOR signaling [49]. Decreased expression levels of SIRT6 found in lung homogenates from COPD patients support the hypothesis that reduced SIRT6 expression with accompanying autophagy insufficiency may be associated with COPD development through the enhancement of cellular senescence, especially in the setting of increased IGF signaling. Furthermore, Decreased SIRT6

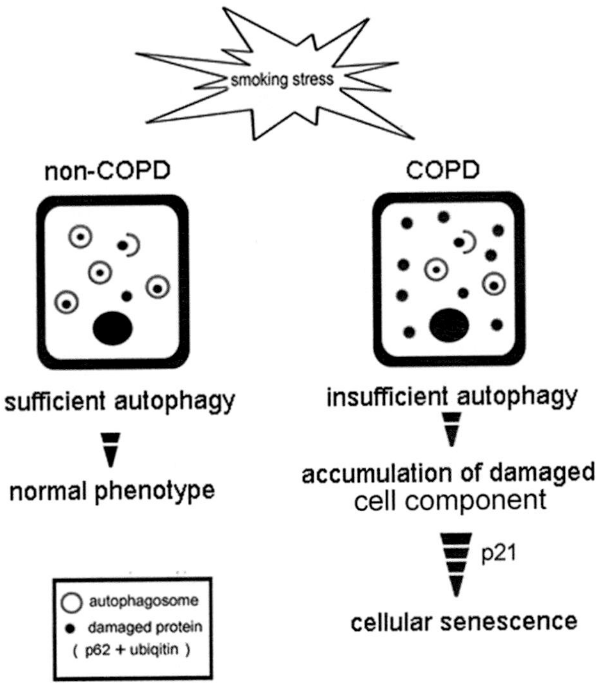

Fig. 6.3 Insufficient autophagic degradation in COPD pathogenesis. We found that baseline autophagy was increased, while autophagy induction was significantly decreased in response to CSE exposure in HBEC isolated from COPD patients compared to those from nonsmokers. We speculate that the mechanism for enhanced baseline autophagy flux may be attributed to increased oxidative stress. It is probable that the attenuation of autophagy flux in response to CSE exposure may reflect an insufficient reserve of autophagy activation in HBEC from COPD patients

expression was significantly correlated with the decrease of $FEV_1\%$ [49]. As IGF-I shares receptors and signaling pathways with insulin, and type II diabetes mellitus with hyperinsulinemia is a common comorbidity in COPD, it may be associated with COPD development via increased IGF/insulin signaling and autophagy inhibition, especially in cases of decreased SIRT6 expression.

Mitochondria are the main organelle producing ATP as well as reactive oxygen species (ROS) and play central roles in cell fate regulation. Mitochondria also release mitochondrial DNA as one of damage-associated molecular pattern. Therefore, maintenance of mitochondrial homeostasis is prerequisite for cellular homeostasis [50]. Mitochondria are dynamic organelles, which continuously change their shape through fission and fusion. Damaged and fragmented mitochondria are removed through mitochondria-specific autophagic degradation (mitophagy). Disruption of mitochondrial dynamics is involved in disease pathology through excessive reactive oxygen species (ROS) production [51] (Fig. 6.4). In electron microscopic examination of lung tissues, we demonstrated that mitochondria in bronchial epithelial cells tended to be fragmented in COPD, suggesting the fission process dominancy of mitochondrial dynamics in COPD pathogenesis [52]. In vitro studies further confirmed that CSE-induced excessive fragmentation of mitochondria is associated with mitochondrial ROS production, resulting in HBEC senescence. Autophagy inducer Torin1 accelerate degradation of damaged mitochondria in autophagosome, resulted in the increase of healthy mitochondria [52].

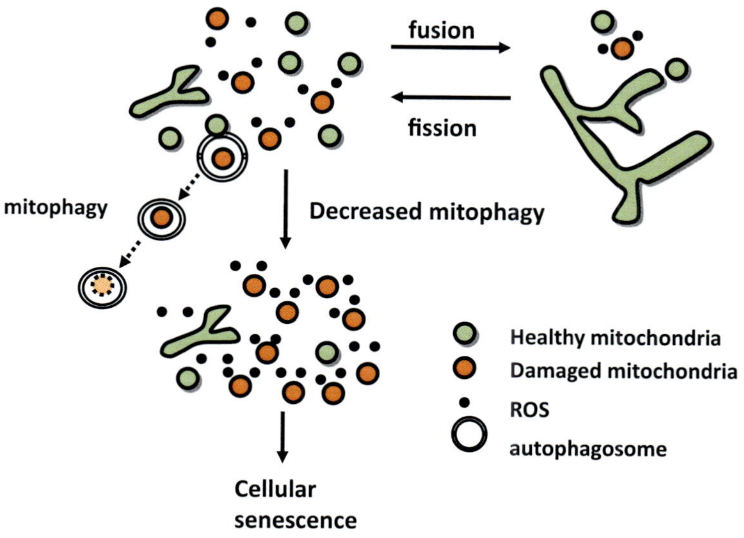

Fig. 6.4 The prevention of cellular senescence by mitophagy through excluding damaged mitochondria. Mitochondria are dynamic organelles, which continuously change their shape through fission and fusion. Damaged and fragmented mitochondria are removed through mitochondria-specific autophagic degradation (mitophagy). Disruption of mitochondrial dynamics is involved in disease pathology through excessive reactive oxygen species (ROS) production

The phosphatase and tensin homolog (PTEN)-induced putative protein kinase 1 (PINK1)-PARK2 pathway has been largely implicated in the removal of damaged mitochondria with depolarized membranes. Stress-induced membrane depolarization stabilizes PINK1, resulting in recruitment of PARK2, an E3 ubiquitin ligase, to mitochondria [53, 54]. We found that PARK2-mediated ubiquitination is crucial for mitophagic degradation in damaged mitochondria in HBEC. Knockdown of PINK1 or PARK2 decreased autophagy activation, the accumulation of damaged mitochondria accompanied by increased ROS production, and cellular senescence in HBEC [55]. PARK2 expression in lung tissue from patients with COPD was significantly decreased compared with that from smokers without COPD. The decreased PARK2 expression was significantly correlated with the decrease of $FEV_1\%$. Immunohistochemistry results showed the expression of PARK2 in bronchial epithelial cells from patients with COPD was significantly decreased compared with that from nonsmokers or smokers without COPD. Therefore, the decrease of PARK2 expression may be associated with the deficiency of mitophagy and cellular senescence in COPD pathogenesis [55] (Fig. 6.5).

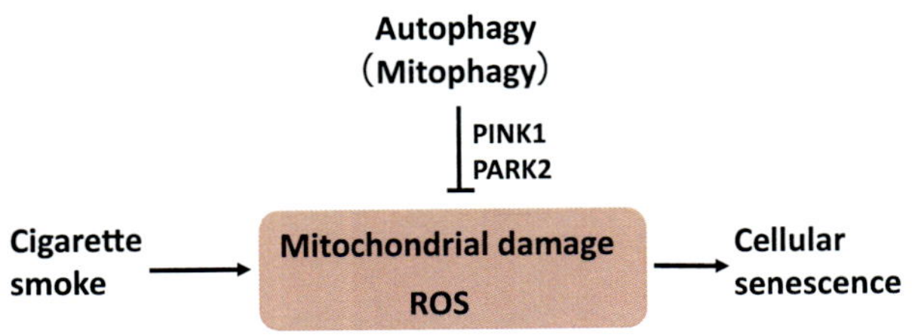

Fig. 6.5 The regulation of damaged mitochondrial removal and ROS production by mitophagy. Cigarette smoke induces mitochondrial damage in association with increased ROS production. This mitochondrial ROS is at least partly involved in cellular senescence. Autophagy suppresses accumulation of damaged mitochondria and ROS production, suggesting that mitochondria-specific autophagy (mitophagy) may play a pivotal role through PINK1 and PARK2 in the regulation of CSE-induced cellular senescence

6.4 Conclusions

An aging society has a problem with various diseases associated with aging. In particular, lung diseases have much attention because COPD, pneumonia, and lung cancer are speculated to be third, fourth, and fifth leading cause of death in the world, respectively. Increased numbers of apoptotic alveolar, bronchiolar, and endothelial cells in lung tissues from patients with COPD were demonstrated. Cigarette smoke induces inflammation, oxidative stress, and protease activation. Protease-antiprotease imbalance and oxidative stress amplify alveolar destruction through inducing apoptosis.

Cellular senescence is the most closely associated with aging processes; therefore, therapies targeting cellular senescence should be important strategies against COPD. Classic “free radical hypothesis” means that ROS induces cellular senescence. Many reports have shown that mitochondrial dysfunction leads to cellular senescence due to excessive ROS production. The treatment strategy against cellular senescence through induction of autophagy, especially mitophagy, may be promising against COPD.

Autophagy is responsible not just for simple homeostatic energy supply but also for elimination of aggregate-prone proteins, damaged organelles, and intracellular microbes. Autophagy is a dynamic process and may rapidly change its status, which can be influenced by not only disease activity but also environmental stresses. Additionally, the regulatory role of autophagy can be dependent on stages in disease development, and the pathogenic involvement may be different in a cell-type-specific manner.

Recent advances in cell death, senescence, and autophagy shed more light on understanding the pathogenesis of COPD and may lead to the development of new therapeutic options. The development of proper biomarkers reflecting status of senescence and autophagy is warranted to precisely evaluate disease progression, and the establishment of novel therapeutic approaches is also warranted to achieve optimal levels of cellular senescence and autophagy status.

References

1. Kroemer G, Reed JC. Mitochondrial control of cell death. Nat Med. 2000;6:513–9.
2. Ferri KF, Kroemer G. Organelle-specific initiation of cell death pathways. Nat Cell Biol. 2001;3:255–63.
3. Tuder RM, Yoshida T, Fijalkowka I, Biswal S, Petrache I. Role of lung maintenance program in the heterogeneity of lung destruction in emphysema. Proc Am Thorac Soc. 2006;3:673–9.
4. Hogg JC, Chu F, Utokaparch S, Woods R, Elliott WM, Buzatu L, et al. The nature of small-airway obstruction in chronic obstructive pulmonary disease. N Engl J Med. 2004;350:2645–53.
5. Aoshiba K, Yokohori N, Nagai A. Alveolar wall apoptosis causes lung destruction and emphysematous changes. Am J Respir Cell Mol Biol. 2003;28:555–62.
6. van der Toorn M, Slebos DJ, de Bruin HG, Leuvenink HG, Bakker SJ, Gans RO, et al. Cigarette smoke-induced blockade of the mitochondrial respiratory chain switches lung epithelial cell apoptosis into necrosis. Am J Physiol Lung Cell Mol Physiol. 2007;292:1211–8.
7. Kasahara Y, Tuder RM, Taraseviciene-Stewart L, Le Cras TD, Abman S, Hirth PK, et al. Inhibition of VEGF receptors causes lung cell apoptosis and emphysema. J Clin Invest. 2000;106:1311–9.
8. Henson PM, Vandivier RW, Douglas IS. Cell death, remodeling, and repair in chronic obstructive pulmonary disease? Proc Am Thorac Soc. 2006;3:713–7.
9. Carnevali S, Petruzzelli S, Longoni B, Vanacore R, Barale R, Cipollini M, et al. Cigarette smoke extract induces oxidative stress and apoptosis in human lung fibroblasts. Am J Physiol Lung Cell Mol Physiol. 2003;284:955–63.
10. López-Otín C, Blasco MA, Partridge L, Serrano M, Kroemer G. The hallmarks of aging. Cell. 2013;153:1194–217. doi:10.1016/j.cell.2013.05.039.
11. Hayflick L. The limited in vitro lifetime of human diploid cell strains. Exp Cell Res. 1965;37:614–36.
12. Campisi J. d'Adda di Fagagna F. Cellular senescence: when bad things happen to good cells. Nat Rev Mol Cell Biol. 2007;8:729–40.
13. Storer M, Mas A, Robert-Moreno A, Pecoraro M, Ortells MC, Di Giacomo V, et al. Senescence is a developmental mechanism that contributes to embryonic growth and patterning. Cell. 2013;155:1119–30. doi:10.1016/j.cell.2013.10.041.
14. van Deursen JM. The role of senescent cells in ageing. Nature. 2014;509:439–46. doi:10.1038/nature13193.
15. Rodier F, Campisi J. Four faces of cellular senescence. J Cell Biol. 2011;192:547–56. doi:10.1083/jcb.201009094.
16. Muñoz-Espín D, Serrano M. Cellular senescence: from physiology to pathology. Nat Rev Mol Cell Biol. 2014;15:482–96. doi:10.1038/nrm3823.
17. Tsuji T, Aoshiba K, Nagai A. Alveolar cell senescence in patients with pulmonary emphysema. Am J Respir Crit Care Med. 2006;174:886–93.
18. Hara H, Araya J, Takasaka N, Fujii S, Kojima J, Yumino Y, et al. Involvement of creatine kinase b in cigarette smoke-induced bronchial epithelial cell senescence. Am J Respir Cell Mol Biol. 2012;46:306–12. doi:10.1165/rcmb.2011-0214OC.
19. Müller KC, Welker L, Paasch K, Feindt B, Erpenbeck VJ, Hohlfeld JM, et al. Lung fibroblasts from patients with emphysema show markers of senescence in vitro. Respir Res. 2006;7:32.
20. Guarente L, Picard F. Calorie restriction–the SIR2 connection. Cell. 2005;120:473–82.
21. Rajendrasozhan S, Yang SR, Kinnula VL, Rahman I. SIRT1, an antiinflammatory and antiaging protein, is decreased in lungs of patients with chronic obstructive pulmonary disease. Am J Respir Crit Care Med. 2008;177:861–70. doi:10.1164/rccm.200708-1269OC.
22. Yao H, Chung S, Hwang JW, Rajendrasozhan S, Sundar IK, Dean DA, et al. Sirt1 protects against emphysema via foxo3-mediated reduction of premature senescence in mice. J Clin Invest. 2012;122:2032–45. doi:10.1172/JCI60132.

23. Mizushima N, Levine B, Cuervo AM, Klionsky DJ. Autophagy fights disease through cellular self-digestion. Nature. 2008;451:1069–75. doi:10.1038/nature06639.
24. Levine B, Kroemer G. Autophagy in the pathogenesis of disease. Cell. 2008;132:27–42. doi:10.1016/j.cell.2007.12.018.
25. Mizushima N, Komatsu M. Autophagy: renovation of cells and tissues. Cell. 2011;147:728–41. doi:10.1016/j.cell.2011.10.026.
26. Rubinsztein DC, Marino G, Kroemer G. Autophagy and aging. Cell. 2011;146:682–95. doi:10.1016/j.cell.2011.07.030.
27. Fujii S, Hara H, Araya J, Takasaka N, Kojima J, Ito S, et al. Insufficient autophagy promotes bronchial epithelial cell senescence in chronic obstructive pulmonary disease. Oncoimmunology. 2012;1:630–41.
28. Ryter SW, Nakahira K, Haspel JA, Choi AM. Autophagy in pulmonary diseases. Annu Rev Physiol. 2012;74:377–401. doi:10.1146/annurev-physiol-020911-153348.
29. Araya J, Kojima J, Takasaka N, Ito S, Fujii S, Hara H, et al. Insufficient autophagy in idiopathic pulmonary fibrosis. Am J Physiol Lung Cell Mol Physiol. 2013;304:L56–69. doi:10.1152/ajplung.00213.2012.
30. Mizumura K, Cloonan SM, Haspel JA, Choi AM. The emerging importance of autophagy in pulmonary diseases. Chest. 2012;142:1289–99. doi:10.1378/chest.12-0809.
31. Kuwano K, Araya J, Nakayama K. Epithelial cell fate following lung injury. Expert Rev Respir Med. 2008;2:573–82. doi:10.1586/17476348.2.5.573.
32. Shimizu S, Kanaseki T, Mizushima N, Mizuta T, Arakawa-Kobayashi S, Thompson CB, et al. Role of bcl-2 family proteins in a non-apoptotic programmed cell death dependent on autophagy genes. Nat Cell Biol. 2004;6:1221–8.
33. Pattingre S, Tassa A, Qu X, Liang XH, Mizushima N, Packer M, et al. Bcl-2 antiapoptotic proteins inhibit beclin 1-dependent autophagy. Cell. 2005;122:927–39.
34. Yousefi S, Perozzo R, Schmid I, Ziemiecki A, Schaffner T, Scapozza L, et al. Calpain-mediated cleavage of atg5 switches autophagy to apoptosis. Nat Cell Biol. 2006;8:1124–32.
35. Young MM, Takahashi Y, Khan O, Park S, Hori T, Yun J, et al. Autophagosomal membrane serves as platform for intracellular death-inducing signaling complex (idisc)-mediated caspase-8 activation and apoptosis. J Biol Chem. 2012;287:12455–68. doi:10.1074/jbc.M111.309104.
36. Rajawat YS, Hilioti Z, Bossis I. Aging: central role for autophagy and the lysosomal degradative system. Ageing Res Rev. 2009;8:199–213. doi:10.1016/j.arr.2009.05.001.
37. Madeo F, Zimmermann A, Maiuri MC, Kroemer G. Essential role for autophagy in life span extension. J Clin Invest. 2015;125:85–93. doi:10.1172/JCI73946.
38. Mizushima N, Levine B. Autophagy in mammalian development and differentiation. Nat Cell Biol. 2010;12:823–30. doi:10.1038/ncb0910-823.
39. Gomes LC, Scorrano L. Mitochondrial morphology in mitophagy and macroautophagy. Biochim Biophys Acta. 1833;2013:205–12. doi:10.1016/j.bbamcr.2012.02.012.
40. Morselli E, Maiuri MC, Markaki M, Megalou E, Pasparaki A, Palikaras K, et al. The life span-prolonging effect of sirtuin-1 is mediated by autophagy. Autophagy. 2010;6:186–8.
41. Gamerdinger M, Carra S, Behl C. Emerging roles of molecular chaperones and co-chaperones in selective autophagy: focus on BAG proteins. Mol Med (Berl). 2011;89:1175–82. doi:10.1007/s00109-011-0795-6.
42. Patschan S, Chen J, Polotskaia A, Mendelev N, Cheng J, Patschan D, Goligorsky MS. Lipid mediators of autophagy in stress-induced premature senescence of endothelial cells. Am J Physiol Heart Circ Physiol. 2008;294:H1119–29.
43. Young AR, Narita M, Ferreira M, Kirschner K, Sadaie M, Darot JF, Tavaré S, Arakawa S, Shimizu S, Watt FM. Narita M Autophagy mediates the mitotic senescence transition. Genes Dev. 2009;23:798–803.
44. Goehe RW, Bristol ML, Wilson EN, Gewirtz DA. Autophagy, senescence, and apoptosis. Methods Mol Biol. 2013;962:31–48. doi:10.1007/978-1-62703-236-0_3.

45. Chen ZH, Lam HC, Jin Y, Kim HP, Cao J, Lee SJ, et al. Autophagy protein microtubule-associated protein 1 light chain-3b (lc3b) activates extrinsic apoptosis during cigarette smoke-induced emphysema. Proc Natl Acad Sci U S A. 2010;107:18880–5. doi:10.1073/pnas.1005574107.
46. Tanaka A, Jin Y, Lee SJ, Zhang M, Kim HP, Stolz DB, et al. Hyperoxia-induced lc3b interacts with the fas apoptotic pathway in epithelial cell death. Am J Respir Cell Mol Biol. 2012;46:507–14. doi:10.1165/rcmb.2009-0415OC.
47. Monick MM, Powers LS, Walters K, Lovan N, Zhang M, Gerke A, et al. Identification of an autophagy defect in smokers' alveolar macrophages. J Immunol. 2010;185:5425–35. doi:10.4049/jimmunol.1001603.
48. Kanfi Y, Naiman S, Amir G, Peshti V, Zinman G, Nahum L, et al. The sirtuin sirt6 regulates lifespan in male mice. Nature. 2012;483:218–21. doi:10.1038/nature10815.
49. Takasaka N, Araya J, Hara H, Ito S, Kobayashi K, Kurita Y, et al. Autophagy induction by SIRT6 through attenuation of insulin-like growth factor signaling is involved in the regulation of human bronchial epithelial cell senescence. J Immunol. 2014;192:958–68. doi:10.4049/jimmunol.1302341.
50. Green DR, Galluzzi L, Kroemer G. Mitochondria and the autophagy-inflammation-cell death axis in organismal aging. Science. 2011;333:1109–12. doi:10.1126/science.1201940.
51. Okamoto K, Kondo-Okamoto N. Mitochondria and autophagy: critical interplay between the two homeostats. Biochim Biophys Acta. 1820;2012:595–600. doi:10.1016/j.bbagen.2011.08.001.
52. Hara H, Araya J, Ito S, Kobayashi K, Takasaka N, Yoshii Y, et al. Mitochondrial fragmentation in cigarette smoke induced-bronchial epithelial cell senescence. Am J Physiol Lung Cell Mol Physiol. 2013;305:L737–46. doi:10.1152/ajplung.00146.2013.
53. Geisler S, Holmstrom KM, Skujat D, Fiesel FC, Rothfuss OC, Kahle PJ, et al. PINK1/Parkin-mediated mitophagy is dependent on VDAC1 and p62/SQSTM1. Nat Cell Biol. 2010;12:119–31. doi:10.1038/ncb2012.
54. Gautier CA, Kitada T, Shen J. Loss of pink1 causes mitochondrial functional defects and increased sensitivity to oxidative stress. Proc Natl Acad Sci U S A. 2008;105:11364–9. doi:10.1073/pnas.0802076105.
55. Ito S, Araya J, Kurita Y, Kobayashi K, Takasaka N, Yoshida M, et al. PARK2-mediated mitophagy is involved in regulation of HBEC senescence in COPD pathogenesis. Autophagy. 2015;11:547–59. doi:10.1080/15548627.2015.1017190.

Part III
Comorbidities

Chapter 7
Pathogenesis of Comorbidities in COPD: By What Mechanism Does Long-Term Smoking Cause Systemic Inflammation?

Yuko Morishima and Nobuyuki Hizawa

Abstract Chronic obstructive pulmonary disease (COPD) is now one of the most common diseases affecting humans worldwide. With the increasing concern about the high mortality in COPD, which is in part attributed to its comorbidities, it has been emphasized that COPD should be considered as a systemic disease rather than a disease localized to the airway. Even though some of the comorbidities are simply age related, shared risk factors such as tobacco smoke may make a significant contribution to their pathogenesis. Tobacco smoke contains thousands of chemicals, free radicals, and reactive oxygen species within its gases and particles. These toxicants cause oxidative stress and immune responses locally in the lungs and/or systemically to trigger the development of extrapulmonary comorbidities. Additionally, other factors, such as genetic susceptibility to inflammation, the clinical symptoms of COPD in themselves, and the adverse effects of medication, may also contribute to the development of comorbidities.

In this chapter, we present an overview of the systemic effects of tobacco smoke and the pathogenesis and clinical manifestations of extrapulmonary comorbidities related to COPD. We encourage clinicians to be aware of the presence of comorbidities in patients with COPD and provide a comprehensive approach for their management.

Keywords Chronic obstructive pulmonary disease • Comorbidity • Smoking • Prevalence • Mortality

---

Y. Morishima (✉) • N. Hizawa
Department of Respiratory Medicine, Division of Clinical Medicine, Faculty of Medicine, University of Tsukuba, 1-1-1 Tennoudai, Tsukuba-shi, Ibaraki 305-8575, Japan
e-mail: mk01a231@md.tsukuba.ac.jp

H. Nakamura, K. Aoshiba (eds.), *Chronic Obstructive Pulmonary Disease*, Respiratory Disease Series: Diagnostic Tools and Disease Managements, DOI 10.1007/978-981-10-0839-9_7

7.1 Introduction

Chronic obstructive pulmonary disease (COPD) is a leading cause of mortality and morbidity worldwide. It is estimated that more than three million people died of COPD and that COPD was the third leading cause of death worldwide in 2012 [1]. In 1990, COPD was the sixth leading cause of death, and researchers warned about the possibility of COPD becoming the third leading cause of death by 2020 if no public interventions were taken [2]. In developed countries, in response to this crisis, tobacco restrictions were tightened, and tobacco consumption began to decline. However, the total number of smokers has risen worldwide, and earlier than expected, COPD has become the third leading cause of death. This is, of course, because of an increase in the number of COPD patients. However, it may also be caused by a characteristic feature of COPD, whereby it manifests with a lot of comorbidities, such as cardiovascular disease, diabetes mellitus, osteoporosis, gastroesophageal reflux (GERD), anxiety and depression, impaired cognitive function, and other pulmonary diseases [3], which could increase the risk of death.

Because COPD is common in the older population, it is obvious that some of the comorbidities are simply age related. However, apart from this, smoking may also explain the link between COPD and its comorbidities. A pathological finding in COPD is an inflammation of the peripheral airways, mainly caused by environmental stimuli such as tobacco smoke and other irritating particles found as a result of indoor and outdoor air pollution. As these inhaled materials have the potential to harm not only the respiratory system but also almost all the organs in the body, it is natural to consider that some of the comorbidities of COPD could be attributed to the systemic inflammation caused by long-term exposure to environmental irritants, especially tobacco smoke.

In contemporary medicine, COPD is regarded as a systemic disease rather than just a disease of the lung [1]. As has been discussed in another chapter, the pulmonary comorbidities in COPD such as lung cancer and pulmonary fibrosis are indicated to have considerable impacts on prognosis and on limitation of the activity of daily living (ADL). The extrapulmonary comorbidities have similar impacts on patient well-being. Therefore, we should be aware of the presence of comorbidities in COPD patients and should manage them during the process of COPD treatment, which would be beneficial in improving patient quality of life (QOL) and survival. Our aim in this chapter is to provide an update on the present knowledge of risk factors for developing systemic inflammation, especially long-term smoking, and to overview the pathogenesis and clinical manifestations of extrapulmonary comorbidities related to COPD.

7.2 Potential Mechanisms Contributing to the Development of Comorbidities in COPD

When patients have one or more comorbidities associated with COPD, questions arise about the pathogenic relationship between these disorders: whether comorbidities occur in a secondary manner to COPD, arise from shared risk factors, or are just present by chance. Because numerous studies have revealed that COPD patients are at higher risk of having multiple comorbidities compared with subjects without COPD, COPD and its comorbidities cannot be assumed to be independent from each other.

7.2.1 Smoking-Induced Airway Inflammation: Is It a First Step in Developing Systemic Inflammation?

It is well established that long-term smoking causes chronic inflammation of the airways, as discussed elsewhere in this book. In brief, in response to exposure to tobacco smoke or other environmental irritants, airway structural and inflammatory cells initially release a wide variety of cytokines, chemokines, and other proinflammatory mediators, leading to subsequent immune reactions (Fig. 7.1) [4]. Recruited macrophages and neutrophils release tissue-destructive enzymes such as matrix metalloproteinases and neutrophil elastase at the inflamed site, causing a protease/antiprotease imbalance, which is considered to be an important process in the development of COPD [5, 6]. Oxidative stress is another key mechanism of airway inflammation. Because tobacco smoke contains many free radicals and reactive oxygen species (ROS) as well as many toxic chemicals in its particulate and gas phases, it is considered to have the potential to directly induce oxidative damage to the lung when the levels are high enough to overcome antioxidant defenses [7, 8]. Oxidants accelerate inflammation by activating the redox-sensitive transcription factor, nuclear factor (NF)-κB, which promotes the expression of multiple inflammatory genes, such as interleukin (IL)-8 and tumor necrosis factor (TNF)-α [9]. Oxidants also activate the NLRP3 inflammasome, which contributes to the maturation of proinflammatory cytokines, including IL-1β and IL-18 [10], and cause a protease/antiprotease imbalance by inactivating the protease inhibitor, α-1-anti-trypsin [11]. Moreover, the IL-1β and TNF-α cytokines are known to have the capacity to activate NF-κB, establishing a positive feedback loop to aggravate inflammation [12].

One of the classical hypotheses to explain the development of systemic inflammation in COPD is the "spillover" theory (Fig. 7.2) [13]. This concept suggests that the inflammatory reaction may initially be local, but thereafter, increased inflammatory mediators may spill over from the inflamed lungs into the circulation to cause systemic inflammation. Because plasma levels of TNF-α, soluble TNF receptor, IL-6, and IL-8 are elevated in patients with COPD [13, 14], an obvious

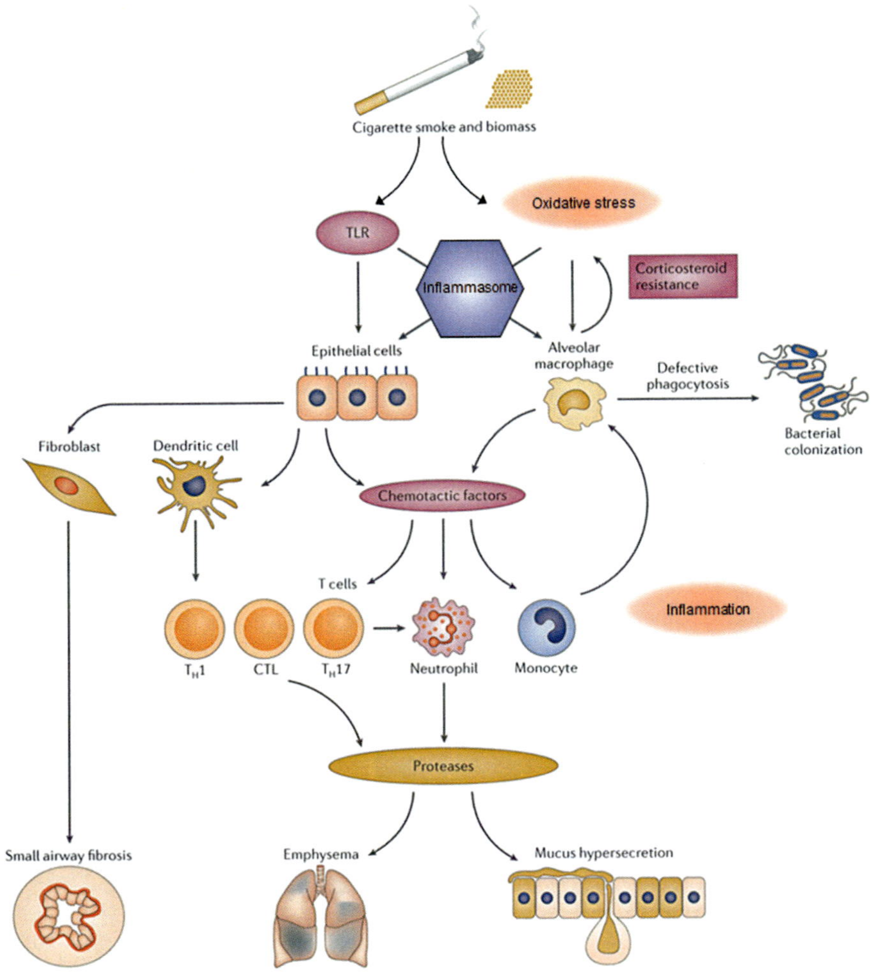

Fig. 7.1 Potential pathways and mechanisms of tobacco smoke in the development of airway inflammation. Tobacco smoke activates macrophages and epithelial cells in the airways via the activation of Toll-like receptors (TLRs) and oxidative stress to cause the release of multiple chemotactic factors. Recruited neutrophils and monocytes, and T lymphocytes as well as structural cells release multiple inflammatory mediators. Some inflammatory and structural cells also release proteases leading to parenchymal destruction and mucus hypersecretion in the airways, and some release fibrogenic mediators leading to small airway fibrosis. Cytotoxic T lymphocytes (CTLs) may also be involved in alveolar wall destruction. Activation of the inflammasome may also be involved, and phagocytic dysfunction of alveolar macrophages may lead to bacterial colonization (Adapted from Barnes 2013 [4])

explanation is that these mediators originate from the airways and accelerate subsequent immune reactions in the extrapulmonary organs. However, this concept remains unclear, as discussed below.

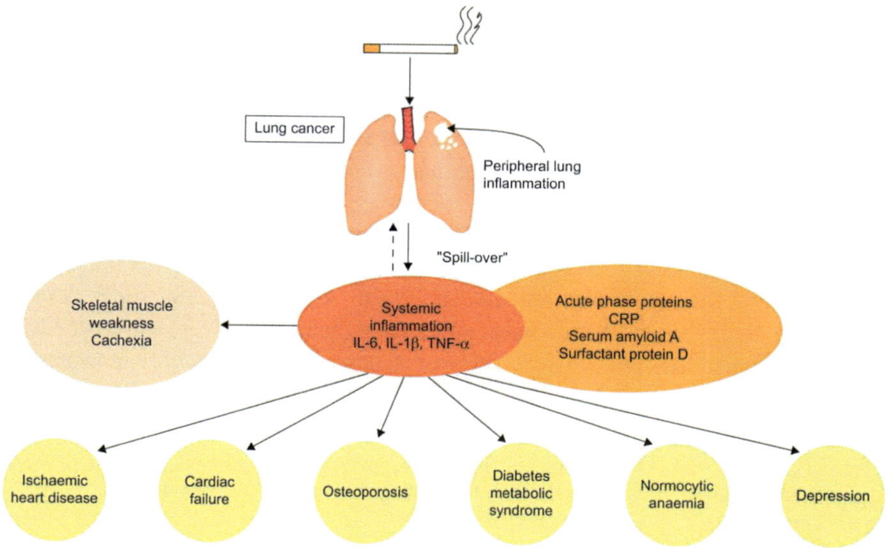

Fig. 7.2 "Spillover" hypothesis. Lung inflammation may cause a "spillover" of cytokines, such as (IL)-6, IL-1β, and tumor necrosis factor (TNF)-α, into the circulation to cause systemic inflammation and subsequent immune reactions within the extrapulmonary organs (Reproduced with permission of the European Respiratory Society ©: European Respiratory Journal May 2009, 33 (5) 1165–1185; DOI: 10.1183/09031936.00128008. This material has not been reviewed by European Respiratory Society prior to release; therefore the European Respiratory Society may not be responsible for any errors, omissions or inaccuracies, or for any consequences arising there from, in the content [13])

7.2.2 The Extrapulmonary Effects of Tobacco Smoke Exposure

Spillover is a clear-cut hypothesis; however, there are some inconsistent findings in previous studies. Wouters et al. reviewed research data from several sources, demonstrating no correlations in the levels of TNF-α, soluble TNF receptor, or IL-8 between sputum and plasma among COPD patients [14]. In addition, a recent study showed that the frequency of comorbid conditions, corresponding to the level of systemic inflammation, was not directly related to COPD severity [15]. In fact, patients with severe COPD demonstrating enhanced airway inflammation do not always develop systemic inflammation, and furthermore, patients with smoking-related cardiovascular disease do not always have COPD. Therefore, extrapulmonary comorbidities may involve an inflammatory process induced by exposure to tobacco smoke, which is independent from that of COPD. When a person inhales tobacco smoke, containing thousands of chemicals, free radicals, and ROS within its gases and particles, toxic substances deposit in the alveoli of the lungs and may rapidly diffuse into the systemic circulation. The toxicants may initially cause oxidative stress and immune responses in vascular endothelial cells and recruited inflammatory cells, similar to those in the airways (Fig. 7.1), and this effect may be further amplified leading to the systemic production of proinflammatory mediators to damage target organs.

The potential mechanisms underlying smoking-related cardiovascular disease are shown in Fig. 7.3. Oxidative stress, enhanced by free radicals and ROS generated from exogenous and endogenous sources, has been attributed a central role in the creation of atherothrombotic conditions, including endothelial dysfunction, inflammation in the vessel walls, a prothrombotic and antifibrinolytic milieu, and lipid peroxidation [16]. However, the causal relationship between airflow limitation and atherosclerosis remains equivocal. A recent clinical study demonstrated that both airflow limitation and endothelial dysfunction were associated with increased atherosclerosis, but were likely to be unrelated and mutually independent [17]. This may suggest that smoking-induced atherosclerosis is not easily explained with a simple linear pathway starting with smoking-induced airway inflammation and ending with the atherosclerotic disease.

Recent experimental studies have also demonstrated that tobacco smoke affects both insulin sensitivity and secretion. Inhaled nicotine has been shown to impair insulin signaling cascades and upregulate lipolysis within the adipose tissue through increased oxidative stress and to increase the levels of circulating free fatty acids in skeletal muscle and liver [18]. It has been also reported to activate mammalian target of rapamycin in skeletal muscle [19]; elevate the levels of circulating TNF-α, cortisol, and sex hormones; and decrease levels of adiponectin [20]. These findings may explain the relationship between nicotine and the impairment of insulin sensitivity. Additionally, tobacco smoke has been shown to suppress insulin secretion because of an alteration in pancreatic function [21]. All these results are consistent with the observation that chronic smokers are insulin resistant and at high risk for diabetes [22, 23].

The relationship between systemic inflammation and bone metabolism has also been characterized. IL-1, IL-6, and TNF-α, potential mediators for inflammation in the airways and extrapulmonary organs in COPD [13], are recognized as stimulators of bone resorption and inhibitors of bone formation [24]. This may correspond to the high prevalence of osteoporosis in patients with COPD.

7.2.3 Other Mechanisms Underlying Comorbidities

Because smoking is indicated as an age-accelerating factor, comorbidities have been associated with both long-term smoking and the consequent altered aging process [25]. However, among older smokers, not all subjects develop comorbidities or COPD. For example, a previous clinical study demonstrated that carotid intima-media thickness, a risk factor for cardiovascular diseases, was not significantly different between smoking and non-smoking control subjects, while it was significantly greater in smokers with airflow limitation than in control smokers without airflow limitation [26]. These data imply that, in addition to environmental

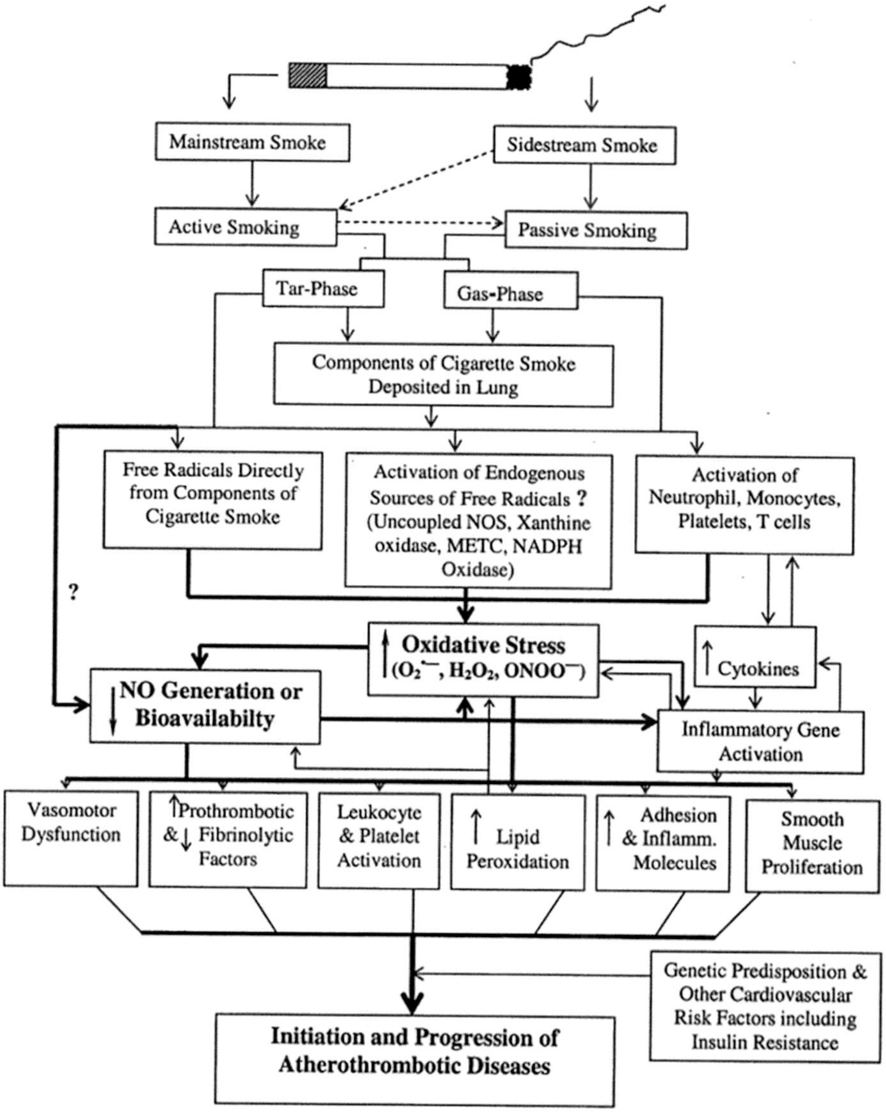

Fig. 7.3 Potential pathways and mechanisms of tobacco smoke in the development of smoking-related cardiovascular disease. Oxidative stress, enhanced by free radicals and reactive oxygen species (ROS) generated from exogenous and endogenous sources, has been attributed a central role in the atherothrombotic conditions caused by tobacco smoke, which include endothelial dysfunction, inflammation in the vessel walls, a prothrombotic and antifibrinolytic milieu, and lipid peroxidation. The *bold boxes* and *arrows* in the flow diagram represent the probable central mechanisms in this complex pathophysiology. H_2O_2, hydrogen peroxide; METC, mitochondial electron transport chain; NADPH, nicotinamide adenine dinucleotide phosphate reduced form; NOS, nitric oxide synthase; $ONOO^-$, peroxinitrite; $O^{\cdot}{}_2{}^-$, superoxide (Reproduced from Ambrose et al. 2004 [16])

factors, host susceptibility to smoke-induced inflammation in the airways and extrapulmonary organs may also be important in the development of COPD and comorbidities. Recent genome-wide association studies have identified several genetic loci responsible for the development of COPD, as discussed in the other chapters [27, 28]. The pathogenic role of these candidate genes in the susceptibility to systemic inflammation needs to be defined in future studies; however, genetic factors could be one possible explanation for a multi-comorbid condition in COPD.

The clinical symptoms and signs of COPD in themselves may be another important factor involved in the development of comorbidities. Feelings of breathlessness upon exertion gradually limit a patient's physical activity, and finally the patient tends to become housebound and develops reduced amounts of vitamin D from the lack of sunlight. This may account for insulin resistance and loss of bone mass, leading to diabetes and osteoporosis. Limitation of the ADL may cause anxiety, depression, and cognitive disorder, and in some cases, the psychological stress may aggravate GERD symptoms by increasing acid production [29]. Furthermore, recent studies reported that percent emphysema was inversely associated with reduced right ventricular (RV) volume, RV mass, and cardiac output [30], and that pharmacological treatment of lung hyperinflation achieved beneficial effects on cardiac structural and functional alterations [31].

From a pharmacological point of view, COPD medications may be a possible risk factor for comorbidities. High-dose and long-term corticosteroid treatment is believed to cause a loss of bone density, and it may also cause peptic ulcer, occasionally associated with gastrointestinal bleeding and perforation. Theophylline, β-adrenergic agonists, and anticholinergics are known to reduce lower esophageal sphincter (LES) pressure, which may lead to gastroesophageal reflux. Theophylline has also been demonstrated to increase production of gastric acid. Treatments for other comorbidities, such as low-dose aspirin or oral anticoagulants for cardiovascular diseases, selective serotonin reuptake inhibitors for psychological problems, and bisphosphonates for osteoporosis, may worsen gastrointestinal symptoms [32, 33]. It is accepted that bronchodilators including β-adrenergic agonists and anticholinergic agents may be associated with an increase in cardiovascular risk. However, it does not necessarily mean that these medications cannot be used for the treatment of COPD. Rather, clinicians should bear the adverse effects of these medications in mind when providing all necessary treatments for both COPD and any comorbidities.

7.3 Etiology of Comorbidities in COPD

Comorbidities in COPD, with a prevalence of 5 % or greater, are presented in Fig. 7.4. Of these, anxiety and/or depression, heart failure, ischemic heart disease, pulmonary hypertension, metabolic syndrome, diabetes, osteoporosis, and GERD are considered particularly important [3]. A large cohort study reported that, compared with control subjects, COPD patients have a high risk of presenting

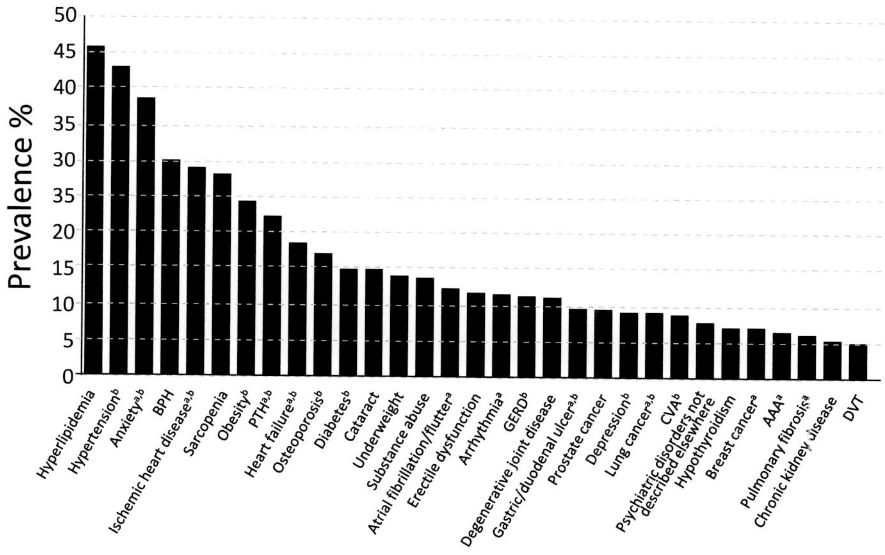

Fig. 7.4 Prevalence of comorbidities in patients with chronic obstructive pulmonary disease (COPD). a, comorbidities which result in a significant increase in the risk of mortality compared with COPD patients without the comorbidity; b, comorbidities with a significantly increased prevalence in COPD patients compared with the general population; AAA, abdominal aortic aneurysm; BPH, benign prostatic hypertrophy; COPD, chronic obstructive pulmonary disease; CVA, cerebrovascular accident; DVT, deep vein thrombosis; GERD, gastroesophageal reflux disease; PHT, pulmonary hypertension (Reproduced from Smith et al. 2014 [3])

with comorbidities. The odds ratios in COPD patients for the prevalence of chronic heart failure, angina, myocardial infarction, atrial fibrillation, hypertension, and diabetes compared with the control subjects were 8.48, 4.38, 4.42, 4.41, 1.76, and 1.51, respectively [34].

With regard to mortality, COPD patients with comorbidities are believed to have a poor prognosis compared with those without comorbidities. Among various causes of death, cardiovascular disease and lung cancer are the two major contributors other than respiratory failure itself (Fig. 7.5) [35]. The proportion of cardiovascular mortality was reported to be 12–37 % of the total death in COPD [36], and the adjusted relative risks for cardiovascular death in COPD are 3.53 for chronic heart failure, 1.81 for myocardial infarction, and 1.25 for stroke, compared with those without COPD [34]. However, interestingly, in mild or moderate COPD, comorbidities such as cardiovascular disease and lung cancer are the main causes of death, while respiratory failure becomes the predominant cause in more advanced COPD [36].

To gain a comprehensive understanding of COPD and its associated comorbidities, the "comorbidome," proposed by Divo et al., is a useful concept. As shown in Fig. 7.6, it is a graphical representation, in which each comorbidity is plotted as a bubble that depicts two values, the prevalence and mortality of that

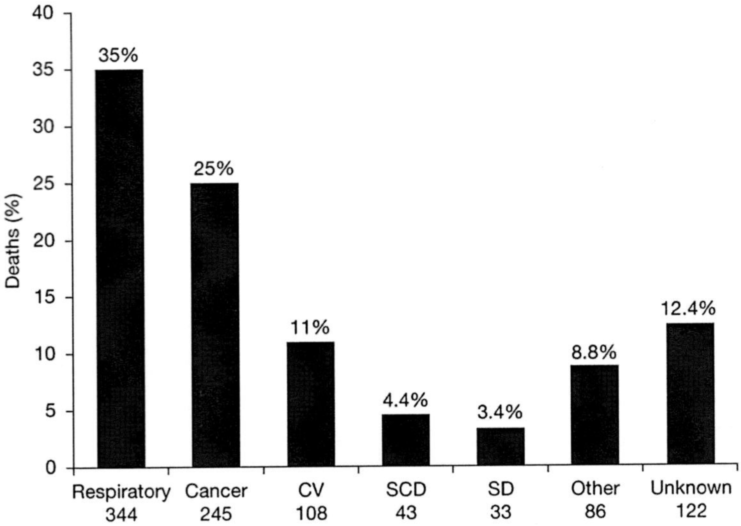

Fig. 7.5 The primary cause of death in patients with chronic obstructive pulmonary disease (COPD). The number of deaths in each category is provided below the cause of death. CV, cardiovascular; SCD, sudden cardiac death; SD, sudden death (Reproduced from McGarvey et al. 2014 [35])

comorbidity, through its size and location [37]. Although it remains contentious because patients at high risk for death were excluded in this study, the idea is simple and visually accessible, to allow us to easily recognize the multiplicity of comorbidities.

It is interesting that most patients with COPD self-reported to have one or more comorbidities, and more than half of patients reported to have four or more comorbidities, even when their COPD was stable (Fig. 7.7) [38]. Additionally, the coexistence of multiple comorbidities, along with respiratory impairment, has been demonstrated to contribute to the risk of hospitalization and death (Fig. 7.8) [39]. These results imply that clinicians must pay attention to the entire spectrum of comorbidities associated with COPD, as well as respiratory symptoms.

7.4 Comorbidities in COPD

As stated previously, and demonstrated in Fig. 7.7, almost all patients with COPD may have some kind of comorbid condition. Comorbidities have pivotal roles in causing poor health and a poor prognosis in COPD patients. It is therefore essential for clinicians to screen patients for the presence of these comorbidities and treat them comprehensively, in addition to treating their COPD. Below are outlines of the major extrapulmonary comorbidities in COPD. However, the presence of

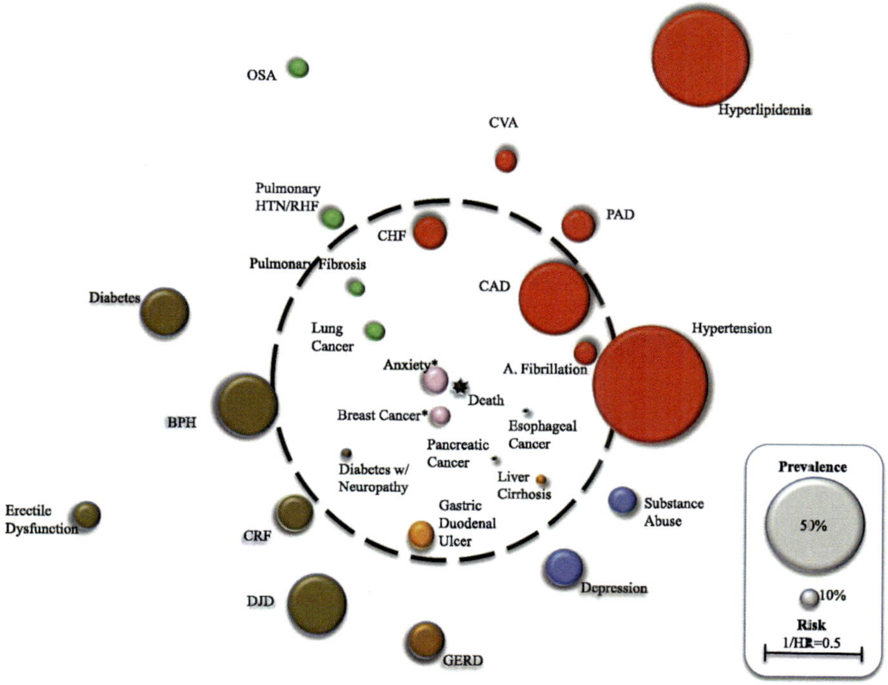

Fig. 7.6 The "comorbidome." Comorbidities associated with chronic obstructive pulmonary disease (COPD), with more than 10 % prevalence, are plotted as bubbles. The diameter of each bubble reflects the prevalence of the disease. The distance to the center (death) is scaled using the inverse of the hazard ratio (HR) (1/HR). All bubbles (comorbidities) with a statistically significant increase in mortality are inside the dotted orbit (1/HR <1). A. fibrillation, atrial fibrillation/flutter; BPH, benign prostatic hypertrophy; CAD, coronary artery disease; CHF, congestive heart failure; CRF, chronic renal failure; CVA, cerebrovascular accident; DJD, degenerative joint disease; GERD, gastroesophageal reflux disease; OSA, obstructive sleep apnea; PAD, peripheral artery disease; pulmonary HTN + RHF, pulmonary hypertension and right heart failure (Reprinted with permission of the American Thoracic Society. Copyright © 2016 American Thoracic Society. Cite: Divo M, et al. /2012/ Comorbidities and risk of mortality in patients with chronic obstructive pulmonary disease. / Am J Respir Crit Care Med /186/155-61. The *American Journal of Respiratory and Critical Care Medicine* is an official journal of the American Thoracic Society [37])

pulmonary comorbidities including lung cancer and pulmonary fibrosis also has a great impact on clinical outcomes in COPD and is discussed in the other chapters.

7.4.1 Cardiovascular Disease

Cardiovascular diseases, such as ischemic heart disease, hypertension, heart failure, atrial fibrillation, and cerebral vessel disease, are the major comorbidities in COPD [3, 39–41]. It is indicated that airflow limitation is associated with atherosclerotic

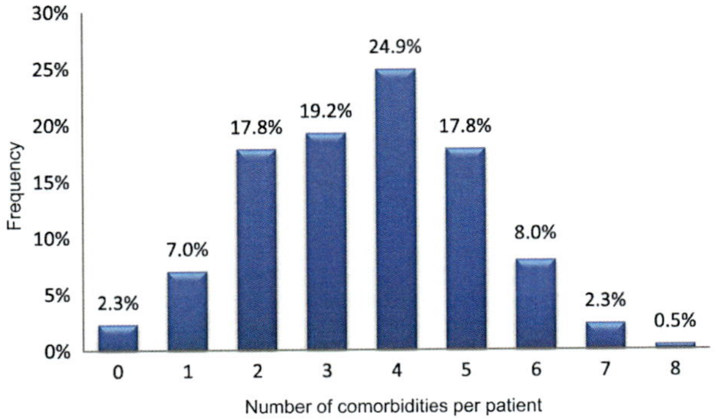

Fig. 7.7 Number of objectively identified comorbidities in patients with chronic obstructive pulmonary disease (COPD) (Reprinted with permission of the American Thoracic Society. Copyright © 2016 American Thoracic Society. Cite: Vanfleteren LE, et al./2013/Clusters of comorbidities based on validated objective measurements and systemic inflammation in patients with chronic obstructive pulmonary disease./Am J Respir Crit Care Med /187/728-35. The *American Journal of Respiratory and Critical Care Medicine* is an official journal of the American Thoracic Society [38])

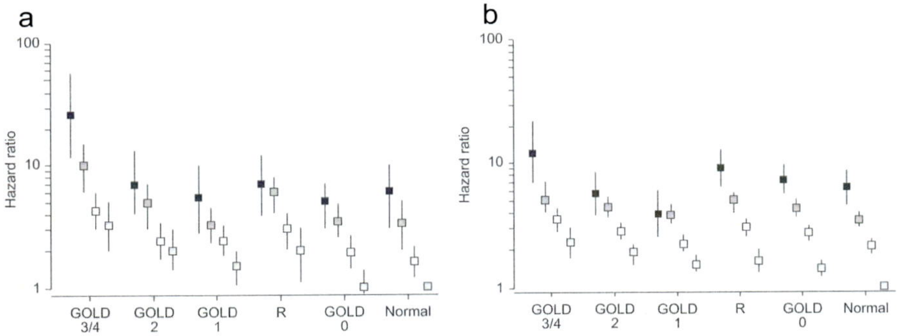

Fig. 7.8 The impact of comorbidities on all-cause mortality and time to first hospitalization in patients with chronic obstructive pulmonary disease (COPD). Cox proportional hazard models were used to predict all-cause death (**a**), and time to first hospitalization (**b**), within 5 years in patients with COPD. The subjects were classified according to their Global Initiative for Obstructive Lung Disease (GOLD) category and the presence of no (□), one (□), two (■), or three (■) comorbidities (diabetes, hypertension, or cardiovascular disease). The control group consisted of subjects with normal lung function for each comorbid disease. GOLD 3/4, forced expiratory volume in one second (FEV_1)/forced vital capacity (FVC) <0.70 and $FEV_1 < 50\,\%$ predicted; GOLD 2, FEV_1/FVC <0.70 and $FEV_1 \geq 50$ to <80 % predicted; GOLD 1, FEV_1/FVC <0.70 and $FEV_1 \geq 80\,\%$ predicted; restricted (R), FEV1/FVC ≥0.70 and FVC <80 % predicted; GOLD 0, presence of respiratory symptoms in the absence of any lung function abnormality and no lung disease (Reproduced with permission of the European Respiratory Society ©: European Respiratory Journal Oct 2008, 32 (4) 962–969; DOI: 10.1183/09031936.00012408. This material has not been reviewed by European Respiratory Society prior to release; therefore the European Respiratory Society may not be responsible for any errors, omissions or inaccuracies, or for any consequences arising there from, in the content [39])

plaque formation in the carotid artery and increased levels of coronary artery calcium [17], and tobacco smoke is an important risk factor for both atherosclerosis and COPD. Therefore, this shared factor is likely to contribute to the increased risk of cardiovascular comorbidities in patients with COPD. Moreover, from the evidence that carotid intima-media thickness is greater in smokers with airflow limitation than in those without airflow limitation [26], COPD patients may be particularly prone to atherosclerosis.

The presence of cardiovascular diseases is associated with a high incidence of death in patients with COPD [39], and therefore, we should be prepared to identify such comorbidities and treat them appropriately. Unnecessary or excessive dosage with β-adrenergic agonists or antagonists in COPD patients with unstable cardiovascular disease or with cardiovascular disease during COPD exacerbation, respectively, can be harmful and should be avoided. In general, when choosing β-adrenergic bronchodilators, inhaled selective β-2 adrenergic agonists, rather than nonselective adrenergic agonists, are recommended in COPD patients with cardiovascular disease. Conversely, cardioselective β-blockers would be safer for patients with cardiovascular disease at risk of COPD exacerbation. In any case, according to an expert consensus, clinicians should always implement all necessary treatments for both COPD and cardiovascular comorbidities.

7.4.2 Diabetes

The high prevalence of diabetes among patients with COPD [3, 39, 40] and, conversely, the high prevalence of COPD among patients with diabetes have been documented [42]. Although the underlying mechanism of smoking-induced hyperglycemia is not yet completely elucidated, the association between COPD and diabetes may be explained by a combination of several factors: tobacco smoking as a shared risk [18, 19, 23, 43], exercise limitation as a result of respiratory symptoms, and/or the adverse effects of oral corticosteroid use. Uncontrolled diabetes in COPD patients may cause unfavorable outcomes, for instance, the occurrence of infectious conditions such as bacterial pneumonia, a delay in the wound-healing process of injured respiratory organs, and the progression of other microvascular and cardiovascular comorbidities. In fact, concomitant diabetes is associated with an increased risk of hospitalization [44] and mortality [45].

It is also important to note that recent studies have revealed that hyperglycemia might have an impact on the decline in pulmonary function, suggesting that the presence of diabetes may worsen the progression of COPD. These studies demonstrated that subjects without any pulmonary dysfunction and with diabetes showed a modest but statistically significant decrease in measures of pulmonary function, including forced vital capacity, forced expiratory volume in 1 s, diffusion capacity of the lungs for carbon monoxide, and 6-min walk distance, compared with those without diabetes [46, 47]. It has also been reported that patients with type 1 diabetes who underwent pancreas and kidney transplantation demonstrated improved pulmonary function, as their blood sugar became well controlled [48]. Four mechanisms have been proposed whereby hyperglycemia could cause an impairment in pulmonary function: (1) reduced lung elasticity caused by nonenzymatic glycosylation-induced alteration of lung connective tissue, (2) reduced pulmonary capillary blood volume because of microangiopathy, (3) more frequent and more severe exacerbation of pulmonary symptoms caused by an increased susceptibility to respiratory infection, and (4) impaired diaphragmatic function caused by phrenic nerve neuropathy [46]. Some of these pathological changes are likely to be irreversible; however, it is important to realize that controlling diabetes has significant benefits for COPD patients in improving QOL and extending survival.

7.4.3 Osteoporosis

The prevalence of osteoporosis in COPD patients is estimated to be quite high, ranging from 50 to 70 % [3]. The incidence of low volumetric bone mineral density has been shown to increase in parallel with the severity of COPD and reached 84 % in patients at a very severe stage. Even after adjustment for smoking, steroid use, age, and exacerbations, COPD, especially with emphysematous changes, was associated with both low volumetric bone mineral density and vertebral fractures [49]. Many contributory factors for osteoporosis have been suggested, but these may vary with the individual. These include increased levels of proinflammatory mediators caused by smoking, limited physical activity because of respiratory symptoms, malnutrition resulting from poor food intake, a hypermetabolic state caused by systemic inflammation, treatment with corticosteroids, and a lack of estrogen after menopause in older women.

It is uncertain whether osteoporosis is a consequence of COPD or actually functions as an aggravating factor. Osteoporosis increases the risk of bone fracture, and because of the consequent pain, this results in a deterioration in the level of physical activity, increases shortness of breath, and creates difficulties in expectorating sputum. These can further be associated with a decline in the ADL and exacerbations in COPD, which limit a patient's physical activities even more. Consequently, patients with both COPD and osteoporosis enter into a negative cycle of losing bone mass and a debilitating respiratory condition. Considering the high prevalence of coexisting osteoporosis and COPD, an evaluation for osteoporosis may have potential implications in the comprehensive management of patients with COPD.

7.4.4 Gastrointestinal Disease

Gastrointestinal diseases, such as peptic ulcer and GERD, are also commonly found in COPD patients [3]. COPD patients tend to take multiple medications for their comorbidities as well as for their COPD. The risk of peptic ulcer and/or gastrointestinal bleeding is higher in those who regularly take corticosteroids, theophylline, low-dose aspirin or other nonsteroidal anti-inflammatory drugs, oral anticoagulants, selective serotonin reuptake inhibitors, or bisphosphonates [32, 33]. Psychological stress, frequently experienced by COPD patients, has also been demonstrated to increase the incidence of peptic ulcer [29]. Furthermore, long-term smoking, hypoxemia, and poor nutrition are considered to delay the wound-healing process in the ulcerated gastrointestinal tissue, and these may be additional contributory factors in peptic ulcer.

The prevalence of GERD in COPD patients ranges from 30 to 60 % [3]. GERD is usually caused by LES dysfunction, resulting in the reflux of gastric acid into the esophagus. COPD may predispose patients to gastroesophageal reflux by the following mechanisms [50]. One involves an enhancement of the pressure gradient between the thorax and abdomen caused by an increased respiratory muscle effort, airway obstruction, and coughing. The other mechanism involves a low-lying diaphragm from lung hyperinflation, whereby the diaphragm may not be able to function as an external sphincter. Medications for COPD, including β-adrenergic agonists, anticholinergics, and theophylline, are also believed to decrease LES pressure. However, as mentioned previously, this does not mean that these medications should not be administered to COPD patients with GERD. It is indisputable that a better control of COPD symptoms, such as breathlessness and coughing, may comprehensively improve gastroesophageal reflux, even if the medication itself has a contrary effect if examined in isolation. Moreover, acid reflux is indirectly implicated in bronchoconstriction and airway inflammation, through a vagally mediated esophagobronchial reflex, and directly following microaspiration of refluxed material into the respiratory tract. Therefore, COPD and gastrointestinal conditions need to be treated simultaneously, given the prospect that they are associated with an increased risk of COPD exacerbation and/or an impaired QOL for patients.

7.4.5 *Psychological Disorders*

Psychological conditions, such as anxiety and depression, are well known to be associated with COPD [51]. Breathlessness is the primary symptom of COPD and often results in exercise limitation. As dyspnea progresses, the patient becomes inactive and housebound, which leads to a deterioration in QOL. Such patients may have feelings of exhaustion, frustration, and discouragement for various reasons, including persistent respiratory symptoms, functional limitation, social isolation, and uncertainty about the future. Therefore, they may experience psychological distress including anxiety or depression. In addition, a recent study demonstrated that there were structural changes in the brains of patients with moderate-to-severe COPD, and of these, a reduction in gray matter volume in the anterior cingulate cortex was correlated with greater disease-specific fears [52].

Concerning cognitive impairment, a population-based longitudinal cohort study has suggested that mild cognitive decline is more common in older adults with COPD than those without COPD [53]. Cognitive impairment, as well as cerebral vessel disease, shares common risk factors with COPD including aging and smoking. Furthermore, physical inactivity, hypoxia caused by reduced gas transfer, enhanced systemic inflammation, and oxidative stress are the other risk factors fueled by COPD [54].

Previous studies demonstrate that, compared with COPD patients with a stable psychological condition, COPD patients with anxiety or depression are likely to be at greater risk for exacerbations, long hospital stays, and a poor prognosis [55, 56]. It has also been shown that the risk of ADL disability and functional limitation is higher when COPD and cognitive impairment occur together, than when COPD presents alone [53]. It is difficult in some cases to detect the psychological symptoms that can accompany COPD; however, clinicians should recognize that patients with COPD frequently demonstrate related psychological problems and should aim to treat those conditions.

7.5 Conclusion

The concept of COPD has changed a great deal over the past 10 years. To date, COPD is regarded not as a disease of peripheral-airway inflammation but as a disease of systemic inflammation associated with a variety of comorbidities including cardiovascular disease, diabetes, osteoporosis, GERD, anxiety and depression, impaired cognitive function, and other pulmonary diseases. Although the exact pathogenesis of comorbidities in COPD has not been fully elucidated, it might be explained by systemic inflammation, accelerated by direct environmental stimuli such as tobacco smoke and/or proinflammatory mediators that spill over from the inflamed lung.

COPD and its comorbidities mutually aggravate each other and may negatively affect QOL and result in a poor prognosis. Therefore, clinicians should consider COPD as a systemic disease, be aware of the presence of comorbidities, and control all COPD-related pathological conditions comprehensively to achieve the best patient outcomes.

References

1. World Health Organization (WHO) Media Centre: the top 10 causes of death. http://www.who.int/mediacentre. Updated May 2014.
2. Murray CJ, Lopez AD. Alternative projections of mortality and disability by cause 1990–2020: Global Burden of Disease Study. Lancet. 1997;349:1498–504.
3. Smith MC, Wrobel JP. Epidemiology and clinical impact of major comorbidities in patients with COPD. Int J Chron Obstruct Pulmon Dis. 2014;9:871–88.

4. Barnes PJ. New anti-inflammatory targets for chronic obstructive pulmonary disease. Nat Rev Drug Discov. 2013;12:543–59.
5. Hautamaki RD, Kobayashi DK, Senior RM, Shapiro SD. Requirement for macrophage elastase for cigarette smoke-induced emphysema in mice. Science. 1997;277:2002–4.
6. Shapiro SD, Goldstein NM, Houghton AM, Kobayashi DK, Kelley D, Belaaouaj A. Neutrophil elastase contributes to cigarette smoke-induced emphysema in mice. Am J Pathol. 2003;163:2329–35.
7. Repine JE, Bast A, Lankhorst I. Oxidative stress in chronic obstructive pulmonary disease. Am J Respir Crit Care Med. 1997;156:341–57.
8. MacNee W, Rahman I. Oxidants and antioxidants as therapeutic targets in chronic obstructive pulmonary disease. Am J Respir Crit Care Med. 1999;160:S58–65.
9. Barnes PJ. Chronic obstructive pulmonary disease. New Engl J Med. 2000;343:269–80.
10. Abais JM, Xia M, Zhang Y, Boini KM, Li PL. Redox regulation of NLRP3 inflammasomes: ROS as trigger or effector? Antioxid Redox Signal. 2015;22:1111–29.
11. MacNee W, Rahman I. Is oxidative stress central to the pathogenesis of chronic obstructive pulmonary disease? Trends Mol Med. 2001;7:55–62.
12. Li Q, Verma IM. NF-kappaB regulation in the immune system. Nat Rev Immunol. 2002;2:725–34.
13. Barnes PJ, Celli BR. Systemic manifestations and comorbidities of COPD. Eur Respir J. 2009;33:1165–85.
14. Wouters EF, Reynaert NL, Dentener MA, Vernooy JH. Systemic and local inflammation in asthma and chronic obstructive pulmonary disease: is there a connection? Proc Am Thorac Soc. 2009;6:638–47.
15. Echave-Sustaeta JM, Comeche Casanova L, Cosio BG, Soler-Cataluña JJ, Garcia-Lujan R, Ribera X. Comorbidity in chronic obstructive pulmonary disease. Related to disease severity? Int J Chron Obstruct Pulmon Dis. 2014;9:1307–14.
16. Ambrose JA, Barua RS. The pathophysiology of cigarette smoking and cardiovascular disease: an update. J Am Coll Cardiol. 2004;43:1731–7.
17. Chandra D, Gupta A, Strollo PJ Jr, Fuhrman CR, Leader JK, Bon J, et al. Airflow limitation and endothelial dysfunction: unrelated and independent predictors of atherosclerosis. Am J Respir Crit Care Med. 2016;194:38–47.
18. Wu Y, Song P, Zhang W, Liu J, Dai X, Liu Z, et al. Activation of AMPKα2 in adipocytes is essential for nicotine-induced insulin resistance in vivo. Nat Med. 2015;21:373–82.
19. Bergman BC, Perreault L, Hunerdosse D, Kerege A, Playdon M, Samek AM, et al. Novel and reversible mechanisms of smoking-induced insulin resistance in humans. Diabetes. 2012;61:3156–66.
20. Tweed JO, Hsia SH, Lutfy K, Friedman TC. The endocrine effects of nicotine and cigarette smoke. Trends Endocrinol Metab. 2012;23:334–42.
21. Milnerowicz H, Sliwinska-Mosson M, Rabczyński J, Nowak M, Milnerowicz S. Dysfunction of the pancreas in healthy smoking persons and patients with chronic pancreatitis. Pancreas. 2007;34:46–54.
22. Facchini FS, Hollenbeck CB, Jeppesen J, Chen YD, Reaven GM. Insulin resistance and cigarette smoking. Lancet. 1992;339:1128–30.
23. Pan A, Wang Y, Talaei M, Hu FB, Wu T. Relation of active, passive, and quitting smoking with incident type 2 diabetes: a systematic review and meta-analysis. Lancet Diabetes Endocrinol. 2015;3:958–67.
24. Pietschmann P, Mechtcheriakova D, Meshcheryakova A, Föger-Samwald U, Ellinger I. Immunology of osteoporosis: a mini-review. Gerontology. 2016;62:128–37.
25. Rutten EP, Gopal P, Wouters EF, Franssen FM, Hageman GJ, Vanfleteren LE, et al. Various mechanistic pathways representing the aging process are altered in COPD. Chest. 2016;149:53–61.

26. Iwamoto H, Yokoyama A, Kitahara Y, Ishikawa N, Haruta Y, Yamane K, et al. Airflow limitation in smokers is associated with subclinical atherosclerosis. Am J Respir Crit Care Med. 2009;179:35–40.
27. Cho MH, McDonald ML, Zhou X, Mattheisen M, Castaldi PJ, Hersh CP, et al. NETT genetics, ICGN, ECLIPSE and COPDGene investigators. Risk loci for chronic obstructive pulmonary disease: a genome-wide association study and meta-analysis. Lancet Respir Med. 2014;2:214–25.
28. Soler Artigas M, Wain LV, Miller S, Kheirallah AK, Huffman JE, Ntalla I, et al. Sixteen new lung function signals identified through 1000 Genomes Project reference panel imputation. Nat Commun. 2015;6:8658.
29. Levenstein S, Rosenstock S, Jacobsen RK, Jorgensen T. Psychological stress increases risk for peptic ulcer, regardless of Helicobacter pylori infection or use of nonsteroidal anti-inflammatory drugs. Clin Gastroenterol Hepatol. 2015;13:498–506.
30. Grau M, Barr RG, Lima JA, Hoffman EA, Bluemke DA, Carr JJ, et al. Percent emphysema and right ventricular structure and function: the multi-ethnic study of atherosclerosis-lung and multi-ethnic study of atherosclerosis-right ventricle studies. Chest. 2013;144:136–44.
31. Stone IS, Barnes NC, James WY, Midwinter D, Boubertakh R, Follows R, et al. Lung deflation and cardiovascular structure and function in COPD: a randomized controlled trial. Am J Respir Crit Care Med. 2016;193:717–26.
32. Andrade C, Sandarsh S, Chethan KB, Nagesh KS. Serotonin reuptake inhibitor antidepressants and abnormal bleeding: a review for clinicians and a reconsideration of mechanisms. J Clin Psychiatry. 2010;71:1565–75.
33. Peng YL, Hu HY, Luo JC, Hou MC, Lin HC, Lee FY. Alendronate, a bisphosphonate, increased upper and lower gastrointestinal bleeding: risk factor analysis from a nationwide population-based study. Osteoporos Int. 2014;25:1617–23.
34. Sidney S, Sorel M, Quesenberry Jr CP, DeLuise C, Lanes S, Eisner MD. COPD and incident cardiovascular disease hospitalizations and mortality: Kaiser Permanente Medical Care Program. Chest. 2005;128:2068–75.
35. McGarvey LP, Magder S, Burkhart D, Kesten S, Liu D, Manuel RC, et al. Cause-specific mortality adjudication in the UPLIFT® COPD trial: findings and recommendations. Respir Med. 2012;106:515–21.
36. Sin DD, Anthonisen NR, Soriano JB, Agusti AG. Mortality in COPD: role of comorbidities. Eur Respir J. 2006;28(6):1245–57.
37. Divo M, Cote C, de Torres JP, Casanova C, Marin JM, Pinto-Plata V, et al. BODE Collaborative Group. Comorbidities and risk of mortality in patients with chronic obstructive pulmonary disease. Am J Respir Crit Care Med. 2012;186:155–61.
38. Vanfleteren LE, Spruit MA, Groenen M, Gaffron S, van Empel VP, Bruijnzeel PL, et al. Clusters of comorbidities based on validated objective measurements and systemic inflammation in patients with chronic obstructive pulmonary disease. Am J Respir Crit Care Med. 2013;187:728–35.
39. Mannino DM, Thorn D, Swensen A, Holguin F. Prevalence and outcomes of diabetes, hypertension and cardiovascular disease in COPD. Eur Respir J. 2008;32:962–9.
40. Chen W, Thomas J, Sadatsafavi M, FitzGerald JM. Risk of cardiovascular comorbidity in patients with chronic obstructive pulmonary disease: a systematic review and meta-analysis. Lancet Respir Med. 2015;3:631–9.
41. Portegies ML, Lahousse L, Joos GF, Hofman A, Koudstaal PJ, Stricker BH, et al. Chronic obstructive pulmonary disease and the risk of stroke: the Rotterdam Study. Am J Respir Crit Care Med. 2016;193:251–8.
42. Ehrlich SF, Quesenberry Jr CP, Van Den Eeden SK, Shan J, Ferrara A. Patients diagnosed with diabetes are at increased risk for asthma, chronic obstructive pulmonary disease, pulmonary fibrosis, and pneumonia but not lung cancer. Diabetes Care. 2010;33:55–60.

43. Foy CG, Bell RA, Farmer DF, Goff Jr DC, Wagenknecht LE. Smoking and incidence of diabetes among U.S. adults: findings from the Insulin Resistance Atherosclerosis Study. Diabetes Care. 2005;28:2501–7.
44. Singh JA, Yu S. Utilization due to chronic obstructive pulmonary disease and its predictors: a study using the U.S. National Emergency Department Sample (NEDS). Respir Res. 2016;17:1.
45. Singanayagam A, Schembri S, Chalmers JD. Predictors of mortality in hospitalized adults with acute exacerbation of chronic obstructive pulmonary disease. Ann Am Thorac Soc. 2013;10:81–9.
46. van den Borst B, Gosker HR, Zeegers MP, Schols AM. Pulmonary function in diabetes: a metaanalysis. Chest. 2010;138:393–406.
47. Kinney GL, Black-Shinn JL, Wan ES, Make B, Regan E, Lutz S, et al. Pulmonary function reduction in diabetes with and without chronic obstructive pulmonary disease. Diabetes Care. 2014;37:389–95.
48. Dieterle CD, Schmauss S, Arbogast H, Domsch C, Huber RM, Landgraf R. Pulmonary function in patients with type 1 diabetes before and after simultaneous pancreas and kidney transplantation. Transplantation. 2007;83:566–9.
49. Jaramillo JD, Wilson C, Stinson DS, Lynch DA, Bowler RP, Lutz S, et al. Reduced bone density and vertebral fractures in smokers. Men and COPD patients at increased risk. Ann Am Thorac Soc. 2015;12:648–56.
50. Lee AL, Goldstein RS. Gastroesophageal reflux disease in COPD: links and risks. Int J Chron Obstruct Pulmon Dis. 2015;10:1935–49.
51. Maurer J, Rebbapragada V, Borson S, Goldstein R, Kunik ME, Yohannes AM, Hanania NA. ACCP workshop panel on anxiety and depression in COPD. Anxiety and depression in COPD: current understanding, unanswered questions, and research needs. Chest. 2008;134:43S–56.
52. Esser RW, Stoeckel MC, Kirsten A, Watz H, Taube K, Lehmann K, et al. Structural brain changes in patients with chronic obstructive pulmonary disease. Chest. 2016;149:426–34.
53. Martinez CH, Richardson CR, Han MK, Cigolle CT. Chronic obstructive pulmonary disease, cognitive impairment, and development of disability: the health and retirement study. Ann Am Thorac Soc. 2014;11:1362–70.
54. Lahousse L, Tiemeier H, Ikram MA, Brusselle GG. Chronic obstructive pulmonary disease and cerebrovascular disease: a comprehensive review. Respir Med. 2015;109:1371–80.
55. Laurin C, Moullec G, Bacon SL, Lavoie KL. Impact of anxiety and depression on chronic obstructive pulmonary disease exacerbation risk. Am J Respir Crit Care Med. 2012;185:918–23.
56. Pumar MI, Gray CR, Walsh JR, Yang IA, Rolls TA, Ward DL. Anxiety and depression-Important psychological comorbidities of COPD. J Thorac Dis. 2014;6:1615–31.

Chapter 8
Assessment of Inflammation in COPD: Are There any Biomarkers that Can be Used to Assess Pulmonary and Systemic Inflammation?

Nobuyuki Horita and Takeshi Kaneko

Abstract Numerous inflammatory substances have been identified as potentially useful biomarkers to evaluate COPD. These substances were derived from sputum, blood, exhaled gas, exhaled breath condensate, and bronchoscopic specimens. However, the majority of these biomarkers are not currently clinically applicable due to the lack of sufficient difference of value between COPD subjects and healthy subjects, insufficient validation in randomized controlled trial, invasive procedure required to obtain specimen directly from the lung, or technical issue preventing reproducible measurements.

Nonetheless, we have biomarkers that can be used to assess pulmonary and systemic inflammation for patients with COPD. Plasma fibrinogen can predict the future incidence of COPD and future FEV_1 decline in COPD and non-COPD subjects. In July 2015, the US Food and Drug Administration approved serum fibrinogen as the first COPD biomarker to identify patients that are at a higher risk of exacerbation or death in clinical trials. Researchers hope this approval will accelerate trials for new medications. Serum C-reactive protein is another widely approved biomarker related to COPD diagnosis, exacerbation diagnosis, and patient prognosis. Sputum/blood eosinophils, fractional exhaled nitric oxide, and the T helper type 2 genes can be candidate predictive biomarkers to pick up the asthma-COPD overlap syndrome cases who are amenable to inhaled corticosteroids. The tumor necrosis factor-α-308 variant is associated with COPD risk and emphysematous change especially in Asians.

Keywords Fibrinogen • C-reactive protein • Eosinophils • Helper T

N. Horita • T. Kaneko (✉)
Department of Pulmonology, Yokohama City University Graduate School of Medicine, 3-9 Fukuura, Kanazawa-ku, Yokohama 236-0004, Japan
e-mail: takeshi@yokohama-cu.ac.jp

H. Nakamura, K. Aoshiba (eds.), *Chronic Obstructive Pulmonary Disease*, Respiratory Disease Series: Diagnostic Tools and Disease Managements,
DOI 10.1007/978-981-10-0839-9_8

8.1 Introduction

Although chronic obstructive pulmonary disease (COPD) was first defined, in 1964, as a disease condition characterized by nonreversible airflow limitation, our understanding of COPD has been greatly modified during the last five decades, and now we focus on systemic inflammation [1]. Systemic inflammation may have spilled over from COPD lungs, or systemic inflammatory condition of multiple organs may lead to pulmonary manifestations. Currently, COPD is regarded as a progressive systematic inflammatory disease characterized by airflow limitation and systemic comorbidities [1]. Thus, evaluation of COPD was expanded from forced expiratory volume in one second (FEV_1) to total body assessment including degree of dyspnea, exercise capacity, history of exacerbation, activities of daily living, comorbidities, and level of systematic inflammation [1]. Historically, FEV_1 almost solely defined the severity of the disease and was a well-known predictor for mortality along with age. Therefore, therapeutic trials in COPD have depended on FEV_1 as a primary outcome when mortality was not suitable as the primary outcome due to limitations of study design. FEV_1 is easily obtainable and highly reproducible. The US Food and Drug Administration indicated, as of 2007, that "with the exception of lung function tests, there are no well-validated biomarkers or surrogate endpoints that can be used to establish efficacy of a drug for COPD [2]." However, FEV_1 has some weak points as a tool to evaluate COPD cases. First, the FEV_1 alone usually does not accurately reflect respiratory and non-respiratory symptoms of COPD. Second, FEV_1 cannot assess short-term change in the COPD patient's condition, unlike in the case of asthma the obstruction of which is easily reversible by administrating bronchodilator. Third, FEV_1 does not reflect an underlying pathologic process or phenotype of COPD. Fourth, decreased FEV_1, or airflow limitation, is not specific to COPD [2, 3].

The World Health Organization has defined a biomarker as "any substance, structure, or process that can be measured in the body or its products and influence or predict the incidence of outcome or disease [4]." Sin et al. proposed five essential questions as biomarkers for COPD [1]: (i) Is there a strong biological plausibility in terms of its role in the pathogenesis of disease? (ii) Is there a strong, consistent, and independent association between the biomarker and chronic obstructive pulmonary disease? (iii) Is there a strong, independent association between the biomarker and hard clinical outcomes such as mortality and hospitalization? (iv) Is there evidence from randomized controlled trials (RCT) that the biomarker is modifiable by interventions? (v) Is there evidence from RCTs that changes in the biomarker status result in changes in an important (and accepted) clinical outcome (e.g., mortality, exacerbation, rate of decline in FEV_1, health status)? In short, a biomarker has to be a consistent independent surrogate for diagnosis, severity, and hard-endpoint treatment effect in RCT that is supported by biological plausibility. Many previous biomarkers had been investigated in an observational manner [5] (Fig. 8.1), though few have been validated in a randomized manner [2, 3, 5, 6].

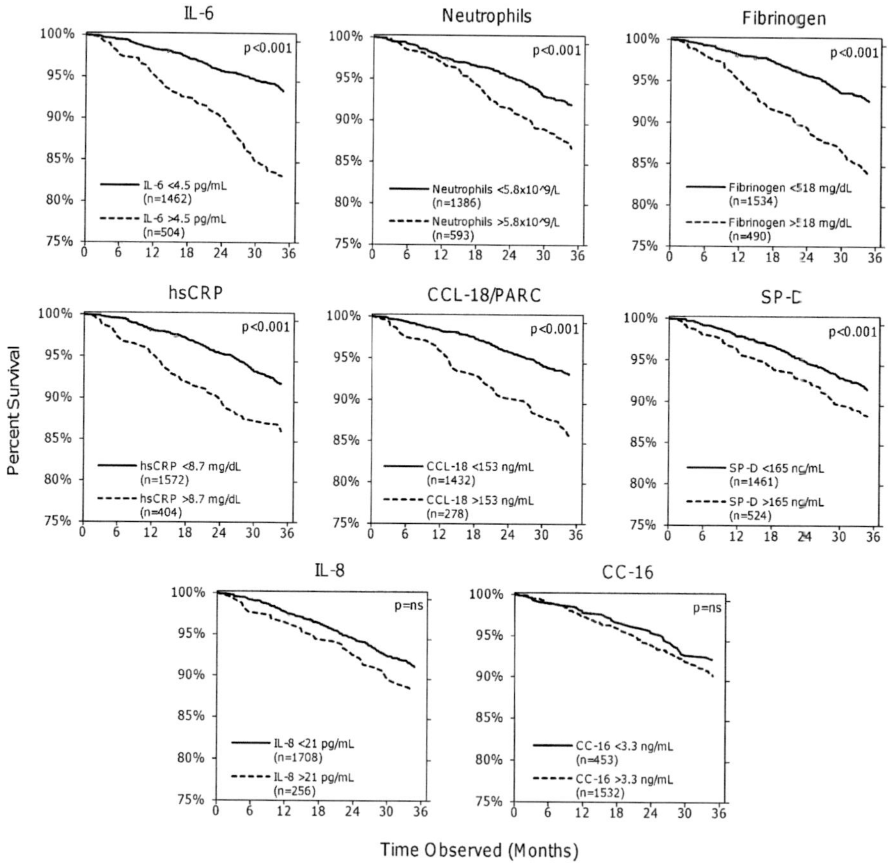

Fig. 8.1 Kaplan–Meier survival curves for the panel of biomarkers analyzed. Cutoff values correspond to the 95 % percentile determined in the nonsmoking control subjects included in the Evaluation of COPD Longitudinally to Identify Predictive Surrogate Endpoints study. *CC-16* Clara cell secretory protein-16, *CCL-18/PARC* chemokine ligand 18/pulmonary and activation-regulated chemokine, *hsCRP* high-sensitivity C-reactive protein, *SP-D* surfactant protein D. This figure was referred with permission from the publisher (Reprinted with permission from the American Thoracic Society. Copyright © 2015 American Thoracic Society. Celli BR, et al. Inflammatory biomarkers improve clinical prediction of mortality in chronic obstructive pulmonary disease. Am J Respir Crit Care Med. 2012;185:1065–72 [5]. The American Journal of Respiratory and Critical Care Medicine is an official journal of the American Thoracic Society)

In addition, a biomarker preferably can guide phenotyping of COPD. It is unlikely that all patients with COPD have the same underlying disease process and the same response to a specific medication. If a biomarker can differentiate a category of patients who have good response to a specific treatment from those with poor response, this is regarded as predictive biomarker [7].

Given the current evidence, it is conclusive that COPD is associated with systemic inflammation. A subgroup of patients with COPD that have persistently raised concentrations of inflammatory biomarkers often have significantly increased all-cause mortality and exacerbation frequency. However, whether persistent systemic inflammation can be a target of pharmacological treatment is far from clear. Some promising systematic anti-inflammatory medications, namely, long-term oral systemic steroids and statins, have failed to improve survival [8, 9].

Biomarkers have often been discussed as a tool to distinguish subtypes of COPD. The Evaluation of COPD Longitudinally to Identify Predictive Surrogate Endpoints (ECLIPSE) study was a large-scale 3 year observational controlled multicenter international study to classify clinically relevant subtypes of COPD and to identify novel biomarkers and genetic factors [6]. ECLIPSE confirmed that many previously known biomarkers truly have relation with COPD. This also revealed some novel biomarkers that required further validation to be used in practice. The ongoing subpopulations and intermediate outcomes in COPD study is another large-scale study that deals both with phenotyping and biomarkers. This is a multicenter longitudinal, observational study to identify novel phenotypes and biomarkers of COPD [2].

In this chapter, we will review COPD biomarkers that can be used for diagnosis, phenotyping, and evaluating severity, prognosis, therapeutic effect, and future risk to develop COPD, focusing on inflammatory substances. In addition, we will review biomarkers that are related to comorbidities.

8.2 Sputum

Patients with COPD usually produce more sputum than healthy persons. Sputum samples were expected to be ideal to investigate the airway inflammation because sputum is produced in the airway, in contrast to blood, which is made in bone marrow, and because sputum can be obtained noninvasively. However, the examination of sputum on inflammatory biomarkers seemed difficult and unreliable until 1992 when the sputum induction technique was established to obtain sputum from healthy subjects and subjects with airway diseases. The sputum analysis technique has been refined to provide reliable results for an increasing number of inflammatory biomarkers. Initially, these biomarkers were studied mainly in patients with asthma and chronic bronchitis. Later, sputum biomarkers were used in research to study the airway inflammation in COPD cases. Sputum induction is required when the sputum cannot be obtained spontaneously or obtained sputum is not of sufficient quality. Sputum induction is usually conducted with a hypertonic saline aerosol in concentrations of 4.5 %. The considerable limitation with sputum induction in patients with COPD and asthma is that the saline aerosol can cause bronchoconstriction. We can obtain sufficient sputum from more than 90 % of patients with COPD. After processing, cellular markers can be analyzed using flow cytometry [10, 11].

In healthy persons, macrophages and neutrophils account for approximately 60 % and 40 % of sputum cell count, respectively. Few bronchial epithelial cells, lymphocytes, eosinophils, and metachromatic cells have been observed [10].

8.2.1 *Sputum Neutrophils*

The number or proportion of neutrophils is labile in both healthy persons and patients with COPD cases depending on many stimuli, such as sputum induction, smoking, air pollutants, endotoxins, occupational exposures, and infections. Although it is well known that sputum neutrophilia is common in COPD subjects, it is not specific to COPD. As smoking itself induce sputum neutrophilia, sputum neutrophilia among non-COPD smokers largely diminishes the diagnostic value of sputum neutrophilia for COPD. However, among smokers with COPD, the degree of sputum neutrophilia relates weakly to the degree of airflow limitation and the degree of disease progression. Leukocyte-specific integrin CD11b/CD18 expressed on neutrophils may also be related to the severity of COPD [10].

Increased numbers of neutrophils have been found in sputum samples of stable COPD cases. Furthermore, a negative correlation has been confirmed between the proportion of neutrophils and FEV_1. The neutrophilic inflammation partially explains why most COPD patients are resistant to steroid treatment.

The effect of drugs on neutrophilic inflammation in COPD was investigated in some studies. One study has reported that the sputum neutrophil count was reduced after 2 months of treatment with inhaled beclomethasone [12]. However, this requires further study, since this result conflicts with the known effect of corticosteroids to prolong the life of neutrophils. In another study, theophylline reduced induced sputum neutrophils [13].

COPD exacerbation is often associated with sputum neutrophilia especially when caused by bacterial infection [10, 11]

8.2.2 *Sputum Eosinophils*

Although sputum samples contain relatively a small number of eosinophils compared to that of neutrophils, the significance of sputum eosinophils for COPD has been extensively investigated. Many studies have demonstrated sputum eosinophilia (sputum eosinophils $> 3\,\%$) in stable COPD patients and an inverse correlation between the number of sputum eosinophils and FEV_1 value [11]. Saetta et al. reported in 1994, sputum eosinophil number increases when COPD patients experience exacerbations [14]. Fujimoto replicated increased sputum eosinophil numbers during exacerbations in Japanese cases [15]. According to Papi et al., sputum eosinophil numbers were increased, especially during virus-associated exacerbations [16].

This biomarker is clinically meaningful since COPD patients with sputum eosinophilia respond better to treatment with inhaled steroids, though controversy exists on whether eosinophils in COPD are actually activated or not. Recently proposed asthma-COPD overlap syndrome (ACOS) is a commonly encountered yet loosely defined clinical entity. Both COPD and bronchial asthma are respiratory diseases with airflow limitation. COPD and bronchial asthma share symptoms, decreased FEV_1, and medications. ACOS accounts for approximately 15–25 % of the obstructive airway diseases. Patients with ACOS experience worse outcomes compared to those with asthma or COPD alone. ACOS patients are generally younger than patients with "lone COPD," have the combined risk factors of smoking and atopy, and experience acute exacerbations with higher frequency and greater severity than lone COPD. However, these characteristics are not sufficiently sensitive or specific to distinguish ACOS from lone COPD. One of the most important reasons why we have to distinguish ACOS and lone COPD is that there are differences in treatment options [17].

The current GOLD documents recommend the first-line use of ICS only for a patient with groups C and D COPD: severe to very severe airflow limitation, $\geq$ 2 exacerbations per year, and/or $\geq$ 1 with hospitalization for exacerbation [1]. However, recent evidence questions whether ICS actually reduces exacerbations and is truly beneficial for COPD cases [18]. Both COPD and asthma are associated with chronic inflammation of the lung accompanied by airflow limitation. However, there are differences in the type of inflammatory cells and mediators involved. While ICS is indicative for bronchial asthma in which IgE and eosinophils play an important role, ICS cannot be so effective on neutrophils observed in the respiratory tract of COPD cases. The importance of ICS treatment for ACOS has been emphasized recently. Schematically, we have two COPD phenotypes. One is non-ACOS COPD characterized by low sputum eosinophils for which ICS does not have a good indication. The other is ACOS, which is accompanied by an increased number of sputum eosinophils for which ICS has good indication [18, 19].

Kitaguchi et al. observed 63 patients with stable COPD, of which 46 had COPD without asthma and 17 had COPD with asthma. A significant correlation was observed between the increases in FEV_1 in response to treatment with ICS and sputum eosinophil counts ($r = 0.42$, $P = 0.0006$). Using 2.5 % as the cutoff value, receiver operating characteristic curve analysis revealed 82.4 % sensitivity and 84.8 % specificity of the sputum eosinophil count for detecting COPD with asthma [20].

Blood eosinophils and T helper type 2 may have a similar meaning, which we will discuss later.

8.2.3 *Sputum Interleukin (IL)-6, IL-8*

Not only inflammatory cells, but also inflammatory mediators in the sputum are associated with COPD exacerbation. Bhowmik et al. collected induced sputum samples from 57 patients with moderate to severe COPD. Median IL-6 and IL-8 levels were significantly higher in patients with ≥ 3 exacerbation a year than those with ≤ 2 exacerbation a year. In addition, the IL-6 levels of patients with exacerbations were associated with the presence of cold symptoms and to the total cell count, eosinophil count, and lymphocyte count. IL-8 level was correlated with all sputum cell counts [21].

8.3 Blood Biomarker

The majority of COPD biomarkers are derived from serum or plasma. This is because blood is easily available from veins with acceptable invasiveness and its measurements can be easily standardized. However, it is not entirely clear how the blood measurements relate to the underlying disease activity in the lungs. Another weakness of serum/plasma biomarkers is that they are often easily affected for non-COPD reasons [3].

Among numerous biomarkers in blood, inflammatory biomarkers play essential role for both stable and exacerbated COPD. According to the ECLIPSE study, systematic inflammation evaluated by white blood cell count, C-reactive protein (CRP), IL-6, IL-8, fibrinogen, and TNF-α levels potentially select a subgroup of COPD cases who may be the target of specific research and treatment [22]. Simultaneously elevated levels of CRP, fibrinogen, and leukocyte count in individuals with COPD were also associated with increased risk of having exacerbations [23]. Among these biomarkers, fibrinogen has become the most solidly established biomarker that can estimate COPD activity [24].

Eosinophil count helps in identifying subgroups that have a good response to ICS. Some other biomarkers derived from blood will be also mentioned.

8.3.1 *Plasma Fibrinogen*

Fibrinogen is a soluble glycoprotein in the plasma that helps in the formation of blood clots by being broken down to fibrin by the enzyme thrombin. It has a rodlike shape and shows a negative net charge at physiological pH. Fibrinogen is primarily synthesized by the hepatocytes. The concentration of fibrinogen in the blood plasma is 200–400 mg/dL in the non-acute phase and can increase threefold higher during an acute phase of stimulation such as IL-6-induced acute inflammatory response [5, 25].

Fibrinogen, which is the most robust biomarker investigated in relation to COPD so far [6], was approved as the first COPD biomarker by the US Food and Drug Administration in July 2015. The use of this biomarker is expected to make it easier to identify patients that are at a higher risk of exacerbation or death in clinical trial [26]. Researchers believe the use of fibrinogen will accelerate development of new COPD drugs.

Many published cross-sectional studies have shown that blood fibrinogen levels are higher in individuals with COPD compared with non-COPD healthy controls. According to a meta-analysis by Gan et al, the fibrinogen level was higher in COPD cases than healthy controls with the standardized mean difference of 0.47 units (95 % CI 0.29–0.65) [25].

As well as in the cross-sectional studies, large-scale general-population cohort studies have revealed that high serum fibrinogen level increased the risk for COPD-specific outcomes, future incidence of COPD, and COPD exacerbation. Valvi et al. studied 20,192 individuals from the atherosclerosis risk in communities study and the cardiovascular health study cohort and showed that fibrinogen levels at entry can predict future incidence of COPD diagnosis and COPD-related hospitalization [25]. A cohort of 5247 men randomly selected from a Malmö birth cohort also revealed that people with higher baseline fibrinogen had more hospital admissions with COPD after 25 years of follow-up, even after adjustment of covariables [25]. Dahl et al. followed up 8955 people in the general population and found that individuals with plasma fibrinogen in the upper, middle, and lower tertiles had COPD hospitalization rates of 93, 60, and 52 per 10,000 person-years [27] (Fig. 8.2). This finding is interesting as it suggests that fibrinogen can predict future COPD admission among a cohort of which most did not have a COPD diagnosis. Notably, fibrinogen is the only marker that can predict future FEV_1 decline [25]. In the same study, smokers and nonsmokers with plasma fibrinogen in the upper tertile had an excess annual decline in FEV_1 of 6 ml (3–9 ml) and 4 ml (2–7 ml) compared with smokers and nonsmokers with fibrinogen in the lower tertile. Based on this study by Dahl et al, fibrinogen may act as a surrogate marker of disease activity in individuals with COPD. Furthermore, fibrinogen indicates risk of COPD among a non-COPD cohort.

A high level of fibrinogen can clearly predict all-cause death. Mannino et al. observed 8507 subjects of which 245 had stage III/IV COPD and 826 had stage II COPD. In this study, an elevated fibrinogen level increased the risk of mortality in subjects with stage III/IV (hazard ratio 2.11, 95 % confidence interval (CI) 1.27–3.50) and stage II (hazard ratio 1.45, 95 % CI 1.08–1.96) COPD [25].

A moderate-scale RCT in 2012 by Lomas et al. investigated whether an oral inhibitor of p38 MAP kinase, losmapimod, affects patients with COPD. In this study, 302 individuals with GOLD stage II COPD were randomized to take 7.5 mg of oral losmapimod twice daily, to take inhaled salmeterol/fluticasone propionate in a 50 μg/500 μg combination, or to take placebo. Only losmapimod was well tolerated, and it reduced plasma fibrinogen by 11 % (ratio of effect of losmapimod/placebo 0.89, 95 % CI 0.83–0.96, $P = .002$) [24]. However,

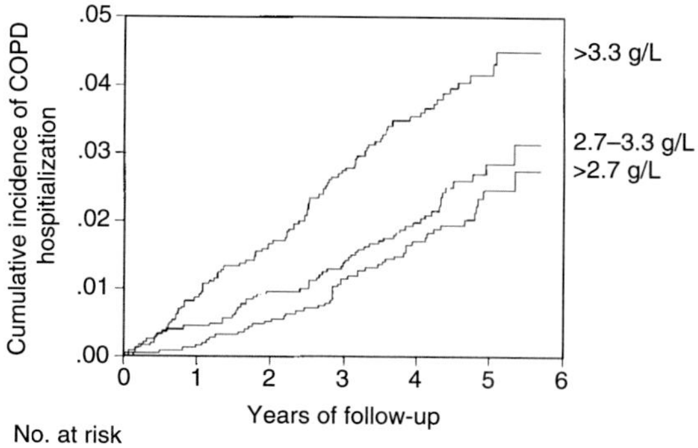

No. at risk						
<2.7 g/L	2985	2916	2884	2825	2298	1051
2.7 – 3.3 g/L	2984	2907	2856	2801	2230	1004
>3.3 g/L	2986	2811	2734	2646	2107	1019

Fig. 8.2 Kaplan–Meier curves showing rate of COPD hospitalizations during follow-up stratified by baseline serum fibrinogen. Number at risk at the beginning of each year is shown below the horizontal axis. $P < 0.001$ for > 3.3 g/L versus < 2.7 g/L, $p = 0.003$ for > 3.3 g/L versus 2.7–3.3 g/L, and $p = 0.31$ for 2.7–3.3 g/L versus < 2.7 g/L on log-rank test (Reprinted with permission from the American Thoracic Society. Copyright © 2015 American Thoracic Society. Dahl M, et al. Elevated plasma fibrinogen associated with reduced pulmonary function and increased risk of chronic obstructive pulmonary disease. Am J Respir Crit Care Med. 2001;164:1008–11 [27]. The American Journal of Respiratory and Critical Care Medicine is an official journal of the American Thoracic Society)

losmapimod did not have significant effect on sputum neutrophilia, which was the primary endpoint.

Fibrinogen may be a tool for distinguishing subgroups of COPD. In a small study with 49 COPD cases, a group with emphysematous lesions involving more than 15 % of the lung parenchyma had higher fibrinogen levels than controls ($n = 25$) [24]. However, fibrinogen is not currently confirmed to guide a specific treatment option.

8.3.2 *Serum CRP*

CRP is an annular, pentameric protein, or pentraxin, which is composed of five identical subunits, found in blood plasma. The levels of CRP rise in response to inflammation, especially when caused by infection [28]. CRP is one of the most commonly used inflammatory biomarkers in practice, thanks to its availability and low cost [29]. CRP was discovered in humans in 1930 as a serum component that binds the C polysaccharide of *Streptococcus pneumoniae*. The reference range of CRP is < 3 mg/L, and its level often surges over 300 mg/L in severe infection when IL-6 and IL-1β trigger its production in the liver [28]. CRP has some actions in response to inflammation. It can also trigger anti-inflammatory immunoglobulin crystallizable fragments gamma inhibitory receptors. In contrast, CRP can also act as a pro-inflammatory agent by activating the classical complement cascade, through binding to the complement fragment. CRP also activates nuclear factor-kB in endothelial cells and mononuclear cells to induce proteases and pro-inflammatory cytokines [28].

In three large population-based case–control studies, levels of CRP were demonstrably higher in stable COPD patients than in controls after adjusting for the confounding factors [24]. In 2012, Zhang et al. conducted a systematic review and a meta-analysis to summarize the association between serum concentration of CRP and COPD. In this meta-analysis from 18 original studies, patients with COPD had higher serum CRP concentrations than healthy controls (mean weighted difference: 4.72 mg/L, 95 % CI 2.98–6.47) [30].

Regarding the positive significant relation between the COPD severity and inflammation, it is thought that inflammatory biomarkers and lung functions may be linked with each other. Although this issue has often been investigated, results are inconsistent partly due to study design [29]. According to a meta-analysis by Zhang et al., patients with severe COPD had higher serum CRP concentrations than those with moderate COPD (mean weighted difference 1.26 mg/L, 95 % CI 0.78–1.73) [30].

Exacerbation of COPD is usually associated with bacterial or viral infection, and CRP is a sensitive inflammatory marker to detect infection. Actually, the serum CRP level has been shown to be very sensitive to change in response to exacerbation. It is also well known that CRP is usually elevated in pneumonia patients. In a study by Lacoma et al. including 318 consecutive COPD patients, wherein 46 were in a stable phase, 217 were undergoing an exacerbation, and 55 had pneumonia, CRP showed significant differences among the three patient groups, being higher in patients with pneumonia, followed by patients with exacerbation ($P < 0.0001$) [31]. According to Soler et al., serum CRP level is also associated with purulent sputum during COPD exacerbation [32]. In addition, serum CRP level is useful as a prognostic marker for stable COPD [33].

Whether serum CRP level can predict a hard endpoint, death is an issue of concern. Man et al. measured serum CRP levels in 4803 participants in the Lung Health Study with mild-to-moderate COPD. The risk of all-cause and disease-specific causes of mortality was determined, adjusting for important covariates such as age, sex, cigarette smoking, and lung function. The CRP level was associated with all-cause, cardiovascular, and cancer-specific causes of mortality. Patients in the highest quintile of CRP had a relative risk of all-cause mortality of 1.79 (95 % CI 1.25–2.56) compared with those in the lowest quintile of CRP [34].

To be an acceptable surrogate biomarker, CRP should correlate with hard endpoints in RCTs. The levels of inflammatory biomarkers are expected to be ameliorated in response to treatment that suppresses inflammation. ICS is currently accepted as one of the first-choice medications for a case with high risk of exacerbation in the belief that ICS prevents future exacerbations [1]. A small observational study with 41 mild-to-moderate COPD patients was performed by Sin et al. The patients took to fluticasone (500 μg twice a day), oral prednisone (30 mg/day), or placebo over 2 weeks, followed by 8 weeks of fluticasone at 500 μg twice a day and another 8 weeks at 1000 μg twice a day. Two weeks with inhaled fluticasone reduced CRP levels by 50 % (95 % CI 9–73 %), while prednisone reduced it by 63 % (95 % CI 29–81 %). No significant changes were observed with the placebo [29]. In another study by Perng et al. 99 subjects were randomized to receive salmeterol/fluticasone, tiotropium/fluticasone, and tiotropium alone. A significant decrease in CRP was observed in all of the three arms; however, there were no statistically significant differences between the three groups. In this study, there was a significant reduction in IL-8 and matrix metalloproteinase (MMP)-9 in the salmeterol/fluticasone group compared with patients treated with tiotropium alone. The authors concluded that the anti-inflammatory effects of salmeterol/fluticasone probably contribute to the clinical benefits seen in COPD patients. This indicated that CRP could not detect the anti-inflammatory effect of tiotropium/fluticasone [29]. In another study in 2008, Sin et al. randomized 289 patients to investigate whether inhaled fluticasone alone or in combination with salmeterol over 4 weeks effect on circulating biomarkers of systemic inflammation. As a result, inhaled fluticasone with/without salmeterol did not reduce serum CRP level [29]. In conclusion, we do not have consistent evidence from RCT that CRP is modifiable by interventions mainly using ICS.

8.3.3 Blood Eosinophils

Assessment of eosinophilic airway inflammation using sputum samples is a method of judging whether a patient will benefit from ICS. However, it is technically demanding and not always successful, which reduces the usefulness of the test in routine clinical practice. Blood eosinophil count might be an alternative strategy, thanks to good correlation between blood and sputum eosinophil count.

Pascoe et al. conducted a post hoc analysis of a large-scale study including 3177 patients in the analyses, with 2083 patients (66 %) having an eosinophil count of 2 % or

higher at entry. Adding ICS reduced exacerbations by 29 % (mean 0.91 vs 1.28 exacerbations per patient per year, $P < 0.0001$) in patients with eosinophil counts of 2 % or higher and by only 10 % (0.79 vs 0.89, $P = 0.2827$) in patients with eosinophil counts lower.

This study suggested that blood eosinophils with a cutoff of 2 % are a simple predictive biomarker to know the responsiveness of ICS [35].

8.3.4 Serum Procalcitonin

Since last decade, several studies featured procalcitonin as promising biomarker for severe bacterial infection. Schuetz et al. performed a systematic review and meta-analysis to compare treatment algorithms with and without procalcitonin for acute respiratory tract infections. This review was not COPD-specific research but included patients with COPD exacerbation and patients with background COPD. They concluded that use of the procalcitonin algorithm shorten the antibiotic treatment duration for acute respiratory infections without increasing mortality or treatment failure [36].

8.3.5 White Blood Cell/Neutrophil Count in Blood

White blood cell and neutrophil counts were weakly associated with persistent systemic inflammation, frequent exacerbations, and mortality in the ECLIPSE cohort. A recent study in the general population has replicated similar observations concerning exacerbations. Similar results were also obtained absolute neutrophil counts [6].

8.3.6 Other Blood Biomarkers

In addition to fibrinogen, CRP, and eosinophils, many inflammatory biomarkers for COPD have been identified. However, the significance of most of these biomarkers as regards COPD diagnosis or COPD-related outcomes has not been sufficiently validated in replicate studies. Even if replicated, the observed relevance between most of these biomarkers and outcomes was weak, thus clinical meaning is often not clear. Although these markers are interesting for future research, they are not regarded as useful biomarkers for practical purposes at present.

CC-Chemokine Ligand-18 (CCL-18)/ Pulmonary and Activation-Regulated Chemokine (PARC) CCL-18, previously known as PARC, is a 7-kD protein that is constitutively expressed by monocytes/macrophages and dendritic cells and is secreted predominantly in the lungs. Although the exact biological role of CCL-18 is still not clear, serum level of CCL-18 is elevated in pulmonary disease, namely, idiopathic pulmonary fibrosis, wherein serum CCL-18 levels seem to reflect fibrotic activity and correlate with survival. Concerning COPD, in one small study of patients with mild-to-moderate disease, serum CCL-18 level was associated with deteriorated FEV_1 and the body mass index, airflow limitation, dyspnea, and exercise capacity index score, and acute exacerbations [37]. According to ECLIPSE and the Lung Health Study data set, serum CCL-18 levels were higher in subjects with COPD than in smokers or never smokers without COPD. Elevated CCL-18 levels were also associated with increased risk of overall mortality in the ECLIPSE cohort [6, 24]. Although these data are plausible, some questions remain unclear regarding the possible use of CCL-18 as an effective biomarker in COPD, including its relationship with clinical outcomes such as hospitalization and mortality and its responsiveness to pharmacological therapy [24]

The 16 kDa Clara Cell Protein (CC16) The Clara cell is one of the most heterogeneous and multifunctional cell types of the mammalian lung, showing a great interspecies variability in abundance and spatial distribution. One of the major proteins secreted by the Clara cells is CC16. Although the exact in vivo function of the CC16 remains to be clarified, CC16 has been suggested to have some role in the defense mechanism against oxidative stress in the airway epithelium and also has anti-inflammatory and immunomodulatory effects [38]. CC16 was weakly associated with lung function decline, emphysema, and comorbid depression in the ECLIPSE cohort [6]. However, serum CC16 did not independently predict overall mortality in the cohort [24]

Surfactant Protein D (SP-D) SP-D is a large multimeric, calcium-binding glycoprotein that belongs to the collectin family. This protein, which is produced predominantly in pneumocytes II in the lungs, serves as an innate immune regulatory molecule. SP-D causes the elimination of pathogens by its ability to recognize carbohydrate structures on the surface of microorganisms such as bacteria, viruses, and fungi. Both genetic and environmental factors have been shown to contribute to SP-D expression. SP-D has an important regulatory effect for innate immunity and is capable of binding pathogens and facilitating phagocytosis. This protein also facilitates direct microbicidal activity on selected microbes. Decreased levels of SP-D caused by cigarette smoking often weaken lung immunity [24, 39]. SP-D has shown a weak association with COPD exacerbations and is sensitive to treatment with oral and inhaled corticosteroids [6].

Although far from a clinical application, the following inflammatory substance biomarkers, besides the markers mentioned above, might be related to COPD diagnosis and/or exacerbation: MMP-9, myeloid progenitor inhibitory factor-1, adipocyte complement-related protein of 30 kD, soluble intercellular adhesion molecule, eotaxin-2, interferon-inducible protein 10, IL-1α, tumor necrosis factor receptor-1, IL-6, serum amyloid A, IL-8, and tumor necrosis factor-α (TNF-α) [2].

8.4 Exhaled Gas

Exhaled gas is completely noninvasive and is particularly suitable for longitudinal studies. It is potentially useful for assessing the efficacy of pharmacological treatment. However, there are inevitable issues about reproducibility and sensitivity that need to be addressed before this approach can be recommended as an outcome measurement.

8.4.1 Fractional Exhaled Nitric Oxide (FeNO)

One of the most important pathogeneses of COPD is oxidative stress associated with inflammatory cellular infiltration. FeNO has been extensively investigated in asthma and has been shown to correlate with airway eosinophilic inflammation. This measurement is acceptably reproducible in normal subjects and in subjects with asthma if properly conducted [40, 41].

FeNO measurements have been regarded as surrogate marker for eosinophilic airway inflammation, especially in asthma. High FeNO has been regarded as an indicator of good steroid responsiveness. Recent GOLD documents recommend adding FeNO monitoring to other measurements since it provides easier detection of eosinophilic airway inflammation and indicates the likelihood of corticosteroid responsiveness. However, in COPD subjects, FeNO seems less useful because the levels of FeNO are usually normal or only slightly elevated in stable COPD subjects. While diagnosis of COPD per se does not greatly affect FeNO level, current smoking and COPD severity meaningfully decrease FeNO levels in COPD patients. Moreover, comorbid pulmonary hypertension leads to declined FeNO value. In contrast, exacerbation of COPD and decompensated heart failure are accompanied by high FeNO level [40, 41].

8.5 Exhaled Breath Condensate (EBC)

EBC is a noninvasive method for evaluating the composition of airway lining fluid, which is formed mainly by water vapor and contains aerosol biomolecule particles. Some inflammatory mediators are elevated in patients COPD. These aerosolized particles are generated from the entire respiratory tract into air which is saturated with water vapor. EBC analysis has many advantages over other examinations for assessing lung inflammation. Measuring EBC biomarker is a very attractive approach to monitoring COPD inflammation, as it is noninvasive and repeated sampling is possible. However, the lack of standardization of the EBC analysis is the primary limitation of this technique. The commonly used EBC methodologies present results with considerable variability concerning both sample collection and analysis. Therefore, it is difficult to establish a universal reference range of each EBC biomarker. Several methodological issues need to be addressed before EBC is considered for clinical use with patients with COPD. In addition, the values of most EBC biomarkers have a large overlap between COPD patients and healthy volunteers: thus, most EBC biomarkers cannot clearly differentiate between COPD patients and healthy individuals. Another limitation of EBC analysis is that this method provides little information on the inflammatory cells involved in the pathophysiology of COPD [42, 43]

8.5.1 EBC pH

Airway acidification is thought to indicate the pathogenesis of obstructive lung disease. One possible mechanism is that protons cause the release of tachykinins, resulting in bronchoconstriction and airway inflammation. The pH of EBC is a general marker of airway inflammation rather than a disease-specific marker. Unlike other EBC mediators, the mean EBC pH observed in healthy subjects from different studies suggested has similar values. This is the overwhelming advantage of EBC pH over other EBC biomarkers. The normal level in healthy subjects, pH = approximately 8.0. However, there is a clear differentiation between the pH of COPD subjects, with pH approximately = 7.0, and normal range [43].

8.5.2 EBC Leukotriene B_4 (LTB_4)

LTB_4 is an eicosanoid inflammatory mediators produced in leukocytes by the oxidation of arachidonic acid by the enzyme arachidonate 5-lipoxygenase. Although it helps in the production of inflammatory cytokines by various immune cells, its primary function is to recruit neutrophils to areas of tissue damage. Increased levels of EBC LTB_4 have been observed in stable COPD patients when compared with healthy smokers. In addition, a high EBC LTB_4 level in healthy smokers compared with nonsmokers has been demonstrated. These observations indicate that EBC LTB_4 level may aid the diagnosis of COPD. However, there is a wide variation in absolute levels of EBC LTB_4 between studies. Furthermore, some studies have indicated that there is a large overlap of EBC LTB_4 levels between healthy subjects and COPD cases. The potential methodological pitfalls associated with LTB_4 collection and analysis, especially oral contamination and lack of enzyme-linked immunosorbent assay sensitivity, may reduce the applicability of this biomarker in a clinical setting [43].

8.5.3 EBC 8-Isoprostane

The EBC mediator 8-isoprostane has been extensively reported. The free radical peroxidation of arachidonic acid forms 8-isoprostane. This is a putative marker of pulmonary oxidative stress. Some studies have shown higher levels of EBC 8-isoprostane in stable COPD patients compared with healthy subjects. However, mean values of 8-isoprostane in COPD patients have varied widely across studies and have often overlapped with those of healthy subjects. Furthermore, the EBC 8-isoprostane level is also increased in smokers and asthma patients. Therefore, the meaning of this biomarker for COPD is far from clear at present [43].

8.6 Bronchoscopic Specimens

Bronchoscopy, which is used to scrutinize airway and to obtain samples from the lungs, is an essential examination for pulmonologists to allow them to find out what is going on in the lungs of patients with pulmonary disease. This technique is very useful to gain a diagnosis or to decide on a therapeutic plan for emergent and critical diseases such as lung cancers, acute exacerbation of interstitial pneumonia, or severe pulmonary infection with unknown etiology. However, COPD can usually be diagnosed through history taking, physical exams, CT scan, and spirometry without using bronchoscopy. Moreover, information gained through bronchoscopy does not greatly affect the treatment plan for COPD. Given the high invasiveness of bronchoscopy, it is not indicated for COPD patients in daily practice [1, 40].

For research purposes, bronchial biopsies may give some pathogenetic inflammation of COPD. Bronchoscopic specimens have shown that there is increased activation of the transcription factor, nuclear factor–kB, in the bronchial epithelial cells of patients with COPD, which increases with disease severity and that there is also a reduction in histone deacetylase activity [40].

Bronchoalveolar lavage (BAL) performed during bronchoscopy is a possible option to gain important information about immunologic, inflammatory, and infectious processes taking place at the alveolar level. The advantage of BAL over bronchial biopsy specimens is that BAL can sample inflammatory cells in the peripheral lung. The cellular composition of BAL of COPD cases is predominantly alveolar macrophages, with some neutrophils and T lymphocytes as for healthy subjects. Macrophages from patients with COPD may have increased expression of inflammatory proteins, such as TNF-α, IL-8, and MMP-9. Levels of the eosinophil cationic protein and myeloperoxidase are also frequently increased in patients with COPD [40].

8.7 Gene

COPD is a multifactorial disorder caused by environmental determinants, mainly smoking. In addition to exposure to smoking, genetic susceptibility to COPD is also believed to play a considerable role in the development of COPD. A genetic variant in the alpha-1 antitrypsin was discovered to be the first reliable etiologic gene for COPD. However, alpha-1 antitrypsin deficiency accounts for only 1–2 % of all COPD cases. Due to the heterogeneous nature of the disease, it has been, for decades, difficult to unravel the genetic predisposition and pathogenetic mechanisms of COPD. In addition, each causal gene has a weak impact as a risk factor for COPD, generally with an odds ratio less than 1.5 [44].

Basic genetic approaches to identify the etiologic gene are the family study and the case–control study. Linkage analysis is also a helpful method for genetic analysis. However, the genome-wide association study and genome sequencing are by far the most powerful way to detect the association between a common disease and novel gene variant. Results from research with these methods and meta-analyses of the published studies have revealed more than 100 candidate gene relating to COPD etiology. These candidate genes are related to numerous pathways such as inflammation (ILs, TNF, leukocyte, etc.), protease/antiprotease (MMP-9, etc.), and oxidative stress (human heme oxygenase-1, etc.).

However, even after genome-wide screening, identified genetic variants can explain only a small part of COPD etiology. Thus, it is hypothesized that other kind of etiologies, such as epigenetics, may cause COPD [44].

8.7.1 Tumor Necrosis Factor-α (TNF-α) Gene

The TNF-α signaling pathway plays an essential role in immune-related diseases and inflammatory lung diseases. Overexpression of TNF-α in the lung induces pulmonary fibrosis and smoking-related emphysema. TNF-α concentration is higher in COPD patients than in smoking and nonsmoking control subjects.

Among hundreds of genes, a single nucleotide polymorphism involving a G-A transition at position −308 within the TNF-α proximal promoter has been the most extensively investigated in recent years. Zhang et al. conducted a systematic review and a meta-analysis that investigated 4975 patients and 6518 control subjects from the 36 studies. [45] According to this meta-analysis, the association between the TNF-α-308G/A SNP and the risk of COPD was significant for Asians (odds ratio 2.36, 95 % CI 1.84–3.02, $P < 0.0001$) but not for Caucasians (odds ratio 1.07, 95 % CI 0.91–1.25, $P = 0.438$). Similarly in the smoker-subgroup analysis, the association between the TNF-α-308G/A SNP and COPD was significant for Asians (odds ratio 1.72, 95 % CI 1.14–2.61, $P = 0.011$) but not for Caucasians (odds ratio = 1.16, 95 % CI 0.86–1.56, $P = 0.33$) [45].

There are two plausible pathogeneses for emphysema. One is the protease–antiprotease hypothesis, and the other is the oxidant–antioxidant hypothesis. Apoptosis may also occur in vascular endothelial and alveolar epithelial cells in COPD patients with emphysematous changes of the lung. TNF-α may contribute to the airway remodeling and alter smooth muscle cell function in lungs affected by COPD. Furthermore, TNF-α activates sphingomyelin hydrolysis, leading to an increase of ceramide levels, in turn leading to apoptosis. Therefore, TNF-α may have a key role in the apoptosis of alveolar epithelial cells. According to an observation of 84 Japanese and Southeast Asian COPD patients by Sakao et al., the TNF-α-308 variant may partly explain the extent of emphysematous changes in patients with COPD [46].

8.7.2 T Helper Type 2 Gene

Besides TNF-α, which is the most frequently researched gene associated with COPD, we here review the T helper type 2 gene as this biomarker potentially promotes personalized pharmacotherapy for COPD. Some patients with COPD present with asthma-like clinical symptoms, which has recently been referred as ACOS. This implies that asthma-associated inflammatory pathways may have a significant role in ACOS. This subgroup is known to be more amenable to ICS. Christenson et al. compared disease-associated airway epithelial gene expression in 105 asthma patients and 237,171 COPD patients. They found that the T helper type 2 gene expression was related to asthma-like symptom. Their data identified molecular and cellular pathways underlying the ACOS population and suggested that the T helper type 2 gene expression may serve as a predictive biomarker to select patients who will benefit from ICS treatment [19].

8.8 Comorbidities

Recent knowledge emphasizes that COPD has many comorbidities caused by systemic inflammation. GOLD listed the main comorbidities of COPD: cardiovascular disease, osteoporosis, depression, lung cancer, infections, metabolic syndrome, and diabetes. [1] Although the levels of most inflammatory substances are commonly elevated in patients with these comorbidities, the mechanism by which these biomarkers bridge between COPD and these conditions have not been comprehensively understood. Some persistent low-grade pulmonary and systemic inflammatory biomarkers can be risk factors for these comorbidities with acceptable biological plausibility [47, 48]. Thomsen et al. observed 8656 patients with COPD from two large Danish population studies and during a median 5 years' follow-up, which showed clear stepwise increase in the absolute 5 year risk of major comorbidities after stratifying smoking status based on three key inflammatory biomarkers, CRP, fibrinogen, and blood leukocyte count. [49] (Fig. 8.3)

8.8.1 Cardiovascular Disease

Cardiovascular disease is one of the leading causes of mortality among COPD patients. Certain molecules can promote the inflammatory process underlying cardiovascular diseases. CRP, which is the most studied inflammatory molecule in relation to cardiovascular disease, can upregulate production of other inflammatory cytokines, activate the complement system, promote uptake of low density lipoprotein by macrophages, and foster leukocyte adhesion to vascular endothelium, thereby, amplifying the risk for cardiovascular diseases [47]

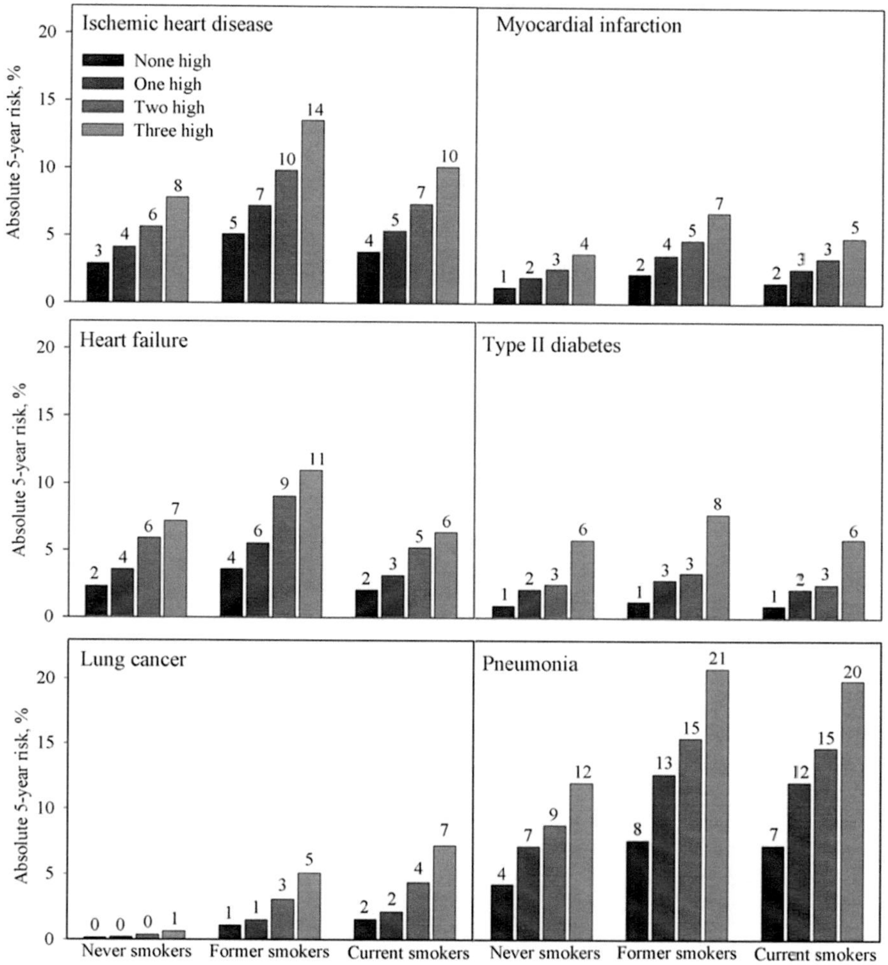

Fig. 8.3 Absolute 5 year risk of ischemic heart disease, myocardial infarction, heart failure, type II diabetes, lung cancer, and pneumonia in percentage, by levels of three inflammatory biomarkers and smoking status. Plasma C-reactive protein, fibrinogen, and blood leukocyte count were defined as high or low according to cut-points of 3 mg/L, 14 mmol/L, and 9 3 109/L, respectively (Reprinted with permission from the American Thoracic Society. Copyright © 2015 American Thoracic Society. Thomsen M, et al. Inflammatory biomarkers and comorbidities in chronic obstructive pulmonary disease. Am J Respir Crit Care Med. 2012;186:982–8 [49]. The American Journal of Respiratory and Critical Care Medicine is an official journal of the American Thoracic Society)

8.8.2 *Osteoporosis*

Osteoporosis is an important systemic feature of COPD. There is a correlation between the emphysema phenotype of COPD and reduced bone mineral density. Some experimental studies indicate that IL-1β, IL-6 and TNF-α, and the osteoprotegerin, receptor activator of nuclear factor-kappa B and receptor activator of nuclear factor-kappa B ligand (OPG/RANK/RANKL) system, may play key roles in the etiology of both osteoporosis and emphysema. According to a study by Bai et al., radiographic emphysema is correlated to low bone mineral density in current and former smokers with COPD. IL-1β, IL-6, TNF-α, and the osteoporosis-related protein system OPG/RANK/RANKL seem to have synergetic effects on emphysema and bone loss in COPD [50].

8.8.3 Depression and Anxiety

Depression is a common psychiatric issue in patients with chronic diseases. However, the incidence and prevalence of depression among COPD patients are higher than among those with other chronic diseases. Recent understanding is that depression may be directly caused by systemic inflammation. A study by Al-shair et al. with 120 moderate COPD cases indicates the association between TNF-α and depression [51]. According to Cote study, anxiety is also a very strong risk factor for death [52].

8.8.4 Lung Cancer

Both COPD and lung cancer are associated with cigarette smoke exposure [1]. However, even after adjusting for the influence of smoking, patients with COPD have high risk for lung cancer [1]. Experimental studies suggest that cigarette smoke upregulates the production of cytokines such as interleukin IL-1β resulting in increased level of cyclooxygenase-2, which can promote an inflammatory response by the lymphocytes, leading to the overproduction of IL-6, IL-8, and IL-10. Some of these cytokines can inhibit apoptosis and interfere with cellular repair, which eventually leads to carcinogenesis [1].

8.8.5 Infection

Pulmonary infection, namely, pneumonia and viral bronchial infection often cause exacerbation. Many inflammatory markers become elevated during infection and/exacerbation. Moreover, high serum fibrinogen level and high neutrophil count increase the risk for COPD exacerbation [25, 27]. Meaning of CRP level, procalcitonin level, and leukocyte count for infection were already discussed previous section.

8.8.6 *Metabolic Syndrome and Diabetes*

A systemic inflammatory process caused by COPD partly explains why patients with COPD have an increased risk for type II diabetes. Fibrinogen and circulating neutrophils predict the development of type II diabetes. Metabolic syndrome is also associated with a pro-inflammatory state, and its central pathophysiological features include acute-phase reactants such as CRP [48]. Patients with chronic bronchitis phenotype have slightly mild inflammation and slightly frequent metabolic syndromes [53].

8.9 Conclusion

Numerous inflammatory substances have been identified as potentially useful biomarkers to evaluate COPD. These substances were derived from sputum, blood, exhaled gas, EBC, and bronchoscopic specimens. However, the majority of these biomarkers are not currently clinically applicable due to the lack of sufficient difference of value between COPD subjects and healthy subjects, insufficient validation in RCT, or technical issue preventing reproducible measurements.

Nonetheless, we have biomarkers that can be used to assess pulmonary and systemic inflammation for patients with COPD. Plasma fibrinogen can predict the future incidence of COPD and future FEV_1 decline in COPD and non-COPD subjects. In July 2015, the FDA approved serum fibrinogen as the first COPD biomarker to identify patients that are at a higher risk of exacerbation or death in clinical trials. Researchers hope this approval will accelerate trials for new medications. Serum CRP is another widely approved biomarker related to COPD diagnosis, exacerbation diagnosis, and patient prognosis. Sputum/blood eosinophils, FeNO, and the T helper type 2 gene can be candidate predictive biomarkers to pick up the ACOS subgroup who are amenable to ICS. The TNF-α-308 variant is associated with COPD risk and emphysematous change especially in Asians.

References

1. The Global Strategy for the Diagnosis, Management and Prevention of COPD, Global Initiative for Chronic Obstructive Lung Disease (GOLD) 2015. Available from: http://www.goldcopd.org/. Accessed on 20 Sept, 2015.
2. Sin DD, Vestbo J. Biomarkers in chronic obstructive pulmonary disease. Proc Am Thorac Soc. 2009;6:543–5.
3. Rosenberg SR, Kalhan R. Biomarkers in chronic obstructive pulmonary disease. Transl Res. 2012;159:228–37.
4. Whorld Health Organization. Biomarkers in Risk Assessment: Validity and Validation. 2001. Available from: http://apps.who.int/bookorders/anglais/detart1.jsp?codlan=1&codcol=16&codcch=222. Accessed on 20 Sept, 2015.

5. Celli BR, Locantore N, Yates J, Tal-Singer R, Miller BE, Bakke P, et al. Inflammatory biomarkers improve clinical prediction of mortality in chronic obstructive pulmonary disease. Am J Respir Crit Care Med. 2012;185:1065–72.
6. ECLIPSE Study Investigators. Lessons from ECLIPSE: a review of COPD biomarkers. Thorax. 2014;69:666–72.
7. Kaneda H, Saito Y. The prognostic factor tumor, node, metastasis classification: how helpful is it as a predictive factor of the success of a specific treatment? J Thorac Oncol. 2014;9, e64.
8. Criner GJ, Connett JE, Aaron SD, Albert RK, Bailey WC, Casaburi R, et al. Simvastatin for the prevention of exacerbations in moderate-to-severe COPD. N Engl J Med. 2014;370:2201–10.
9. Horita N, Miyazawa N, Morita S, Kojima R, Inoue M, Ishigatsubo Y, et al. Evidence suggesting that oral corticosteroids increase mortality in stable chronic obstructive pulmonary disease. Respir Res. 2014;15:37.
10. Crapo RO, Jensen RL, Hargreave FE. Airway inflammation in COPD: physiological outcome measures and induced sputum. Eur Respir J Suppl. 2003;41:19s–28.
11. Tsoumakidou M, Tzanakis N, Siafakas NM. Induced sputum in the investigation of airway inflammation of COPD. Respir Med. 2003;97:863–71.
12. Confalonieri M, Mainardi E, Della Porta R, Bernorio S, Gandola L, Beghè B, et al. Inhaled corticosteroids reduce neutrophilic bronchial inflammation in patients with chronic obstructive pulmonary disease. Thorax. 1998;53:583–5.
13. Kanehara M, Yokoyama A, Tomoda Y, Shiota N, Iwamoto H, Ishikawa N, et al. Anti-inflammatory effects and clinical efficacy of theophylline and tulobuterol in mild-to-moderate chronic obstructive pulmonary disease. Pulm Pharmacol Ther. 2008;21:874–8.
14. Saetta M, Di Stefano A, Maestrelli P, Turato G, Ruggieri MP, Roggeri A, et al. Airway eosinophilia in chronic bronchitis during exacerbations. Am J Respir Crit Care Med. 1994;150:1646–52.
15. Fujimoto K, Yasuo M, Urushibata K, Hanaoka M, Koizumi T, Kubo K. Airway inflammation during stable and acutely exacerbated chronic obstructive pulmonary disease. Eur Respir J. 2005;25:640–6.
16. Papi A, Bellettato CM, Braccioni F, Romagnoli M, Casolari P, Caramori G, et al. Infections and airway inflammation in chronic obstructive pulmonary disease severe exacerbations. Am J Respir Crit Care Med. 2006;173:1114–21.
17. Global Initiative For Asthma. Asthma, COPD and Asthma-COPD Overlap Syndrome (ACOS). Available from: http://www.ginasthma.org/documents/14. Accessed on 20 Sept, 2015.
18. Horita N, Miyazawa N, Tomaru K, Inoue M, Kaneko T. Long-acting muscarinic antagonist + long-acting beta agonist versus long-acting beta agonist + inhaled corticosteroid for COPD: a systematic review and meta-analysis. Respirology. 2015;20:1153–9.
19. Christenson SA, Steiling K, van den Berge M, Hijazi K, Hiemstra PS, Postma DS, et al. Asthma-COPD overlap. Clinical relevance of genomic signatures of type 2 inflammation in chronic obstructive pulmonary disease. Am J Respir Crit Care Med. 2015;191:758–66.
20. Kitaguchi Y, Komatsu Y, Fujimoto K, Hanaoka M, Kubo K. Sputum eosinophilia can predict responsiveness to inhaled corticosteroid treatment in patients with overlap syndrome of COPD and asthma. Int J Chron Obstruct Pulmon Dis. 2012;7:283–9.
21. Bhowmik A, Seemungal TA, Sapsford RJ, Wedzicha JA. Relation of sputum inflammatory markers to symptoms and lung function changes in COPD exacerbations. Thorax. 2000;55:114–20.
22. Agustí A, Edwards LD, Rennard SI, MacNee W, Tal-Singer R, Miller BE, et al. Persistent systemic inflammation is associated with poor clinical outcomes in COPD: a novel phenotype. PLoS One. 2012;7, e37483.
23. Thomsen M, Ingebrigtsen TS, Marott JL, Dahl M, Lange P, Vestbo J, et al. Inflammatory biomarkers and exacerbations in chronic obstructive pulmonary disease. JAMA. 2013;309:2353–61.

24. Lock-Johansson S, Vestbo J, Sorensen GL. Surfactant protein D, Club cell protein 16, Pulmonary and activation-regulated chemokine, C-reactive protein, and Fibrinogen biomarker variation in chronic obstructive lung disease. Respir Res. 2014;15:147.
25. Duvoix A, Dickens J, Haq I, Mannino D, Miller B, Tal-Singer R, et al. Blood fibrinogen as a biomarker of chronic obstructive pulmonary disease. Thorax. 2013;68(7):670–6.
26. COPD Foundation. FDA Approves First COPD Biomarker: Paving Way for New, Improved Treatments and Cures. Available from: http://www.copdfoundation.org/About-Us/Press-Room/Press-Releases/ID/303/FDA-Approves-First-COPD-Biomarker-Paving-Way-for-New-Improved-Treatments-and-Cures.aspx. Accessed on 20 Sept, 2015.
27. Dahl M, Tybjaerg-Hansen A, Vestbo J, Lange P, Nordestgaard BG. Elevated plasma fibrinogen associated with reduced pulmonary function and increased risk of chronic obstructive pulmonary disease. Am J Respir Crit Care Med. 2001;164:1008–11.
28. Anderson GP. COPD, asthma and C-reactive protein. Eur Respir J. 2006;27:874–6.
29. Heidari B. The importance of C-reactive protein and other inflammatory markers in patients with chronic obstructive pulmonary disease. Caspian J Intern Med. 2012;3:428–35.
30. Zhang Y, Bunjhoo H, Xiong W, Xu Y, Yang D. Association between C-reactive protein concentration and chronic obstructive pulmonary disease: a systematic review and meta-analysis. J Int Med Res. 2012;40:1629–35.
31. Lacoma A, Prat C, Andreo F, Lores L, Ruiz-Manzano J, Ausina V, et al. Value of procalcitonin, C-reactive protein, and neopterin in exacerbations of chronic obstructive pulmonary disease. Int J Chron Obstruct Pulmon Dis. 2011;6:157–69.
32. Soler N, Esperatti M, Ewig S, Huerta A, Agustí C, Torres A. Sputum purulence-guided antibiotic use in hospitalised patients with exacerbations of COPD. Eur Respir J. 2012;40:1344–53.
33. Lahousse L, Loth DW, Joos GF, Hofman A, Leufkens HG, Brusselle GG, et al. Statins, systemic inflammation and risk of death in COPD: the Rotterdam study. Pulm Pharmacol Ther. 2013;26:212–7.
34. Man SF, Connett JE, Anthonisen NR, Wise RA, Tashkin DP, Sin DD. C-reactive protein and mortality in mild to moderate chronic obstructive pulmonary disease. Thorax. 2006;61:849–53.
35. Pascoe S, Locantore N, Dransfield MT, Barnes NC, Pavord ID. Blood eosinophil counts, exacerbations, and response to the addition of inhaled fluticasone furoate to vilanterol in patients with chronic obstructive pulmonary disease: a secondary analysis of data from two parallel randomised controlled trials. Lancet Respir Med. 2015;3:435–42.
36. Schuetz P, Müller B, Christ-Crain M, Stolz D, Tamm M, Bouadma L, et al. Procalcitonin to initiate or discontinue antibiotics in acute respiratory tract infections. Cochrane Database Syst Rev. 2012;9, CD007498.
37. Sin DD, Miller BE, Duvoix A, Man SF, Zhang X, Silverman EK, et al. Serum PARC/CCL-18 concentrations and health outcomes in chronic obstructive pulmonary disease. Am J Respir Crit Care Med. 2011;183:1187–92.
38. Broeckaert F, Bernard A. Clara cell secretory protein (CC16): characteristics and perspectives as lung peripheral biomarker. Clin Exp Allergy. 2000;30(4):469–75.
39. Bowler RP. Surfactant protein D as a biomarker for chronic obstructive pulmonary disease. COPD. 2012;9:651–3.
40. Barnes PJ, Chowdhury B, Kharitonov SA, Magnussen H, Page CP, Postma D, et al. Pulmonary biomarkers in chronic obstructive pulmonary disease. Am J Respir Crit Care Med. 2006;174:6–14.
41. Malerba M, Radaeli A, Olivini A, Damiani G, Ragnoli B, Montuschi P, et al. Exhaled nitric oxide as a biomarker in COPD and related comorbidities. Biomed Res Int. 2014;2014:271918.
42. Montuschi P. Exhaled breath condensate analysis in patients with COPD. Clin Chim Acta. 2005;356:22–34.
43. Borrill ZL, Roy K, Singh D. Exhaled breath condensate biomarkers in COPD. Eur Respir J. 2008;32:472–86.

44. Berndt A, Leme AS, Shapiro SD. Emerging genetics of COPD. EMBO Mol Med. 2012;4:1144–55.
45. Zhang S, Wang C, Xi B, Li X. Association between the tumour necrosis factor-α-308G/A polymorphism and chronic obstructive pulmonary disease: an update. Respirology. 2011;16:107–15.
46. Sakao S, Tatsumi K, Igari H, Watanabe R, Shino Y, Shirasawa H, et al. Association of tumor necrosis factor-alpha gene promoter polymorphism with low attenuation areas on high-resolution CT in patients with COPD. Chest. 2002;122:416–20.
47. Sin DD, Anthonisen NR, Soriano JB, Agusti AG. Mortality in COPD: role of comorbidities. Eur Respir J. 2006;28:1245–57.
48. Fabbri LM, Luppi F, Beghé B, Rabe KF. Complex chronic comorbidities of COPD. Eur Respir J. 2008;31:204–12.
49. Thomsen M, Dahl M, Lange P, Vestbo J, Nordestgaard BG. Inflammatory biomarkers and comorbidities in chronic obstructive pulmonary disease. Am J Respir Crit Care Med. 2012;186:982–8.
50. Bai P, Sun Y, Jin J, Hou J, Li R, Zhang Q, Wang Y. Disturbance of the OPG/RANK/RANKL pathway and systemic inflammation in COPD patients with emphysema and osteoporosis. Respir Res. 2011;12:157.
51. Al-shair K, Kolsum U, Dockry R, Morris J, Singh D, Vestbo J. Biomarkers of systemic inflammation and depression and fatigue in moderate clinically stable COPD. Respir Res. 2011;12:3.
52. Divo M, Cote C, de Torres JP, Casanova C, Marin JM, Pinto-Plata V, et al. Comorbidities and risk of mortality in patients with chronic obstructive pulmonary disease. Am J Respir Crit Care Med. 2012;186:155–61.
53. Watz H, Waschki B, Kirsten A, Müller KC, Kretschmar G, Meyer T, et al. The metabolic syndrome in patients with chronic bronchitis and COPD: frequency and associated consequences for systemic inflammation and physical inactivity. Chest. 2009;136:1039–46.

Part IV
Management and Treatment

Chapter 9
Exercise Therapy for COPD: How Is Exercise Therapy Significant?

Takashi Motegi

Abstract Exercise training is the most common form of non-pharmacologic therapy prescribed to chronic obstructive pulmonary disease (COPD) patients. In the pathogenesis of COPD, only ventilation limitation is not a problem, and many patients have also caused muscle dysfunction. Therefore, the treatment for the muscle dysfunction is required. Pulmonary rehabilitation has been shown to be as highly effective as pharmacotherapy for improving lung function as evidenced by contributing to improvements in shortness of breath, quality of life, exercise capacity, depression, and rates of hospitalization. In addition, it has also been recommended that the patients who fail to clinically improve solely with pharmacotherapy undergo pulmonary rehabilitation.

Since it has been recognized that physical activity is associated with a better prognosis in patients with COPD, incorporating more physical activity into daily life has drawn much attention recently. Thus, the improvement and maintenance of physical activity has become one of the objectives of pulmonary rehabilitation. To date, the evidence that rehabilitation directly improves physical activity is poor quality. In the daily life management of patients with COPD, we work on the support of self-management, the maintenance of exercise training, and the improvement of physical activity.

Keywords Exercise • Rehabilitation • Physical activity

9.1 What Is Pulmonary Rehabilitation?

9.1.1 Introduction

The Japanese population is the world's fastest aging society. There is a growing emphasis on the measures of the bedridden as well as preventative care of elderly

T. Motegi (✉)
Respiratory Care Clinic, Nippon Medical School, 4-7-15 Kudanminami, Chiyoda-ku, Tokyo, Japan
e-mail: mo-dr@nms.ac.jp

H. Nakamura, K. Aoshiba (eds.), *Chronic Obstructive Pulmonary Disease*,
Respiratory Disease Series: Diagnostic Tools and Disease Managements,
DOI 10.1007/978-981-10-0839-9_9

people in health policy. Studies show that the first, second, and third highest risk factors for Japanese adult death are preventable, and they include smoking, hypertension, and lack of exercise, respectively [1]. Thus, it has become a popular belief that our focus should be placed on these three factors to encourage the prevention of lifestyle-related diseases. As a result, the second term of the National Health Promotion Movement in the twenty-first century [Health Japan 21 (the second term)] has proposed that there be an increase in physical activity for all nations [2].

The number of patients affected by chronic obstructive pulmonary disease (COPD) increases each year in Japan, and there are particularly many elderly patients. Furthermore, we can regard COPD as one of the lifestyle-related diseases associated with cigarettes and smoking. In recent years, increasing physical activity has been recognized as an important preventative measure against lifestyle-related diseases, including COPD. It has been shown that there is a low incidence of chronic disease in middle-aged adults who have a high amount of daily activity [3]. The method for enhancing the physical activity of people has been attracting attention recently.

This chapter explains why rehabilitation is important in patients with COPD, and the relationship between physical activity level and exercise training is mentioned.

9.1.2 The Definition of Pulmonary Rehabilitation and the Evidence

The American Thoracic Society (ATS) and the European Respiratory Society (ERS) have adopted the following definition of pulmonary rehabilitation: "Pulmonary rehabilitation is a comprehensive intervention based on a thorough patient assessment followed by patient tailored therapies that include, but are not limited to, exercise training, education, and behavior change, designed to improve the physical and psychological condition of people with chronic respiratory disease and to promote the long-term adherence to health-enhancing behaviors." [4] By this definition, rehabilitation does not merely suggest that exercise is all that is needed but that it must include healthy interventions that encompass all aspects of everyday life in order to promote health as a whole.

Because the need for clinical management of tuberculosis remained prominent in Japan for a long time after World War II, lung physiotherapy had been the leading empirical treatment. Since Japan was so focused on solely lung physiotherapy, it fell behind Europe and the United States when it came to a concept of interdisciplinary comprehensive intervention. It was not until 2002 when the Japan Society for Respiratory Care and Rehabilitation and other related academic societies made a statement regarding pulmonary rehabilitation, and shortly thereafter, recommendations for exercise therapy and an educational manual for patients were finally published based on this statement. Subsequently, in April of 2006, pulmonary rehabilitation started to be reimbursed by public medical insurance in Japan.

Table 9.1 Main outcomes of pulmonary rehabilitation in GOLD guideline [5]

Outcome	Strength of evidence
Improvement of exercise performance	A
Dyspnea relief	A
Improves health-related quality of life	A
Reduces number of hospitalizations and days in hospital	A
Reduces anxiety and depression	A
Upper limbs strength/endurance training improves arm function	B
Benefits persist beyond training period	B
Improves survival	B
Improves recovery after hospitalization for exacerbation	B
Enhance the effect of long-acting bronchodilators	B
Respiratory muscle training can be beneficial, especially when combined with general exercise training	C

A randomized controlled trials (rich body of data), *B* randomized controlled trials (limited body of data), *C* nonrandomized controlled trials (observational studies)

The Global Initiative for Chronic Obstructive Lung Disease (GOLD) guideline presents a collection of firm evidence that supports the positive effects of pulmonary rehabilitation (Table 9.1) [5]. Evidence proving the improvement of dyspnea, exercise capacity, and health-related quality of life (HRQOL) with pulmonary rehabilitation are the most well established. In regard to HRQOL, in particular the St. George's Respiratory Questionnaire (SGRQ) and Chronic Respiratory Disease Questionnaire (CRQ), there is improvement to significantly surpass minimal clinically important difference (MCID). Another advantageous benefit of pulmonary rehabilitation is that it can naturally relieve the symptoms of depression and thus possibly avoid the use of medicinal antidepressants.

9.1.3 Why Should the Treatment of the COPD Be more than Mono-pharmacotherapy and Include a Multidisciplinary Approach?

The basic pathogenesis of COPD is small airway disease and emphysema, which creates limited airflow. This limitation in airflow, in turn, causes ventilatory impairment by the dynamic hyperinflation on exertion and hypoxemia [5]. This results in the characteristic symptoms of COPD, such as shortness of breath and physical limitation on exertion. Due to these conditions, it becomes necessary to reduce dynamic hyperinflation to treatment and to increase inspiratory capacity (IC) via the use of a bronchodilator. The bronchodilator relieves shortness of breath by relaxing the bronchial smooth muscle which in turn expands the bronchial airways to eliminate the airflow restriction and hyperinflation. Therefore, since the mechanism of action of a bronchodilator directly acts to counter the pathophysiology of the COPD, it is an appropriate treatment regimen.

Since the limitation in bronchial airflow greatly contributes to shortness of breath, COPD patients are often considered unable to exercise. However, the symptoms of COPD patients are not simply limited to ventilatory impairment since many COPD patients also experience muscle fatigue [6]. Killian et al. examined the factors that limited exercise in 97 patients with COPD and 320 healthy subjects. They found that only 26 % of COPD patients and 22 % of healthy subjects reported dyspnea as a limiting factor, while 43 % and 36 %, respectively, reported lower limb fatigue as a limiting factor [7]. Hamilton et al. conducted incremental exercise testing in COPD, CHF, and healthy subjects and determined the reasons for discontinuation of exercise in each group. In all of the groups, the combination of dyspnea and lower limb fatigue was a more common reason than dyspnea alone as the patients' reported reason for the discontinuation of exercise [8].

In exercise, the skeletal muscle contributes to acidosis via the production of lactic acid which leads to an increase in the respiratory center's ventilation drive. This abnormal hyperventilation is regarded as an important factor in perpetuating pathologic dyspnea in COPD. COPD patients also attempt to increase their ventilatory drive during exertion; however, due to their dynamic hyperinflation, this results in shortness of breath secondary to inadequate ventilation. To exacerbate this situation, most patients with COPD naturally avoid moving and exertion due to their dyspnea; thus, this results in vicious circle that accelerates their deconditioning (Fig. 9.1) [9].

There are two methods to prevent the dynamic hyperinflation of patients with COPD. The first is a method that reduces airway resistance to quicken the expiratory phase. The second is a method that reduces the respiratory rate, thus increasing the total time for expiration. The current mainstream therapeutic drug is the bronchodilator that reduces hyperinflation primarily by the mechanism of action we previously described. In addition, the inhalation of oxygen also contributes to the reduction of dynamic hyperinflation through the oxygen-sensing

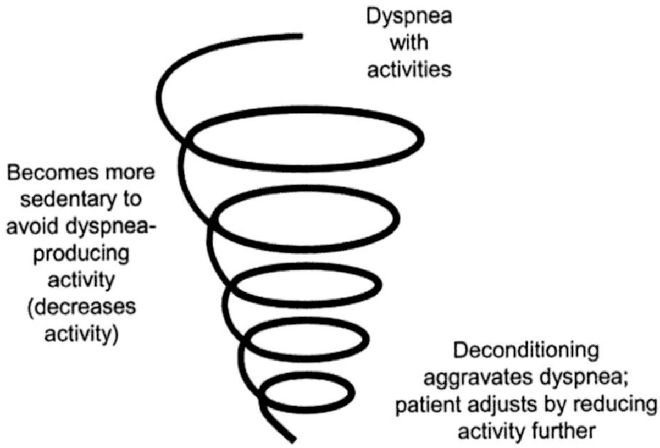

Fig. 9.1 The cycle of decline in the dyspnea spiral (Reproduced by permission from Reference [9])

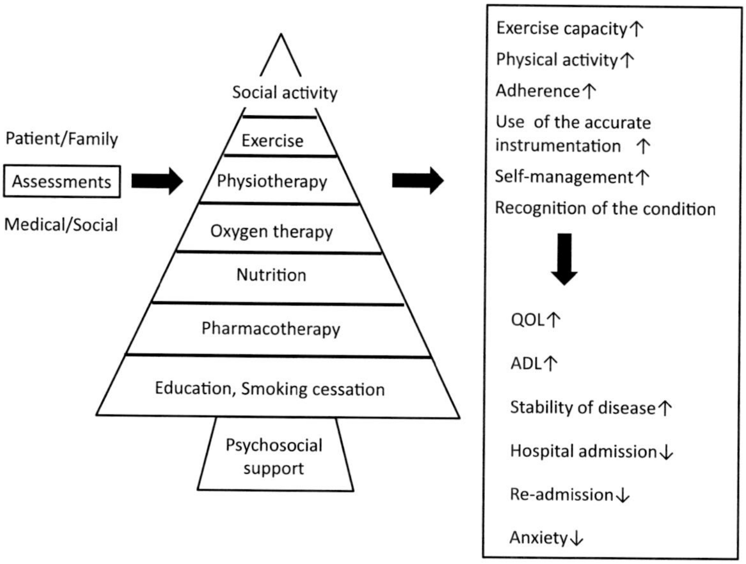

Fig. 9.2 Concept of comprehensive pulmonary rehabilitation in COPD guideline in Japan [11]

chemoreceptors and signaling of the carotid body. In addition, the inhalation of oxygen is thought to reduce dynamic hyperinflation through a mechanism that reducing respiratory rate involves signaling from the carotid body. Furthermore, exercise training will acclimate the skeletal muscle to exercise, which will decrease its production of lactic acid. This decrease in lactic acid production improves hyperinflation because the ventilatory drive is now inhibited, which in turn reduces the respiratory rate [10]. In addition, the muscle itself displays changes induced by exercise, which we will discuss later.

Because dyspnea in COPD, as mentioned above, is a phenomenon that involves multiple factors, a multidisciplinary approach to treatment is beneficial because it targets the multiple mechanisms of COPD and not just any single mechanism. Therefore, most patients require both pharmacotherapy and non-pharmacologic therapies (e.g., exercise therapy, oxygen therapy, nutritional therapy, and patient education). Management of the patients with COPD according to the guidelines of Japan [11] is based on these concepts (Fig. 9.2).

9.1.4 When to Start Rehabilitation?

As for many COPD patients, initial treatment is usually pharmacotherapy, but the question remained as to when it should be initiated and at what point exercise rehabilitation should be added to the regimen. GOLD 2010 initially addressed this question by recommending that rehabilitation should target patients with stage II or more (% $FEV_1 < 80$). However GOLD 2011 has outlined a new set of patient management recommendations which modifies the target of exercise rehabilitation to those who are equal to or greater than Group B. Group B encompasses patients with strong subjective symptoms (CAT > 10 or modified MRC scale ≥ 2) and patients with a risk of progression (exacerbation frequency is more than twice a year or % $FEV_1 < 50$). GOLD 2011 maintains the enforcement of physical activity for patients in Group A, who have mild symptoms and a low risk of future exacerbation [5]. On the other hand, the Japanese COPD guidelines do not contain a similar outline of specific criteria [5]. Patients with symptoms and disabilities of all stages are targeted. However, the guideline that does exist involves insurance; insurance does not cover services for pulmonary rehabilitation unless patients have greater than COPD stage II or modified MRC scale ≥ 2.

Compared to severe COPD, there is little data available to determine the effect of exercise rehabilitation in mild-to-moderate COPD. In the INTERCOM study, which was a randomized controlled trial (RCT) conducted over a 2-year period in the Netherlands, rehabilitation made accessible by offering it within the patients' local communities proved to be beneficial even for patients with mild-to-moderate COPD (mean % $FEV_1 \geq 60$ %). These patients displayed a significant improvement in quality of life, exercise tolerance, and shortness of breath when compared to the non-rehabilitation group [12].

In addition, the already decreased intramuscular oxidation capacity decreases further in mild COPD at a stage where muscle consumption of oxygen is not clear. In addition, it is also noted that exercise duration is shorter than that of a healthy subject [13]. The results of these studies also suggest that muscle training by pulmonary rehabilitation is not just necessary for the critically ill patients, but it is also beneficial when introduced at an early stage of COPD. At the very least, pulmonary rehabilitation is an intervention that is considered a standard of care for individuals who have COPD and remain symptomatic despite optimal bronchodilator therapy.

9.1.5 *What Kind of Contribution Does Exercise Training Make?*

Variations in exercise training can produce a difference in clinical effects. The different aspects of an exercise training regimen that can differ include the setting (inpatient vs. outpatient vs. home based), duration (short term vs. long term), and intensity (high vs. low intensity), which can all influence the observed clinical response. The high-intensity load refers to around 60–80 % of exercises that require maximum oxygen uptake, and the low-intensity load usually points to 40–60 % of exercises that require maximum oxygen uptake. The international guidance for pulmonary rehabilitation recommends a program that consists of 6–12 weeks, 2–3 sessions/week of 30–60 min duration at moderate-to-high exercise intensities [4].

Exercise of the high strength load and intensity has been said to be effective in the guidelines for a long time. However, for the elderly patients who have severe dyspnea, it is actually often difficult to perform exercise of the high-intensity training. Furthermore, there is the problem of the difficulty with the continuation of these high-intensity exercises. Also, the problem of costs and the access affects the ability for continuity in the exercise plan. It has recently been reported that even low-intensity training is beneficial. Baumann et al. conducted an RCT of a 26 week outpatient rehabilitation for 100 patients with moderate to severe cases of COPD. Associated with low-intensity exercise was a dyspnea severity score of 4–6 points on the Borg Scale. These results were compared to another exercise intervention group and a control group without a rehabilitation intervention. The intervention group had a significant improvement in 6MD (+59 m), HRQOL (SGRQ −5 points) [14]. Since it took a long time to see results, continuity of the program was ensured. Low-intensity load exercise is believed to be particularly suitable for the elderly and critically ill patients.

Endurance training has two modes: continuous exercise and interval exercise. High-intensity training has more effect on exercise capacity than low-intensity training, but in patients with severe COPD, it can be difficult to sustain high intensity by the continuous exercise. Although dynamic lung hyperinflation increases progressively during continuous exercise, interval exercise reported to induce less dynamic hyperinflation than continuous exercise in patients with COPD [15]. Beauchamp et al. reported that interval and continuous training modalities did not differ in their effect on measures of exercise capacity or HRQOL. They concluded that interval training may be considered as an alternative to continuous training in patients with varying degrees of COPD severity [16].

9.1.6 What Are the Problems Encountered While Undergoing Rehabilitation?

There are several problems associated with pulmonary rehabilitation. First, there is a low implementation rate of rehabilitation. According to the questionnaire survey for the certification facility of the Japanese Respiratory Society, only 57.3 % of facilities have implemented pulmonary rehabilitation. A number of hospitals that have implemented pulmonary rehabilitation differ regionally. When institutions that had not implemented rehabilitation were questioned as to why, 80 % reasoned lack of manpower, while 30 % reasoned lack of profit [17]. According to the questionnaire results of patients with the Japanese White Paper on Home Respiratory Care, 49 % were rehabilitated at the first investigation in 2005, but only 53 % of those maintained rehabilitation when reexamined in 2010.

In regional community facilities, there is also a new attempt to provide a maintenance program in cooperation with the exercise instructor; however, this is not done at the large medical institutions [18]. The teaching methods of COPD patients included an exercise instructor and exercise training of COPD patients in the community facilities of the region rather than a hospital (twice a week, 1 h or more once) for 6 months. After 6 months and 12 months, 6-min walk distance (6MWD) improved (pre-intervention, 385 m; after 6 months of intervention, 441 m; 12 months, 454 m; $P < 0.001$), and HRQOL was also significantly improved. The study attracted attention despite being carried out in a small regional program because there was a general exercise instructor, who was not a healthcare worker, working with them. Another problem with the rehabilitation is maintenance of the program over a long period of time has not been established. According to the results of the meta-analysis of maintenance of rehabilitation, the intervention group with 9–15 months of maintenance was significantly better than the usual care group after 6 months of building exercise tolerance. However, there was no significant difference when the program continued for 12 months. In addition, between the usual care groups, there was no significant difference in HRQOL after 6 or 12 months. Furthermore continuation rate of these maintenance programs was only 60 % [19]. Determining how to provide programs that enhance continuity has become the problem.

9.2 Does Exercise Affect the Muscle of COPD Patients?

9.2.1 Muscle Structure in the COPD and Metabolic Change

The disordered muscle function in patients with COPD affects muscular strength and decreases the endurance of the muscle. The muscular strength is decided by size and the thickness of the muscle, but the muscular endurance is decided by the amount of glycogen stored. Factors that influence the function of the muscle include intramuscular capillary density, oxygen delivery, and oxidative capacity of the myofibers. Table 9.2 presents the structural and functional abnormalities of the muscle found in COPD. According to a European study, in about 1/3 of patients only possess about 25 % of the average strength of healthy adults [20]. In addition, recent meta-analysis concludes that there is also a decrease of the quadriceps femoris muscle when compared to a healthy control [21].

Biopsies of a COPD patient's femoral muscle (vastus lateralis) show that when compared to healthy controls, there is a decrease in type I muscle fibers (slow-twitch fibers) and an increase in type IIx fibers (fast-twitch fibers). Because oxidative metabolism is dominant in the type I fiber, these are characteristics of fibers for endurance and are thus the less-fatigable muscle fibers. On the other hand, type IIx muscle fibers predominantly utilize glycolytic metabolism, which contributes to agility, but are easily fatigued muscle fibers. These fibers are often mixed, and the proportion at which they are mixed varies according to the site of the

Table 9.2 Structural and functional abnormalities of muscles in COPD

(1) Muscle fiber distribution change
↓ Type I fibers (slow twitch, oxidative)
↑ Type IIx fibers (fast twitch, glycolytic)
(2) Reduced muscle fiber size
(3) Reduction in the capillary numbers and contacts
(4) Decreased oxidative capacity (reduced mitochondrial content)
(5) Early lactic acidosis increases ventilator demands at lower exercise intensity

muscle. The muscle fibers of patients with severe COPD are thin, thus contributing to a decrease in muscle mass [22].

Jobin et al. compared muscle biopsies from COPD and healthy subjects and found that capillary number per unit area in COPD was significantly less than healthy subjects (92.6 ± 16.1 and 213.3 ± 33.5, $P < 0.001$), and the ratio of capillaries per muscle fiber was reduced (0.83 ± 0.05 in COPD and 1.56 ± 0.10 in healthy subjects, $p < 0.001$) [23]. Oxygenation thereby decreases because contact with the muscle fiber decreases when the size of an intramuscular capillary decreases [24].

The aerobic metabolism in the skeletal muscle increases on exercise, but this metabolism usually depends on enough oxygen being supplied and adequate ATP production by the intramuscular mitochondria. As for patients with COPD, they have a higher rate of anaerobic metabolism when compared to healthy controls, as noted by the hyperventilation at an early stage of exercise associated with the increase in blood lactic acid concentrations, thus contributing to a decrease in muscular endurance. This is associated with a decreased mitochondrial content in the skeletal muscle [25].

It is thought that the change of these muscles in a COPD patient is caused by disuse, systemic inflammation, oxidative stress, hypoxemia, undernutrition, and a side effect of steroid treatment. Recently Natanek et al. reported that a reduction of phospho-AMPK is involved in the reduction of oxidative capacity and endurance of COPD patients [26].

9.2.2 *Change of the Muscle by the Exercise*

Exercise training is found to not only improve muscle composition, but it also improves exercise capacity and the quality of life. Vogiatzis et al. studied patients with COPD (GOLD stages II, III, and IV) who underwent comprehensive pulmonary rehabilitation three times a week of high-intensity exercise training for 10 weeks and then examined the changes in muscle composition by vastus lateralis muscle percutaneous biopsy. As a result, type I fiber or type IIa increased after rehabilitation, and type IIb decreased (Fig. 9.3). Moreover, the capillary ratios for the muscular fiber increased. Furthermore, they concluded that because the changes

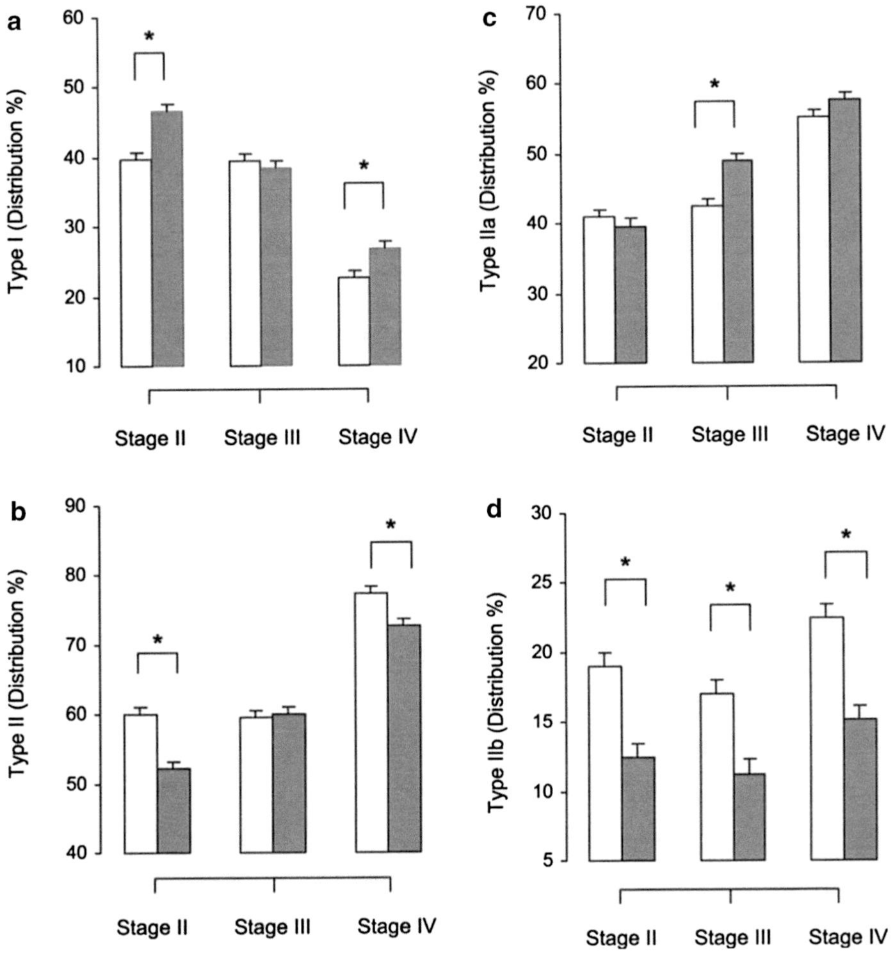

Fig. 9.3 Fiber-type distribution of the vastus lateralis muscle before (*open bars*) and after (*solid bars*) rehabilitation in patients with COPD in GOLD stages II, III, and IV. (**a**) Type I. (**b**) Type II. (**c**) Type IIa. (**d**) Type IIb. Data are represented as means ± SEM. Asterisks denote significant differences between before and after training ($P < 0.01$) (Reproduced by permission from Reference [27])

of these muscles were found to be independent on the severity of COPD, then they could expect that severity of COPD would also have no effect on exercise training [27].

Puente-Maestu et al. reported that exercise training sessions in pulmonary rehabilitation programs produced a significant decrease in the number of mitochondrial DNA in skeletal muscle of patients with COPD, as well as overexpression of peroxisome proliferator-activated receptor-γ coactivator-1α (PGC-1α) mRNA, most likely associated with the enhanced oxidative stress [28].

9.3 Physical Activity and Exercise

9.3.1 The Importance of Physical Activity

Exercise capacity and physical activity are different concepts. Physical activity has been traditionally defined as "any bodily movement produced by skeletal muscles that results in energy expenditure," and this definition has been adapted to physical activity in daily life as "the totality of voluntary movement produced by skeletal muscles during every day functioning" [29]. On the other hand, the exercise capacity is described by how well and how much. The exercise capacity is commonly evaluated by 6-min walk test (6MWT) or a shuttle walk test.

Recently, it has been shown that physical activity in the patients with COPD is decreased when compared to a healthy control. Even if it was a patient with mild illness, the physical activity was still found to be decreased. Furthermore, reduction of physical activity had a deeper association with prognosis than forced expiratory volume in one second (FEV_1) or HRQOL. Waschki et al. measured the degree of physical activity with a multisensory armband and showed that each 0.14 increase in physical activity level was associated with a lower risk of death (hazard ratio [HR], 0.46; 95 % CI, 0.33–0.64; $p < 0.001$). It was also the strongest predictor of all-cause mortality in patients with COPD [30]. Thus, the maintenance of or increase in the level of physical activity is recommended during the early stage of COPD to promote a better prognosis [31]. In response to these results, the ATS/ERS statement on pulmonary rehabilitation included a recommendation to increase physical activity in everyday life [4].

9.3.2 Does Exercise Training Improve Physical Activity?

There are positives and negatives in regard to whether exercise rehabilitation intervention improves physical activity. Table 9.3 lists papers that describe the effects of the relationship between physical activity and rehabilitation. The common thread of these papers was an improvement in exercise capacity. There was an increase in the ability to exercise, but the physical activity did not have change. The cause of no change in physical activity is dependent on that fact that it is affected by a variety of factors. Soicher et al. reported a study that followed the changes in physical activity for 1 year after a 3 month rehabilitation program intervention [32]. The characteristics of the patients who were able to maintain physical activity was that they previously exercised habitually, they experienced a small amount of disorder (ensured time for exercise, compromise with work, access to the exercise location) of continuous exercise, and they were highly self-efficacious. There was much disorder to continuous exercise in the patients who had decreased physical activity after 1 year and low self-efficacy.

Table 9.3 Effects of pulmonary rehabilitation on physical activity in patients with chronic obstructive pulmonary disease

Effect of rehabilitation	Author, year	Number of pts.	COPD severity	Study design	Rehabilitation program	Main effect on physical activity level	Type of activity monitor	Duration of activity monitoring
Positive study	Sewell L, 2005 [41]	180	FEV_1 mean 0.95 ± 0.4 L	RCT	Twice weekly for 7 weeks conventional program vs. individually targeted program	Conventional program +29 %, individually program +41 %	U	2 consecutive days
	Mercken EM, 2005 [42]	11	$\%FEV_1$ $39.4 \pm 4.1\ \%$	Non-RCT	Inpatient pulmonary rehabilitation program on weekdays over 8 weeks	Increased PA +19 %	U	9 consecutive days
	Walker PP, 2008 [43]	24	$\%FEV_1$ $36.4 \pm 11.6\ \%$	Non-RCT	8 weeks outpatient rehabilitation program	Improved mean activity ($p = 0.001$), spent more time moving ($p = 0.014$)	T	7 consecutive days
Intermediate study	Pitta F, 2008 [44]	41	$\%FEV_1$ $46 \pm 16\ \%$	Non-RCT	12–24 weeks hospital-based outpatient PR; 12 weeks, 3 sessions/week, followed by 12 weeks, 2 sessions/week	Movement intensity improved significantly after 3 months, further improvement after 6 months. Walking time did not improve at 3 months, but improved at 6 months	T	5 consecutive weekdays
	Demeyer H, 2014 [45]	57	$\%FEV_1$ $46 \pm 17\ \%$	Non-RCT	12 weeks, 3 sessions/week, outpatient PR	Number of steps per day increased significantly 12 weeks after PR Mean metabolic equivalents of task level did not change	B	7 consecutive days

Negative study	Steele BG, 2003 [46]	41	%FEV_1 $39 \pm 17\,\%$	Non-RCT	8 weeks outpatient	PA did not change	T	5 days before entry and final week of rehabilitation
	Coronado M, 2003 [47]	15	%FEV_1 $54 \pm 16\,\%$	Non-RCT	3 weeks inpatient program, 6–7 sessions/week	No significant increase	U	One day, pre- and post-rehabilitation
	Dalls MI, 2009 [48]	54	%FEV_1 $45 \pm 18\,\%$	Non-RCT	6–12 weeks outpatient rehabilitation program	Mean pedometer counts did not change significantly, increased activity only low baseline PA	P	7 consecutive days, first and last weeks of rehabilitation
	Mador MJ, 2011 [49]	24	%FEV_1 $44 \pm 18\,\%$	Non-RCT	8 weeks, 3 sessions/week	Vector magnitude units per minute did not change	T	5 days before and after rehabilitation
	Eagan C, 2012 [50]	47	%FEV_1 $46.8 \pm 16.6\,\%$	Non-RCT	7 weeks, 2 sessions/week hospital-based outpatient PR	Number of steps, time spent sedentary activity, and METs did not change	B	5 consecutive days per week for 3 months

RCT randomized controlled trial, *U* uniaxial accelerometer, *T* triaxial accelerometer, *B* biaxial accelerometer, *P* pedometer

Michie et al. divided behavior change into three large factors: capability (physical or psychological), opportunity (physical and social environment), and motivation (volitional and automatic processes) [33]. Although pulmonary rehabilitation improves exercise capacity, the reason that physical activity could not be improved significantly was attributed to these three factors. Comprehensive rehabilitation is not simply to carry out an exercise regimen, but it has many different facets. For the first time, we present data in Fig. 9.2 showing that we were able to influence the physical activity of the patients by intervening with a comprehensive regimen involving a multifaceted approach.

9.4 Pulmonary Rehabilitation and COPD Exacerbation

The COPD exacerbation in one of the most serious respiratory conditions is very likely to require hospitalization. It raises mortality and negatively influences the quality of life. Therefore one important point of COPD management is to prevent exacerbation.

COPD exacerbation has been defined as an event in the natural course of the disease characterized by a baseline change in the patient's dyspnea, cough, and/or sputum that is beyond the normal day-to-day variations, has an acute in onset, and may warrant a change in regular medication in a patient with underlying COPD [5].

Recent guidelines for preventing COPD exacerbations have become an important objective for disease management. Various therapeutic agents have been demonstrated to be effective for prevention of exacerbation. Hopefully, in addition to medical management, exercise therapy proves to be effective for the prevention of an exacerbation.

When pulmonary rehabilitation was performed after exacerbation, it was confirmed by meta-analysis that the subsequent rate of hospitalization decreased. In this study, the number needed to treat was four [34], meaning in order to prevent one COPD exacerbation, four people need to undergo pulmonary rehabilitation. This suggests that pulmonary rehabilitation may be more effective than medication.

According to Spruit et al., muscular strength rapidly fell when patients with COPD were hospitalized with exacerbation, and quadriceps femoris muscle power (quadriceps peak torque) decreased an average of 5 % after hospitalization from day 3 to day 8 [35]. This report suggests that exercise therapy should be initiated as soon as possible after a COPD exacerbation.

However, we have yet to discern the precise timing at which exercise therapy should be initiated. Greening et al. reported exercise intervention to start very early within 48 h from hospitalization for 385 COPD exacerbation inpatients. However, after 1 year, no difference in readmission rate was found (intervention group 62 % vs. control group 58 %). The mortality 1 year later had unexpected results where it was found to be higher in the intervention group than in the control group (odds ratio 1.74, 95 % confidence interval 1.05–2.88, $P = 0.03$) [36]. It is speculated that this could be attributed to the intervention period in the hospital being shorter (median = 5 days) and that the exercise situation at home was unknown.

Puhan et al. reported a comparison with the rehabilitation intervention from an early stage within 2 weeks after the exacerbation and that of the late stage which was 6 months after the exacerbation. There was no difference in exacerbation frequency 18 months later in both groups, but shortness of breath and the quality of life showed a moderate improvement in early rehabilitation group [37]. This study was limited due to size (target number of patients: 36). A large-scale randomized controlled trial will be necessary in the future.

The American College of Chest Physicians (CHEST) and Canadian Thoracic Society (CTS) jointly commissioned an evidence-based guideline on the prevention of COPD exacerbations (AECOPD guideline) [38]. In this guideline, they recommended pulmonary rehabilitation starting less than 4 weeks from exacerbation (Grade 1c = strong recommendation, low- or very-low-quality evidence). However, they do not recommend the rehabilitation of the case beyond 4 weeks from exacerbation (Grade 2B = weak recommendation, moderate-quality evidence).

9.5 Pulmonary Rehabilitation Except the Exercise Training

If seen for the purpose of improving the exercise capacity of patients with COPD, exercise training is a main axis of pulmonary rehabilitation. However, the most important aspect to rehabilitation is the actual patient and how well they self-manage their rehabilitation program, including properly handling a therapeutic agent. It is necessary for the patients to take over their own care and master their action plan for the exacerbation. In addition, many of the COPD patients must also have their anxiety and depression treated as well. Health status does not completely improve with only exercise training.

Most pulmonary rehabilitation programs include education on self-management along with their exercise therapy. According to the COPE-II study that combined exercise therapy and a self-care into one program in hopes of a positive behavior modification, no significant difference was observed at 24 months in exercise capacity between the experimental and control groups. However, there was an increase in physical activity of the intervention group when compared to the control group, as measured by a pedometer (1193 steps/day (95 % CI: 203–2182)). In addition CRQ only showed improvement on the CRQ dyspnea score only and not in any other facet [39].

Self-management is the driving force for maintaining treatment as part of the daily life of the patient. The aim of the self-care program is to guide the patient in choosing the appropriate behavior and practices, and it is the role of the medical professional to support the desirable behavior modifications in the patients.

Beneficial results of successful self-management include improvement of dyspnea as measured by modified MRC scale and HRQOL and prevention of respiratory-related hospital admissions [40]. However, the most effective form of intervention to promote self-management has yet to be determined.

9.6 Conclusion

Exercise therapy represents an important form of non-pharmacologic therapy, while pharmacotherapy is an important therapeutic approach in patients who cannot tolerate exercise therapy. Pulmonary rehabilitation, which includes exercise therapy, results in increased exercise tolerability of patients with COPD and improvement of the health-related quality of life. However, improvement in physical activity requires not only exercise training but also a comprehensive pulmonary rehabilitation regimen.

References

1. Ikeda N, Inoue M, Iso H, et al. Adult mortality attributable to preventable risk factors for non-communicable diseases and injuries in Japan: a comparative risk assessment. PLoS Med. 2012;9(1), e 1001160.
2. Ministry of Health, Labour and Welfare. http://www.mhlw.go.jp/seisakunitsuite/bunya/kenkou_iryou/kenkou/kenkounippon21/en/kenkounippon21/
3. Willis BL, Gao A, Leonard D, et al. Midlife fitness and the development of chronic conditions in later life. Arch Intern Med. 2012;172:1333–40.
4. Spruit MA, Singh SJ, Garvey C, et al. An official American thoracic society/European respiratory society statement: key concepts and advances in pulmonary rehabilitation. Am J Respir Crit Care Med. 2013;188:e13–64.
5. Vestbo J, Hurd SS, Agusti AG, et al. Global strategy for the diagnosis, management, and prevention of chronic obstructive pulmonary disease: GOLD executive summary. Am J Respir Crit Care Med. 2013;187:347–65.
6. Casaburi R, ZuWallack R. Pulmonary rehabilitation for management of chronic obstructive pulmonary disease. N Engl J Med. 2009;360:1329–35.
7. Killian KJ, et al. Exercise capacity and ventilatory, circulatory, and symptom limitation in patients with chronic airflow limitation. Am Rev Respir Dis. 1992;146:935–94.
8. Hamilton AL, Killian KJ, Summers E, et al. Symptom intensity and subjective limitation to exercise in patients with cardiorespiratory disorders. Chest. 1996;110:1255–63.
9. Reardon JZ, Lareau SC, ZuWallack R. Functional status and quality of life in chronic obstructive pulmonary disease. Am J Med. 2006;119:32–7.
10. Casaburi R. Combination therapy for exercise intolerance in COPD. Thorax. 2006;61:551–2.
11. The Japanese Respiratory Society. Guidelines for the diagnosis and treatment of COPD. 4th ed. Tokyo: Medical Review; 2013.
12. van Wetering CR, Hoogendoorn M, Mol SJ, et al. Short- and long-term efficacy of a community-based COPD management programme in less advanced COPD: a randomised controlled trial. Thorax. 2010;65:7–13.

13. van den Borst B, Schols AM, de Theije C, et al. Characterization of the inflammatory and metabolic profile of adipose tissue in a mouse model of chronic hypoxia. J Appl Physiol (1985).2013; 14:1619–28
14. Baumann HJ, Kluge S, Rummel K, et al. Low intensity, long-term out-patients rehabilitation in COPD: a randomized controlled trial. Respir Res. 2012;13:86.
15. Vogiatzis I, Nanas S, Kastanakis E, et al. Dynamic hyperinflation and tolerance to interval exercise in patients with advanced COPD. Eur Respir J. 2004;24:385–90.
16. Beauchamp MK, Nonoyama M, Goldstein RS, et al. Interval versus continuous training in individuals with chronic obstructive pulmonary disease: a systematic review. Thorax. 2010;65:157–64.
17. Motegi T, Yamada K, Ishii T, et al. Long-term management of chronic obstructive pulmonary disease: a survey of collaboration among physicians involved in pulmonary rehabilitation in Japan. Respir Inv. 2012;50:98–103.
18. Beauchamp MK, Francella S, Romano JM, et al. A novel approach to long-term respiratory care: results of a community-based post-rehabilitation maintenance program in COPD. Respir Med. 2013;107:1210–6.
19. Beauchamp MK, Evans R, Janaudis-Ferreira T, et al. Systematic review of supervised. Chest. 2013;144:1124–33.
20. Seymour JM, Spruit MA, Hopkinson NS, et al. The prevalence of quadriceps weakness in COPD and the relationship with disease severity. Eur Respir J. 2010;36:81–8.
21. Evans RA, Kaplovitch E, Beauchamp MK, et al. Is quadriceps endurance reduced in COPD? Chest. 2015;147:673–84.
22. Fermoselle C, Rabinovich R, Ausin P, et al. Dose oxidative stress modulate limb muscle atrophy in severe COPD patients? Eur Respir J. 2012;40:851–62.
23. Jobin J, Maltais F, Doyon JF, et al. Chronic obstructive pulmonary disease: capillarity and fiber-type characteristics of skeletal muscle. J Cardiopulm Rehabil. 1998;18:432–7.
24. Saey D, Michaud A, Couillard A, et al. Contractile fatigue, muscle morphometry, and blood lactate in chronic obstructive pulmonary disease. Am J Respir Crit Care Med. 2005;171:1109–15.
25. Puente-Maestu L, Lazaro A, Humanes B. Metabolic derangements in COPD muscle dysfunction. J Appl Physiol. 2013;114:1282–90.
26. Natanek SA, Gosker HR, Slot IGM, et al. Pathways associated with reduced quadriceps oxidative fibers and endurance in COPD. Eur Respir J. 2013;41:1275–83.
27. Vogiatzis I, Terzis G, Stratakos G, et al. Effect of pulmonary rehabilitation on peripheral muscle fiber remodeling in patients with COPD in GOLD stages II to IV. Chest. 2011;140:744–52.
28. Puente-Maestu L, Lazaro A, Tejedor A, et al. Effects of exercise on mitochondrial DNA content in skeletal muscle of patients with COPD. Thorax. 2011;66:121–7.
29. American College of Sports Medicine, Chodzko-Zajko WJ, Proctor DN, et al. American college of sports medicine position stand. Exercise and physical activity for older adults. Med Sci Sports Exerc. 2009;41:1510–30.
30. Waschki B, Kirsten A, Holz O, et al. Physical activity is the strongest predictor of all-cause mortality in patients with COPD. Chest. 2011;140:331–42.
31. Vaes AW, Garcia-Americh J, Marott JL, et al. Changes in physical activity and all-cause mortality in COPD. Eur Respir J. 2014;44:1199–209.
32. Soicher JE, Mayo NE, Gauvin L, et al. Trajectories of endurance activity following pulmonary rehabilitation in COPD patients. Eur Respir J. 2011;39:272–8.
33. Michie S, van Stralen MM, West R. The behaviour change wheel: a new method for characterising and designing behaviour change interventions. Implement Sci. 2011;6:42.
34. Puhan M, Scharplatz M, Troosters T, et al. Pulmonary rehabilitation following exacerbations of chronic obstructive pulmonary disease. Cochrane Database Syst Rev. 2011;10, CD005305.

35. Spruit MA, Gosselink R, Troosters T, et al. Muscle force during an acute exacerbation in hospitalised patients with COPD and its relationship with CXCL8 and IGF-I. Thorax. 2003;58:752–6.
36. Greening NJ, Williams JEA, Hussain SF, et al. An early rehabilitation intervention to enhance recovery during hospital admission for an exacerbation of chronic respiratory disease: randomised controlled trial. BMJ. 2014;349:g4315.
37. Puhan MA, Spaar A, Frey M, et al. Early versus late pulmonary rehabilitation in chronic obstructive pulmonary disease patients with acute exacerbations: a randomized trial. Respiration. 2012;83:499–506.
38. Criner GJ, Bourbeau J, Diekemper RL, et al. Prevention of acute exacerbations of COPD American college of chest physicians and Canadian thoracic society guideline. CHEST. 2015;147:894–942.
39. Zwerink M, van der Palen J, Kerstjens HA, et al. A community-based exercise programme in COPD self-management: two years follow-up of the COPE-II study. Respir Med. 2014;108:1481–90.
40. Zwerink M, Brusse-Keizer M, van der Valk PDLPM. Cochrane database of systematic reviews. 2014, Issue 3. Art. No.: CD002990.
41. Sewell L, Singh SJ, Williams JE, et al. Can individualized rehabilitation improve functional independence in elderly patients with COPD? Chest. 2005;128:1194–200.
42. Mercken EM, Hageman GJ, Schols AM, et al. Rehabilitation decreases exercise-induced oxidative stress in chronic obstructive pulmonary disease. Am J Respir Crit Care Med. 2005;172:994–1001.
43. Walker PP, Burnett A, Flavahan PW, et al. Lower limb activity and its determinants in COPD. Thorax. 2008;63:683–9.
44. Pitta F, Troosters T, Probst VS, et al. Are patients with COPD more active after pulmonary rehabilitation? Chest. 2008;134:273–80.
45. Demeyer H, Burtin C, Van Remoortel H, et al. Standardizing the analysis of physical activity in patients with COPD following a pulmonary rehabilitation program. Chest. 2014;146:318–27.
46. Steele BG, Belza B, Hunziker J, et al. Monitoring daily activity during pulmonary rehabilitation using a triaxial accelerometer. J Cardiopulm Rehabil. 2003;23:139–42.
47. Coronado M, Janssens JP, de Muralt B, et al. Walking activity measured by accelerometry during respiratory rehabilitation. J Cardiopulm Rehabil. 2003;23:357–64.
48. Dalls MI, McCusker C, Haggerty MC, et al. Using pedometers to monitor walking activity in outcome assessment for pulmonary rehabilitation. Chron Respir Dis. 2009;6:217–24.
49. Mador MJ, Patel AN, Nadler J. Effects of pulmonary rehabilitation on activity levels in patients with chronic obstructive pulmonary disease. J Cardiopulm Rehabil Prev. 2011;31:52–9.
50. Eagan C, Deering BM, Blake C, et al. Short term and long term effects of pulmonary rehabilitation on physical activity in COPD. Respir Med. 2012;106:1671–9.

Chapter 10
Nutritional Therapy for COPD: What Is the Present State of Nutritional Therapy and Is There a Possibility of Developing New Drugs?

Takao Tsuji

Abstract Cachexia associated with advanced lung disease has been recognized as "pulmonary cachexia syndrome." Manangement for pulmonary cachexia syndrome is important in COPD, because cachexia is an independent predictor of mortality. In meta-analysis reported in 2012, nutritional support is effective to improve anthropometric measures and exercise capacity in patients with COPD. COPD is treatable disease, but its airflow limitation is not fully reversible, therefore, nutritional therapy preventive to COPD is warranted. In the study reported in 2015, the Alternate Healthy Eating Index 2010 diet score was associated with a lower risk of newly diagnosed COPD.

A better approach would be to incorporate multimodal therapy, which would target simultaneously multiple underlying pathophysiological processes. Important management adjunct to nutritional supports is integrated disease management (IDM). IDM is to establish a program of different components of care in which several healthcare providers collaborate to provide efficient and good quality of care. IDM will help to develop new drugs targeting pulmonary cachexia syndrome in patients with COPD. Integrated nutritional therapy including bronchodilator and exercise program is warranted to answer the question: "Is there a possibility of developing new drugs for cachexia in COPD?"

Keywords Cachexia • Pulmonary cachexia syndrome • Nutrition • AHEI-2010 • Integrated nutritional therapy

T. Tsuji, M.D (✉)
Department of Respiratory Medicine, Institute of Geriatrics, Tokyo Women's Medical University, 2-15-1 Shibuya, Shibuya-ku, 150-0002 Tokyo, Japan
e-mail: tsuji.takao@twmu.ac.jp

H. Nakamura, K. Aoshiba (eds.), *Chronic Obstructive Pulmonary Disease*, Respiratory Disease Series: Diagnostic Tools and Disease Managements,
DOI 10.1007/978-981-10-0839-9_10

10.1 Introduction

Cachexia is an independent predictor of mortality in patients with COPD. Among patients with COPD who meet the definition of cachexia based on a low lean body mass index, the median survival is reduced by almost half from about 4 to 2 years. Manangement for cachexia is important in patients with COPD, and nutritional support is expected to improve cachexia. In 2000, a meta-analysis of randomized controlled trials showed nutritional support had no effect on improving anthropometric measures, lung function, or functional exercise capacity in patients with COPD [1]. However, in meta-analysis reported in 2012, nutritional support is effective to improve anthropometric measures and exercise capacity in patients with COPD [2, 3].

To answer the question "What is the present state of nutritional theapy and is there a possibility of developing new drugs?", we refer to the mechanism of pulmonary cachexia syndrome in COPD and mention the nutritional theapy and medication.

10.2 Pulmonary Cachexia Syndrome in COPD

Cachexia associated with advanced lung disease has been recognized as "pulmonary cachexia syndrome." Pulmonary cachexia syndrome is estimated to occur in 20–40 % of individuals with COPD [4]. Pulmonary cachexia syndrome characterized by loss of fat-free body mass has been determined by a weight <90 % of ideal body weight or BMI <20. A more precise determination would ideally include loss of lean body mass (LBMI) by measurement of percent body fat [5]. A LBMI <17 in men or <14 in women indicates the presence of pulmonary cachexia syndrome.

10.3 Factors That Influence Pulmonary Cachexia Syndrome in COPD

A number of factors contribute to pulmonary cachexia syndrome in COPD, although the exact pathogenesis of pulmonary cachexia syndrome remains unclear.

10.3.1 Genetics

There are some reports to render genetic polymorphisms that underlie the susceptibilities for pulmonary cachexia syndrome. A cross-sectional study was performed in 99 patients with COPD, who were stratified by cachexia based on fat-free mass index. There was a significant difference in the distribution of the SNP at -511 in the IL-1β gene that was seen between cachectic patients with COPD and control subjects [6].

10.3.2 Metabolism

Patients with COPD have ten times increase in energy expenditure for respiratory muscles compared with healthy individuals, because of increasing work of breathing [7]. The basal metabolism declines with aging in normal individuals but not in patients with COPD. Although the normal response to semistarvation is a reduced metabolic rate and depressed whole-body protein turnover, cachectic patients with COPD display an elevated energy expenditure and increased whole-body protein turnover. In cachectic patients with COPD, decreased efficiency of lower-limb muscle contraction and decreased ventilatory efficiency contribute to elevated daily energy requirements.

10.3.3 Calorie Intake

In patients with COPD, fatigue and dyspnea interfere with food preparation and consumption. Chronic sputum production alters the taste of food. Flattening of the diaphragm due to hyperinflation causes less capacity of stomach and early satiety. Depression reduces appetite. Generally, COPD patients have a reduced dietary intake, and the levels of systemic inflammation are inversely correlated with calorie intake in patients with COPD [8].

10.3.4 Aging

Aging is a risk factor for COPD. With aging, body composition changes as individuals progressively lose lean body mass and progressively increase fat stores. The net result of these alterations is a reduction in exercise capacity, contributing a reduced dietary intake.

10.3.5 Oxidative Stress

Oxidative damage due to oxidant-antioxidant imbalance has been proposed as a cause of COPD. Analysis of skeletal muscle from patients with COPD shows a shift in muscle fiber from type I to type II and a decrease in oxidative capacity

[9]. Muscle wasting in patients with COPD is partially due to oxidative stress. These changes are associated with increased oxidative stress, which may render the muscle more susceptible to the toxic effects of free radicals and cause muscle wasting, contributing to pulmonary cachexia syndrome in COPD.

10.3.6 Chronic Inflammation

Elevated levels of plasma TNF-α was detected in patients with COPD who lost weight during the previous year compared with those whose weight had not changed during the same period, although patients of two groups had no cause known to elevate TNF-α serum levels and had similar chronic airflow obstruction and arterial blood gas impairment [10].

In patients with COPD that have $>5\ \%$ weight loss during the preceding year, the release of TNF-α from circulating monocytes after LPS stimulation were increased, compared with those whose body weight fluctuated $\leq 5\ \%$ and age-matched healthy individuals [11]. These data suggested that pulmonary cachexia syndrome in COPD may be related to systemic inflammation, though uncertain whether the increased TNF- α is a cause or effect of weight loss.

10.4 Nutritional Therapy for Pulmonary Cachexia Syndrome in COPD

Optimization of lung function by bronchodilator to alleviate work of breathing would reduce calorie expenditure in patients with COPD. Optimized lung function would enable adherence to an exercise program. Regular exercise can stimulate appetite and improve the effectiveness of nutritional therapy. Therefore, integrated nutritional therapy including bronchiodilator and exercise program is necessary for pulmonary cachexia syndrome in COPD.

10.4.1 Nutritional Intervention

The social benefits of eating at the dining table with other family members should be encouraged. The pleasure of tasting food should be emphasized over total calorie intake. To overcome problems about calorie intake in pulmonary cachexia syndrome (written in 10.3.3), some recommendations about taking meals have been considered (Table 10.1).

Table 10.1 Recommendations for nutritional repletion

Adequate calories to exceed basal energy expenditure slightly
Small, frequent meal
Timing the main meal to corresponed to the time requiring high energy
More protein and fat and less carbohydrate
Meal requiring little preparation
Rest before and after meals

10.4.2 Oral Nutritional Supplements

In 2012, the meta-analysis reported including the Cochrane Airways Group register showed nutritional support is effective to improve anthropometric measures and exercise capacity in patients with COPD [2, 3]. COPD is treatable disease, but its airflow limitation is not fully reversible. Therefore, nutritional therapy preventive to COPD is warranted. In 2015, Varraso, et al. reported that the Alternate Healthy Eating Index 2010 (AHEI-2010) diet score was associated with a lower risk of newly diagnosed COPD [12]. AHEI-2010, a measure of diet quality, is based on 11 components (Table 10.2): six components for which the highest intakes were supposed to be ideal (vegetables, fruit, whole grains, nuts and legumes, long-chain omega-3 fats, and polyunsaturated fatty acids), one component for which moderate intake was supposed to be ideal (alcohol), and four components for which avoidance or lowest intake were supposed to be ideal (sugar-sweetened drinks and fruit juice, red and processed meat, trans fat, and sodium). Each component is given a minimal score of 0 and a maximal score of 10, with intermediate values scored proportionally, and has the potential to contribute 0–10 points to the total score. All the component scores are summed to obtain a total AHEI-2010 score, which ranges from 0 to 110, with a higher score representing a healthier diet. Varraso, et al. investigated 73,228 female from 1984 to 2000 and 47,026 men from 1986 to 1998. Over the study period, 723 cases of newly diagnosed COPD occurred in women and 167 in men. In the pooled analysis, a significant negative association was seen between the risk of newly diagnosed COPD and fifths of the AHEI-2010: hazard ratios were 0.81 for the second fifth, 0.98 for the third fifth, 0.74 for the fourth fifth, and 0.67 for participants who ate the healthiest diet according to the AHEI-2010, compared with those who ate the less healthy diet (Table 10.3) [12]. In this section, components of AHEI-2010 and amino acids, vitamins, and antioxidants are reviewed as oral nutritional supplements.

10.4.2.1 The Highest Intakes Were Supposed to Be Ideal

Vegetables

Two hundred seventy-eight patients with COPD diagnosed within the past 4 years and 340 community-based controls were investigated in Japan. The mean vegetable

Table 10.2 11 components of AHEI-2010

Highest intakes to be ideal	
	Vegetables
	Fruits
	Whole grains
	Nuts and legumes
	Long-chain omega-3 fats
	Polyunsaturated fatty acids
Moderate intake to be ideal	
	Alchol
Lowest intake to be ideal	
	Suga-sweetened drinks and fruit juice
	Red and processed meat
	Trans fat
	Sodium

intakes of patients with COPD were significantly lower than healthy controls (155.62 vs 199.14 g/day). A substantial reduction in COPD risk was found by increasing daily total vegetable intake. This study provided evidence of an inverse association between vegetable consumption and the risk of COPD [13].

Whole Grains, Fruit, Nuts, and Legumes

Whole grains including cereal, fruit, and food grains contain many fibers and antioxidant components. A study from Japan showed fruit intake is lower in COPD patients compared with healthy individuals (248.32 vs 304.09 g/day), and less consumption of dietary fiber is associated with more prevalence of COPD [13]. Investigation of fiber intake with risk of COPD in 11,897 US men and women showed odds ratios of COPD for the highest versus lowest quintiles of intake were 0.85 for total fiber, 0.83 for cereal fiber, and 0.72 for fruit fiber. Dietary fiber in whole grains and fruit is independently associated with reduced risk of COPD [14].

Investigation of 832 cases of COPD showed total dietary fiber intake was negatively associated with risk of newly diagnosed COPD. Particullarly, cereal fiber was significantly associated with newly diagnosed COPD independently of other fiber sources, indicating a diet high in fiber, and possibly specifically cereal fiber, may reduce risk of developing COPD [15].

Long-Chain Polyunsaturated Fatty Acids

The anti-inflammatory activity of long-chain n-3 polyunsaturated fatty acids (PUFAs) has been established. In the cross-sectional associations between the dietary intake of n-3 fatty acid and risk of COPD in 8960 current or former smokers, higher fish consumption, and especially higher intake of PUFAs, was associated

Table 10.3 Association between AHEI-2010 and risk of newly diagnosed COPD

AHEI-2010	Women			Men			Total			
	No	Person years	Hazard ratio (95 % CI)[a]	No	Person years	Hazard ratio (95 % CI)[a]	No	Hazard ratio (95 % CI)[a]	P value[b]	I^2[c]
Lowest fifth[d]	198	221 312	1.00 (referent)	53	103 567	1.00 (referent)	251	1.00 (referent)		
Second fifth	168	226 830	0.98 (0.80–1.21)	27	104 165	0.61 (0.38–0.97)	195	0.81 (0.51–1.29)	0.07	81.0
Third fifth	161	228 007	1.01 (0.81–1.25)	34	104 398	0.85 (0.55–1.33)	195	0.98 (0.80–1.18)	0.50	0.0
Fourth fifth	104	229 754	0.70 (0.54–0.89)	33	104 817	0.90 (0.57–1.43)	137	0.74 (0.59–0.92)	0.33	0.0
Highest fifth[d]	92	231 204	0.69 (0.53–0.90)	20	104 818	0.60 (0.34–1.03)	112	0.67 (0.53–0.85)	0.63	0.0
P for trend			<0.001			0.27		<0.001		

[a]Multivariable hazard ratios adjusted for age, physical activity, body mass index, total energy intake, smoking status, pack years of smoking, pack years^2 of smoking, secondhand tobacco exposure (only in Nurses' Health Study), race/ethnicity, physician visits, US region, spouse's highest educational attainment (only in Nurses' Health Study), and menopausal status (only in Nurses' Health Study)

[b]Test for between studies heterogeneity

[c]Degree of heterogeneity between studies expressed as percentage of total variance

[d]Lowest fifth corresponds to least healthy diet according to AHEI-2010 diet score; highest fifth corresponds to healthiest diet

with lower odds for COPD. In this study, three case definitions of COPD were used: symptoms of chronic bronchitis, physician-diagnosed emphysema reported by the subject, and spirometrically detected COPD. The adjusted odds ratio for the highest quartile of intake as compared with the lowest quartile was 0.66 for chronic bronchitis, 0.31 for physician-diagnosed emphysema, and 0.50 for spirometrically detected COPD [16].

10.4.2.2 Moderate Intake Was Supposed to Be Ideal

Alcohol

One thousand eighty-two COPD patients completed baseline alcohol questionnaires and were included in analysis mainly to evaluate the relationship between alcohol consumption and COPD. In this study, there were small but statistically significant differences in FEV1 among the alcohol intake categories. Heavy alcohol users (>60 drinks/month) have more FEV1, though a higher mean smoking pack-year history. This data suggested some protective role of alcohol in patients with COPD, though the number of patients reporting heavy alcohol intake was small and further study is needed to determine the effect of heavy alcohol intake [17].

10.4.2.3 Lowest Intake Were Supposed to Be Ideal

Sugar-Sweetened Soft Drinks

There was a statistically significant correlation between intake of soft drinks and prevalence of chronic bronchitis. Intake of soda $\geq$5 times a week was associated with nearly twice the likelihood of having chronic bronchitis. Since this study is cross-sectional analysis for adults aged 20–55 y, soft drink intake may contribute to the risk of future COPD [18].

Red and Processed Meat

In 111 self-reported cases of newly diagnosed COPD among 42,915 men, the consumption of cured meats was positively associated with the risk of newly diagnosed COPD for highest versus lowest intake (relative risk = 2.64). Interstingly, the consumption of cured meats was not associated with the risk of adult-onset asthma [19]. Cured meats contain a lot of nitrites which generate reactive nitrogen species and may worsen the adverse effects of smoking on risk of COPD.

Sodium

In a study from Japan with participants including 278 COPD patients, FEV1 and FEV1% predicted were positively correlated with calcium, iron, potassium, and selenium but negatively correlated with sodium. This data suggested sodium intake may have some deleterious effect in patients with COPD [20].

10.4.2.4 Essential Amino Acid

Protein depletion is a hallmark of cachexia. Whole-body protein breakdown and synthesis is elevated in patients with stable severe COPD compared with healthy individuals. Eighty-eight COPD outpatients were randomized to receive essential amino acid (EAA) or placebo for 12 weeks. After 12 weeks, the physical performance and muscle strength were significantly increased versus baseline only in patients who received EAA. Similarly, the SGRQ score improved significantly in patients who received EAA, and changes were significantly different from those measured in the placebo group [21]. These data suggested intake of EAA may be benefical in patients with COPD.

10.4.2.5 Vitamins

Vitamin D deficiency is associated with reduced lung function. A cross-sectional survey using data from the Third National Health and Nutrition Examination Survey that included 14,091 people found that the mean FEV and mean FVC were 126 and 172 mL greater, respectively, for the highest quintile cf serum 25-hydroxy vitamin D level compared to the lowest quintile [22]. In 50 patients with COPD who followed a rehabilitation program randomized to comparing a monthly dose of 100.000 IU of vitamin D with placebo, Vitamin D intervention resulted in significantly larger improvements in inspiratory muscle strength (-11 ± 12 cmH_2O vs 0 ± 14 cmH_2O). However, improvements in quadriceps strength or 6-min walking distance were not significantly different from the effects in the placebo group [23]. Further studies are necessary to determine whether supplementation with vitamin D is of any benefit in patients with COPD.

Vitamin E is important of dietary antioxidants. As a fat-soluble antioxidant, Vitamin E stops the production of oxidative stress formed when fat undergoes oxidation. A post hoc analysis of 38,597 women without chronic lung disease at baseline was randomized double-blind placebo-controlled factorial trial of vitamin E (600 IU every other day) and aspirin (100 mg every other day). The effect of randomized vitamin E assignment on self-reported physician-diagnosed chronic lung disease including COPD was evaluated. During 10 years of follow-up, 760 first occurrences of chronic lung disease were reported in the vitamin E arm compared with 846 in the placebo arm (HR 0.90; 10 % reduction in the risk of incident chronic lung disease) [24]. This study suggested intake of Vitamin E may have protective effect in the risk of COPD.

10.4.2.6 Antioxidants

Oxidative stress results from an oxidant/antioxidant imbalance, an excess of oxidants, and/or a depletion of antioxidants. Oxidative stress plays an important role in the pathogenesis of COPD. One of the potent antioxidants in nutrients includes polyphenols, which are charactrized by the presence of one or more hydroxyl groups with varying structural complexities. Resveratrol, curcumin, quercetin, and catechins are most commonly studied dietary polyphenols. Flavonoids are polyphenolic phytonutrients that occur naturally in many plant-based foods and possess profound effects on human health. Flavan-3-ols are the most common flavonoid to be found in red wine, grean tea, apple, and grapes. Due to antioxidants and anti-inflammatory properties, they may prevent disease progression of COPD. In 13,651 adults from three Dutch cities of MORGEN study, intake of catechins, flavonols, and flavones in relation to pulmonary function and COPD symptoms were examined. Average catechin, flavonol, and flavone intake was 58 mg/day with tea and apples as main sources. Total catechin, flavonol, and flavone intake was positively associated with FEV1 and inversely associated with chronic cough and breathlessness [25].

Nrf2 (nuclear factor erythroid-related factor 2) is a transcription factor that has a key role in the regulation of genes that encode multiple antioxidant proteins and is functionally defective in patients with COPD. Sulforaphane, whose precursor is found naturally in cruciferous vegetables such as broccoli, inhibits generation of oxidative stress and exerts anti-inflammatory activities through activation of Nrf2. A clinical trial of sulforaphane is currently in progress in patients with COPD (ClinicalTrials.gov identifier, NCT01335971). Sulforaphane can also denitrosylate HDAC2, restoring corticosteroid sensitivity in alveolar macrophages from patients with COPD [26]. Although many polyphenols are either less bioavailable, dietary sulforaphane in cruciferous vegetqables is expected to be a novel therapy for overcoming steroid resistance in the management of COPD.

10.5 Medications

While clinical therapies for cachexia in COPD have mainly been oral nutritional supplements, several clinical trials are underway to determine the effect of medications.

10.5.1 Progesterone Analogs

Double-blind, randomized, placebo-controlled trial of either 800 mg/day oral megestrol acetate or placebo to underweight COPD patients for 8 weeks showed that body weight significantly increased in the megestrol acetate group compared with in the placebo group (3.2 vs 0.7 kg). However, anthropometric and dual-energy radiograph absorptiometry assessments confirmed that weight gain was mainly due to fat tissue. Spirometry and maximal voluntary ventilation showed no significant changes from baseline in either group, and the difference in the change in maximum inspiratory pressure between groups was not significant [27].

10.5.2 Anabolic Steroids

Open-label, 4-month clinical trial of oral oxandrolone, 10 mg bid to moderate-to-severe COPD along with significant involuntary weight loss showed that 84 % had significantly gained a mean of 6.0 +/−5.83 lb and the weight gain is primarily lean body mass. Oxandrolone is effective adjunct to facilitate weight restoration in patients with COPD-associated weight loss [28].

10.5.3 Ghrerin

Ghrerin acts by increasing the release of the appetite inducing neuropeptide Y in the hypothalamus. Ghrelin is a growth hormone-releasing peptide that induces a positive energy balance by decreasing fat utility and stimulating feeding. Although open-label pilot study for just seven cachectic patients with COPD, an intravenous administration of ghrelin for 3 weeks resulted in a significant increase in mean body weight, lean body mass, and peripheral and respiratory muscle strength. Food intake was significantly increased during ghrelin therapy. Ghrelin significantly improved QOL of patients with COPD and the distance walked in 6 min, although it did not significantly alter pulmonary function [29].

10.6 Respiratory Failure in Advanced COPD

Respiratory failure results from disturbances of gas exchange due to impairments in either oxygenation or elimination of carbon dioxide or both. Respiratory failure is defined by an arterial oxygen tension (PaO_2) of less than 60 mmHg and/or an arterial carbon dioxide tension ($PaCO_2$) greater than 45 mmHg. In healthy individuals, carbon dioxide retention begins when respiratory muscle strength is <50 % of normal. In patients with COPD, mechanical abnormalities including airflow limitation increase the work of breathing; therefore, hypercapnic respiratory failure occurs with lesser degrees of respiratory muscle weakness. Adequate tissue oxygenation requires appropriate matching of oxygen demand and delivery at the cellular level. In patients with COPD, the increased work of breathing further increases oxygen demand, while the ability to respond to these increased demands is limited. In patients with respiratory failure, supplemental nutrition can increase oxygen consumption and carbon dioxide production. The limited ability to augment ventilation in COPD patients with respiratory failure has raised concern that increased oxygen consumption (VO_2) and carbon dioxide production (VCO_2). In order to avoid excess VCO_2, COPD patients with respiratory failure should receive a calorie intake that matches estimated energy expenditure. VCO_2 is nutritionally determined by the carbohydrate-to-fat ratio. The respiratory quotient is 0.7 for fats and 1.0 for carbohydrates. High-carbohydrate diets lead to greater CO_2 production (VCO_2) than high-fat diets due to the higher respiratory quotient of carbohydrate. Thus, low-carbohydrate/high-fat enteral nutrition was recommended with the intention of reducing the work of breathing. It is difficult to improve muscle function and quality of life in malnourished patients with respiratory failure; however, multimodal nutritional rehabilitation may improve. Trail of 122 patients with chronic respiratory failure (94 patients (77 %) have COPD) on long-term oxygen therapy and/or noninvasive ventilation showed that multimodal nutritional rehabilitation combining health education, oral nutritional supplements, exercise, and oral testosterone for 90 days improved BMI (+0.56 kg/m^2), FFMI (+0.60 kg/m^2), peak workload (+7.2 W), quadriceps isometric force (+28.3 N), and endurance time (+5.9 min), compared with home health education as controls [30].

10.7 Conclusion

While a meta-analysis in 2000 reported nutritional support had no effect, meta-analyses in 2012 showed that nutritional support can lead to improvements in nutritional intake, body weight, muscle mass, fat mass, and peripheral muscle strength in patients with COPD. In contrast with meta-analyses in 2000, those in 2012 did examine nutritional intake and found that current nutritional support resulted in a significantly greater increase in both protein and energy intakes [3]. Since the underlying mechanism of pulmonary cachexia syndrome in COPD is complex, an argument has been made that a single therapeutic agent such as an appetite stimulant would be ineffective in reversing weight loss. A better approach would be to incorporate multimodal therapy, which would target simultaneously multiple underlying pathophysiological processes. Important management adjunct to nutritional supports is integrated disease management (IDM). IDM is to establish a program of different components of care (i.e., self-management, exercise, nutrition) in which several healthcare providers (i.e., nurses, general practitioners,

Table 10.4 Summary of the effect by IDM in patients with COPD

Outcomes	Illustrative comparative risks[a] (95 % CI)		Relative effect (95 % CI)	No of Participants (studies)	Quality of evidence (GRADE)	Comments
	Assumed risk (control)	Corresponding risk (disease management)				
Disease-specific quality of life on the SGRQ, total score (follow-up, 3–12 months)	The mean change in the SGRQ (total score) ranged from 3.4 lower to 6.24 higher	The mean SGRQ in the intervention groups was **3.71 lower** (5.83–1.59 lower)	**MD −3.71** (−5.83 to −1.59)	1425 (13 studies)	**High**[b]	Minimal clinically important difference (MCID) = −4 points, lower score means improvement
Disease-specific quality of life on the CRQ dyspnea domain (follow-up, 3–12 months)	The mean change in the CRQ (dyspnea domain) ranged from 0 to 0.2 lower	The mean CRQ dyspnea domain in the intervention groups was **1.02 higher** (0.67–1.36 higher)	**MD 1.02** (0.68–1.36)	160 (4 studies)	**Moderate**[c]	MCID = 0.5 points. Results on the other domains of the CRQ (fatigue, emotion, mastery) were also all statistically and clinically relevant
Functional exercise capacity (6 min walking distance (6MWD)) (follow-up, 3–12 months)	The mean change in the 6MWD ranged from 38 lower to 36 higher	The mean functional exercise capacity in the intervention groups was **43.86 higher** (21.83–65.89 higher)	**MD 43.86** (21.83–65.89)	838 (14 studies)	**Moderate**[d]	MCID = 35 m. Sensitivity analysis showed there was inconsistency in the effect. After removing the low quality studies, the MD was 15.15 m (95 % CI 6.37–23.93, $p < 0.001$)
Respiratory-related hospital admissions (follow-up, 3–12 months)	**27 per 100 patients**	20 per 100 patients (15–27)	**OR 0.68** (0.47–0.99)	1470 (7 studies)	**High**	
Number of hospital days per patient (all causes) (follow-up, 3–12 months)	The mean change in hospital days ranged from 1.6 to 11.9 higher	The mean number of hospital days per patient in the intervention groups was	**MD −3.78** (−5.9 to −1.67)	741 (6 studies)	**High**	

(continued)

Table 10.4 (continued)

Outcomes	Illustrative comparative risks[a] (95 % CI)		Relative effect (95 % CI)	No of Participants (studies)	Quality of evidence (GRADE)	Comments
	Assumed risk (control)	Corresponding risk (disease management)				
		3.78 lower (5.9–1.67 lower)				

This table is based on a Cochrane Review published in the *Cochrane Database of Systematic Reviews* 2013[1] (see http://www.thecochranelibrary.com for information)

Disease management compared to control for patients with COPD. Patient or population = patients with COPD. Settings: 8 studies in primary care, 12 studies in secondary care, 1 study in tertiary care, 5 studies each in primary and secondary care. Intervention: integrated disease management. Comparison: control (usual care)

GRADE Working Group grades of evidence are as follows. High quality: further research is very unlikely to change our confidence in the estimate of effect. Moderate quality: further research is likely to have an important impact on our confidence in the estimate of effect and may change the estimate. Low quality: further research is very likely to have an important impact on our confidence in the estimate of effect and is likely to change the estimate. Very low quality: we are very uncertain about the estimate

MD mean difference, *CRQ* chronic respiratory questionnaire, *SGRQ* St. George Respiratory Questionnaire

[a]The basis for the assumed risk (e.g., the median control group risk across studies) is provided in footnotes. The corresponding risk (and its 95 % CI) is based on the assumed risk in the comparison group and the relative effect of the intervention (and its 95 % CI)

[b]We did not downgrade due to risk of bias, as studies contributing more than 2.7 % to the meta-analysis had a low risk of bias. Sensitivity analysis on high-risk studies did not change the effect or significance of the effect

[c]We downgraded by one as there was considerable risk of bias in two studies on allocation concealment and two studies did not blind the outcome assessor

[d]We downgraded by one as all included studies were of moderate-to-low quality. If we removed studies that scored high or unclear risk of bias on allocation concealment, the effect decreased to 15 m

physiotherapists, pulmonologists) collaborate to provide efficient and good quality of care. A total of 26 RCTs were included, involving 2997 patients from 11 different countries with a follow-up varying from 3 to 24 months, which showed that patients with COPD treated by an IDM program improved significantly on quality of life scores and reported a clinically relevant improvement of 44 m on 6 min walking distance, compared to controls (Table 10.4) [31]. To answer the question, "Is there a possibility of developing new drugs?", IDM will help to develop new drugs targeting pulmonary cachexia syndrome in patients with COPD.

References

1. Ferreira IM, Brooks D, Lacasse Y, et al. Nutritional support for individuals with COPD: a meta-analysis. Chest. 2000;117:672–8.
2. Ferreira IM, Brooks D, White J, et al. Nutritional supplementation for stable chronic obstructive pulmonary disease. Cochrane Database Syst Rev. 2012;12:Cd000998.
3. Collins PF, Stratton RJ, Elia M. Nutritional support in chronic obstructive pulmonary disease: a systematic review and meta-analysis. Am J Clin Nutr. 2012;95:1385–95.
4. Schols AM. Pulmonary cachexia. Int J Cardiol. 2002;85:101–10.
5. Schols AM, Wouters EF, Soeters PB, et al. Body composition by bioelectrical-impedance analysis compared with deuterium dilution and skinfold anthropometry in patients with chronic obstructive pulmonary disease. Am J Clin Nutr. 1991;53:421–4.
6. Broekhuizen R, Grimble RF, Howell WM, et al. Pulmonary cachexia, systemic inflammatory profile, and the interleukin 1beta -511 single nucleotide polymorphism. Am J Clin Nutr. 2005;82:1059–64.
7. Manaker S, Burke F. Pulmonary disease. In: Morrison G, Hark L, editors. Medical nutrition and disease. Boston: Blackwell Science; 1996. p. 279.
8. Creutzberg EC, Schols AM, Weling-Scheepers CA, et al. Characterization of nonresponse to high caloric oral nutritional therapy in depleted patients with chronic obstructive pulmonary disease. Am J Respir Crit Care Med. 2000;161:745–52.
9. Gosker HR, Zeegers MP, Wouters EF, et al. Muscle fibre type shifting in the vastus lateralis of patients with COPD is associated with disease severity: a systematic review and meta-analysis. Thorax. 2007;62:944–9.
10. Di Francia M, Barbier D, Mege JL, et al. Tumor necrosis factor-alpha levels and weight loss in chronic obstructive pulmonary disease. Am J Respir Crit Care Med. 1994;150:1453–5.
11. de Godoy I, Donahoe M, Calhoun WJ, et al. Elevated TNF-alpha production by peripheral blood monocytes of weight-losing COPD patients. Am J Respir Crit Care Med. 1996;153:633–7.
12. Varraso R, Chiuve SE, Fung TT, et al. Alternate Healthy Eating Index 2010 and risk of chronic obstructive pulmonary disease among US women and men: prospective study. BMJ. 2015;350: h286.
13. Hirayama F, Lee AH, Binns CW, et al. Do vegetables and fruits reduce the risk of chronic obstructive pulmonary disease? A case-control study in Japan. Prev Med. 2009;49:184–9.
14. Kan H, Stevens J, Heiss G, et al. Dietary fiber, lung function, and chronic obstructive pulmonary disease in the atherosclerosis risk in communities study. Am J Epidemiol. 2008;167:570–8.
15. Varraso R, Willett WC, Camargo Jr CA. Prospective study of dietary fiber and risk of chronic obstructive pulmonary disease among US women and men. Am J Epidemiol. 2010;171:776–84.

16. Shahar E, Folsom AR, Melnick SL, et al. Dietary n-3 polyunsaturated fatty acids and smoking-related chronic obstructive pulmonary disease. Atherosclerosis Risk in Communities Study Investigators. N Engl J Med. 1994;331:228–33.
17. Wetherbee EE, Niewoehner DE, Sisson JH, et al. Self-reported alcohol intake and risk of acute exacerbations of chronic obstructive pulmonary disease: a prospective cohort study. Int J Chron Obstruct Pulmon Dis. 2015;10:1363–70.
18. DeChristopher LR, Uribarri J, Tucker KL. Intake of high fructose corn syrup sweetened soft drinks is associated with prevalent chronic bronchitis in U.S. Adults, ages 20–55 y. Nutr J. 2015;14:107.
19. Varraso R, Jiang R, Barr RG, et al. Prospective study of cured meats consumption and risk of chronic obstructive pulmonary disease in men. Am J Epidemiol. 2007;166:1438–45.
20. Hirayama F, Lee AH, Oura A, et al. Dietary intake of six minerals in relation to the risk of chronic obstructive pulmonary disease. Asia Pac J Clin Nutr. 2010;19:572–7.
21. Dal Negro RW, Testa A, Aquilani R, et al. Essential amino acid supplementation in patients with severe COPD: a step towards home rehabilitation. Monaldi Arch Chest Dis. 2012;77:67–75.
22. Black PN, Scragg R. Relationship between serum 25-hydroxyvitamin d and pulmonary function in the third national health and nutrition examination survey. Chest. 2005;128:3792–8.
23. Hornikx M, Van Remoortel H, Lehouck A, et al. Vitamin D supplementation during rehabilitation in COPD: a secondary analysis of a randomized trial. Respir Res. 2012;13:84.
24. Agler AH, Kurth T, Gaziano JM, et al. Randomised vitamin E supplementation and risk of chronic lung disease in the Women's Health Study. Thorax. 2011;66:320–5.
25. Tabak C, Arts IC, Smit HA, Heederik D, Kromhout D. Chronic obstructive pulmonary disease and intake of catechins, flavonols, and flavones: the MORGEN Study. Am J Respir Crit Care Med. 2001;164:61–4.
26. Malhotra D, Thimmulappa RK, Mercado N, Ito K, Kombairaju P, Kumar S, Ma J, Feller-Kopman D, Wise R, Barnes P, Biswal S. Denitrosylation of HDAC2 by targeting Nrf2 restores glucocorticosteroid sensitivity in macrophages from COPD patients. J Clin Invest. 2011;121:4289–302.
27. Weisberg J, Wanger J, Olson J, et al. Megestrol acetate stimulates weight gain and ventilation in underweight COPD patients. Chest. 2002;121:1070–8.
28. Yeh SS, DeGuzman B, Kramer T. Reversal of COPD-associated weight loss using the anabolic agent oxandrolone. Chest. 2002;122:421–8.
29. Nagaya N, Itoh T, Murakami S, et al. Treatment of cachexia with ghrelin in patients with COPD. Chest. 2005;128:1187–93.
30. Pison CM, Cano NJ, Cherion C, et al. Multimodal nutritional rehabilitation improves clinical outcomes of malnourished patients with chronic respiratory failure: a randomised controlled trial. Thorax. 2011;66:953–60.
31. Kruis AL, Smidt N, Assendelft WJ, et al. Integrated disease management interventions for patients with chronic obstructive pulmonary disease. Cochrane Database Syst Rev. 2013;10, CD009437.
32. Kruis AL, Smidt N, Assendelft WJ, Gussekloo J, Boland MR, Rutten-van Mölken M, Chavannes NH. Cochrane corner: is integrated disease management for patients with COPD effective? Thorax. 2014;69:1053–5.

Chapter 11
Long-Term Oxygen Therapy (or Home Oxygen Therapy) for COPD: The Present State and Future Problems

Keisaku Fujimoto

Abstract The purpose of long-term oxygen therapy, which has been called home oxygen therapy (HOT) in Japan, for chronic respiratory failure is to prevent severe hypoxemia and the development of pulmonary hypertension, and improve mortality. The recommendations for HOT are based on the MRC and NOTT studies performed over 30 years ago. The indications for HOT based on the two studies may not necessarily be representative of today's COPD patients. There is no concrete evidence concerning the effects of HOT on the prevention of pulmonary hypertension, improvement of ADL, QOL, and physical activity, and little beneficial evidence for patients with mild to moderate hypoxemia at rest or daytime, except for exercise-induced severe hypoxemia, nocturnal oxygen desaturation, comorbidities such as cardio- and cerebrovascular comorbidities, or severe breathlessness on exertion. Further examination will be necessary in the future during the development of a new oxygen supplying device. At the time of HOT prescription, we let the patients and their family understand the need for HOT and educate them in the directions for use. We should explain and guide them in how to use the oxygen supply apparatus safely, the confirmation of the prescribed oxygen flow, the management and maintenance of the oxygen supplying device, communication for a disaster and emergency, concerns about daily life, the prevention and correspondence of the exacerbation, the use of the welfare system, and medical expenses.

Keywords Home oxygen therapy • Survival • Pulmonary hemodynamics • Activity of daily life (ADL) • Nocturnal oxygen desaturation

---

K. Fujimoto (✉)
Department of Clinical Laboratory Sciences, Shinshu University School of Health Sciences, 3-1-1, Asahi, Matsumoto, Nagano 390-8621, Japan
e-mail: keisaku@shinshu-u.ac.jp

H. Nakamura, K. Aoshiba (eds.), *Chronic Obstructive Pulmonary Disease*, Respiratory Disease Series: Diagnostic Tools and Disease Managements, DOI 10.1007/978-981-10-0839-9_11

11.1 Introduction

It was reported in Japan as of 2010 that COPD occupied 45 % of the underlying diseases of long-term oxygen therapy (LTOT), usually called home oxygen therapy (HOT) in Japan [1]. The purpose of HOT for chronic respiratory failure is to prevent severe hypoxemia and the development of pulmonary hypertension, and improve mortality [2, 3]. In the mid to late twentieth century two randomized trials were performed almost simultaneously which have had a profound effect on the management of chronic obstructive pulmonary disease (COPD) over the last three decades. The two large-scale trials, the UK Medical Research Council (MRC) study [2] and the US Nocturnal Oxygen Therapy Trial (NOTT) [3], showed that LTOT when given for greater than 15 h/day improved survival for 3 years in patients with COPD and chronic hypoxemia ($PaO_2 \leqq$ 55–60 mmHg), with or without hypercapnia, and oxygen therapy for more than 18 h improved survival further than did oxygen therapy for 12–15 h/day (Fig. 11.1) [3]. The improved survival by the treatment of HOT has been suggested to be mainly due to attenuated pulmonary hypertension [4]. These results significantly altered the treatment of hypoxemic COPD and HOT is the only therapy confirmed as evidence apart from smoking cessation that has been shown to reduce mortality in COPD.

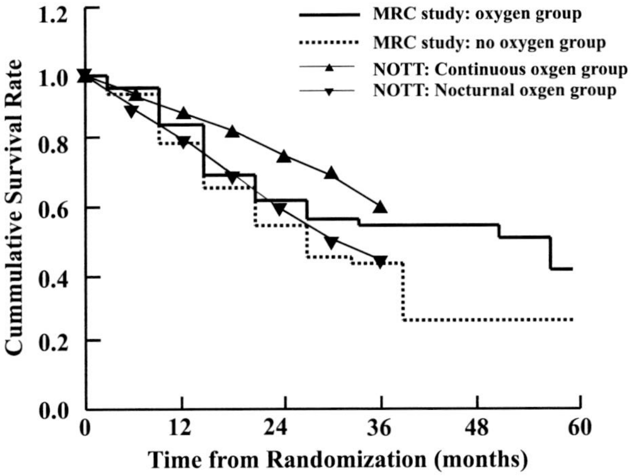

Fig. 11.1 Comparison of cumulative survival rate in the UK Medical Research Council (MRC) study and the US Nocturnal Oxygen Therapy Trial (NOTT). Long-term oxygen therapy for greater than 15 h daily significantly improved survival for 3 years in patients with COPD compared with no oxygen (MRC study), and oxygen therapy for more than 18 h further improved survival more than oxygen therapy for 12–15 h/ day (NOTT) (Figure drawn from Refs. [2] and [3])

11.2 Effects of Long-Term Oxygen Therapy on Survival

The MRC study [2] included 87 hypercapnic patients with severe hypoxemia (PaO_2: 40–55 mmHg). The patients received oxygen via concentrator for 15 h/day or no oxygen at all. Portable oxygen cylinders were not provided and those patients who continued smoking were not excluded. The mortality at 3 years was 45.2 % in the oxygen-treated group and 66.7 % in controls. The MRC study showed that LTOT when given for greater than 15 h/day significantly improved survival in patients with hypoxic COPD. The NOTT study [3] enrolled 203 patients with stable hypoxemia ($PaO_2 \leqq 55$ mmHg or $55 < PaO_2 \leqq 59$ mmHg in the presence of cor pulmonale, hematocrit $\geqq 55$ %, or electrocardiographic evidence of P pulmonale) on two measurements over a 3-week exacerbation-free period. The patients received continuous or nocturnal oxygen and were also followed for a period of 3 years or until death. The continuous oxygen flow rate was sufficient to increase PaO_2 to 60–80 mmHg, with flow rates increased by 1 L/min during sleep and exercise. The mortality rates at 24 months and 3 years were 27 and 32 % for the continuous group and 41 and 50 % for the nocturnal group, respectively. The NOTT study demonstrated a significant survival advantage in the continuous oxygen group, in whom the average oxygen usage was 18 h/day, compared with the nocturnal oxygen only group. Also, the survival advantage was prominent in patients with carbon dioxide retention and also present in patients with relatively poor lung function, low mean nocturnal oxygen saturation, more severe brain dysfunction, and prominent mood disturbances. Continuous O_2 therapy also appeared to benefit patients with low mean pulmonary artery pressure (Ppa) and pulmonary vascular resistance (PVR) and those with relatively well-preserved exercise capacity.

In a similar investigation, the result of a 5-year Japanese international survey from 1986, it has been reported that the patients receiving HOT for 5 years showed a significant improvement in cumulative survival rates compared with a patient not prescribed HOT [5]. Figure 11.2 shows the cumulative survival rates in patients with severe hypoxemic pulmonary emphysema who were prescribed HOT (red circle) or not prescribed HOT due to personal reasons although adapted for HOT (black circle) ($PaO_2 \leqq 55$ mmHg at rest under breathing room air or $55 < PaO_2 \leqq$ 60 mmHg at rest under breathing room air associated with pulmonary hypertension or with severe hypoxemia ($PaO_2 \leqq 55$ mmHg) during exercise or sleep). It was also reported that the cumulative survival rate for female patients was better than that for male patients among the patients receiving continuous oxygen therapy [6] which was the same as in the NOTT study [4], however, according to the report from Sweden, female COPD patients adversely showed a lower survival rate compared with males [7].

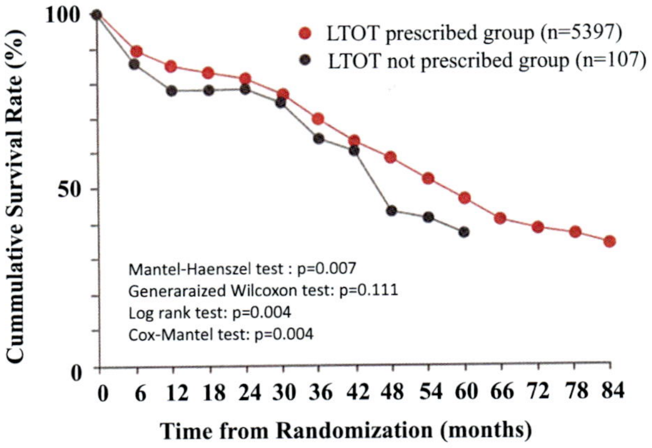

Fig. 11.2 Cumulative survival rates in patients prescribed long-term oxygen therapy (LTOT) compared with the patient not prescribed LTOT due to personal reasons although the patient fulfilled criteria for LTOT (from the result of a 5-year Japanese international survey from 1986). The patients receiving LTOT for 5 years showed a significant improvement in cumulative survival rates compared with the patient not prescribed LTOT (Figure modified from Ref. [5])

11.3 Other Benefits of Long-Term Oxygen Therapy

Acute beneficial effects of oxygen inhalation on dyspnea, exercise tolerance, and pulmonary hemodynamics are well known in patients with moderate to severe COPD, especially in patients who show desaturation below 88 % during exercise [8]. However, there is little convincing evidence from studies to date that LTOT has significant benefits other than on survival. Indeed, the mechanism for the improvement in survival with oxygen therapy still remains unclear, despite the observation of small improvements in some hemodynamic parameters in the NOTT [4].

Cooper et al. [9] have evaluated the effects of receiving LTOT for at least 15 h/day for 12 years in 72 patients (53 male) with a mean age of 60 years presenting with chronic obstructive airways disease and hypoxic cor pulmonale. The mean PaO_2 and $PaCO_2$ were 46 mmHg and 52 mmHg, respectively. All patients had a $PaO_2 \leqq 60$ mmHg and 57 patients had a $PaCO_2 \geqq 45$ mmHg. Pulmonary hemodynamics were measured in 45 patients before and 12–18 months after the induction of LTOT. There were no significant changes in mean Ppa (from 28.3 ± 10.2 (mean $\pm$ SD) to 26.1 ± 11.0 mmHg), cardiac output (from 5.9 ± 1.8 to 6.7 ± 2.8 L/min), and total PVR (from 59.2 ± 25.3 to 51.1 ± 24.7 kPa/L/s); overall 5-year survival was 62 %, but the 10-year survival was only 26 %, indicating an acceleration in death rate at 10 years despite continuing LTOT whereas the cumulative survival rates at 5 years were superior to those in the continuous oxygen group of NOTT (53 % in NOTT). Zielifiski et al. [10] also demonstrated the effects of 6 years of domiciliary oxygen therapy on pulmonary hemodynamics in 95 patients with COPD (72 men, 23 women, mean age: 58 ± 9 years, FEV_1: 0.84 ± 0.31 L, PaO_2:55 ± 6 mmHg, $PaCO_2$: 48 ± 9 mmHg, Ppa: 28 ± 11 mmHg, PVR:

353 ± 172 dyn $\times$ s $\times$ cm^{-5}). After initial assessment, all patients were started on a regimen of LTOT. Pulmonary artery catheterization was repeated every 2 years. The mean Ppa in 39 patients fell from 25 ± 8 to 23 ± 6 mmHg, which was no significant difference, and resulted in a small reduction of pulmonary hypertension after the first 2 years followed by a return to initial values and subsequent stabilization of Ppa over 6 years (in 12 patients who completed 6 years of LTOT, Ppa was 25 ± 7 at entry, and 21 ± 4, 26 ± 7, and 26 ± 6 mmHg at 2, 4, and 6 years, respectively; $p < 0.01$ for 2 vs. 6 years). The long-term stabilization of pulmonary hypertension occurred despite progression of the airflow limitation and of hypoxemia. These findings suggest that the effect of LTOT on pulmonary hemodynamics is temporary and the disturbances of pulmonary hemodynamics may no longer be important determinants of survival.

Neuropsychological function and quality of life (QOL) were assessed in both continuous and nocturnal oxygen therapy groups at baseline and 6 months in the NOTT. Only 42 % of patients showed improvements of the decreased neuropsychological function at 6 months and there were no differences between the continuous and nocturnal groups [11], but a small improvement of the QOL was found in NOTT. Okubadejo et al. [12] examined the relationships between ADL, quality of life, mood state, and airway obstruction in patients using LTOT and in patients not requiring LTOT. They found no significant difference between groups in health status using the St. George's Respiratory Questionnaire (SGRQ), and the patients using LTOT were less independent in activities of daily living than those not requiring long-term oxygen therapy. On the other hand, Eaton et al. [13] evaluated the effects of LTOT on QOL as the manner of prospective longitudinal interventional study by comparing between the LTOT group fulfilling criteria and commenced on LTOT and the non-LTOT group not fulfilling criteria and continued on standard care.

Significant improvements in QOL assessed by using the Chronic Respiratory Questionnaire (CRQ), total generic Dartmouth COOP Charts, and anxiety domain of the Hospital Anxiety and Depression scale were noted at 2 and 6 months in the LTOT group. Conversely the non-LTOT group demonstrated a progressive decline in QOL. They concluded that the introduction of LTOT to patients with severe COPD fulfilling standard criteria was associated with early significant improvements in HRQL with sustained or further response at 6 months. It is difficult to determine whether the improvements of QOL were due to more than placebo effect because of the lack of placebo, that is, compressed air instead of oxygen. Also, the control subjects were a non-LTOT group enrolled from the subjects not fulfilling criteria for LTOT in the above two studies. The control subjects should be enrolled from the patients adapted to LTOT at random, and different results might be found. We cannot assert that oxygen improves QOL at present. However, daily life is limited by sustained oxygen treatment for LTOT and patients felt uneasy and the QOL decreased. The effects of LTOT may be dependent on the individual style of daily life. If the portable oxygen devices were developed to be smaller, lighter weight, and easy to carry, the effects of LTOT on ADL and QOL would become clear.

11.4 Application of HOT

Most international guidelines for the management of oxygen therapy in COPD recommended that LTOT should be considered for patients with stable COPD, who show PaO_2 consistently less than or equal to 55 mmHg at rest when awake and breathing room air and for patients with PaO_2 56–59 mmHg with polycythemia (hematocrit > 0.55) or clinical, electrocardiographic, or echocardiographic evidence of pulmonary hypertension and/or right heart failure [14, 15, 16]. In Japan, for severe hypoxemia, with PaO_2 are ≦ 55 Torr at rest or 55 < PaO_2 ≦ 60 mmHg with severe desaturation during sleep or exercise under breathing room air, continuing in a stable state for more than one month providing enough medical therapy and pulmonary rehabilitation and a doctor judges the necessity, HOT is prescribed. Also, subjects having pulmonary hypertension are adapted for HOT regardless of cause. All of the guidelines generally recommended that oxygen should be used for as many hours of the day as possible, ideally a minimum of 15 h. Górecka et al. [17] examined the benefit of LTOT on survival in COPD patients with moderate hypoxemia. One hundred and thirty-five patients with COPD who showed their PaO_2 were 56–65 mmHg, borderline severe hypoxemia at rest, and advanced airflow limitation (mean FEV_1: 0.83 L) were randomly allocated to a control and LTOT group. The patients were followed every 3 months for at least 3 years or until death. The cumulative survival rate was 88 % at 1 year, 77 % at 2 years, and 66 % at 3 years. No significant differences were found in survival rates between patients treated with LTOT and controls, nor did longer oxygen use (over 15 h/day) improve survival (Fig. 11.3). They concluded that domiciliary oxygen treatment does not prolong survival in patients with COPD with moderate hypoxemia. It has been suggested that LTOT should be prescribed earlier for patients who complain of severe dyspnea on effort where their PaO_2 are ≧ 60 mmHg at rest. However, it has been demonstrated that there was little improvement of dyspnea, QOL, and neuropsychological dysfunction for the patients who complained of dyspnea on effort and showed mild hypoxemia of PaO_2 71.4 mmHg as mean values at rest [18]. At the present time, HOT is not approved as the treatment for dyspnea on effort if the patient does not show severe hypoxemia.

11.5 HOT for Patients with COPD Showing Only During Exercise

Most patients with COPD show more hypoxemia (desaturation) and increased Ppa during exercise, and the supplemental oxygen improves desaturation and increased Ppa [19]. Therefore, the oxygen supply needs to be increased in order to maintain the SpO_2 ≧ 90 % during exercise in patients who were prescribed supplemental oxygen at rest. On the other hand, the use of ambulatory oxygen during exercise or with exertion in patients with mild hypoxemia at rest and unfulfilled criteria for

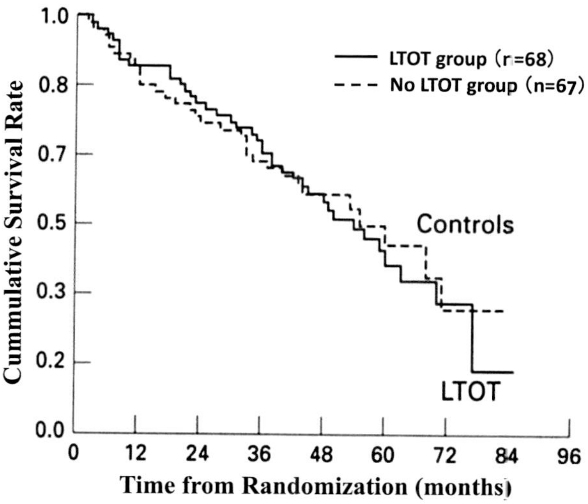

Fig. 11.3 Effect of long-term oxygen therapy (LTOT) on the cumulative survival rate in COPD patients who showed moderate hypoxemia (PaO_2 at rest: 56–65 mmHg) and advanced airflow limitation. The cumulative survival rate was 88 % at 1 year, 77 % at 2 years, and 66 % at 3 years. No significant differences were found in survival rates between patients treated with LTOT and controls (Referred from Ref. [17])

LTOT remains controversial. Meta-analysis about acute efficacy of supplemental oxygen revealed that the supplemental oxygen improved dyspnea and exercise tolerance especially in moderate to severe COPD patients with mild hypoxemia at rest [20]. The acute efficacy is dose-dependent and is suggested to be partly related to a reduction in dynamic hyperinflation and reduced breathing frequency [21]. Also, COPD patients with mild hypoxemia at rest, whose SpO_2 decreased lower than 90 % during the 6-min walking test (6MWT) have been demonstrated to have a poor prognosis [22]. The moderate to severe patients with COPD, whose SpO_2 decreased lower than 90 % within one minute after starting the walk, have a tendency to be prescribed supplemental oxygen at an earlier time [23]. There is no large-scale study about the long-term efficacy of ambulatory supplemental oxygen therapy for patients with COPD who show severe hypoxemia only during exercise.

A 12-week, double-blind, randomized crossover study of O_2 versus cylinder-compressed air in 41 COPD patients with breathlessness and mild hypoxemia at rest but showing exertional desaturation ($SpO_2 \leqq 88\ \%$) was examined. Improvements were seen in all domains of the CRQ for cylinder oxygen compared with compressed air [24]. Significant improvements were also noted in anxiety and depression and in certain domains of the SF-36. These benefits cannot be predicted by baseline characteristics or acute response supplemental oxygen. On the other hand, Moore et al. [18] examined a 12-week, parallel, double-blinded, randomized, placebo-controlled trial of cylinder air versus cylinder oxygen trial in 143 patients with COPD, having $PaO_2 > 60$ mmHg at rest breathing room air and moderate to severe exertional dyspnea including 50 patients with exertional desaturation to $\leq 88\ \%$. The oxygen or compressed air was provided at 6 L/min intranasally for use during any activity provoking breathlessness. However, no significant differences in any outcome were found between groups receiving air or oxygen (Fig. 11.4).

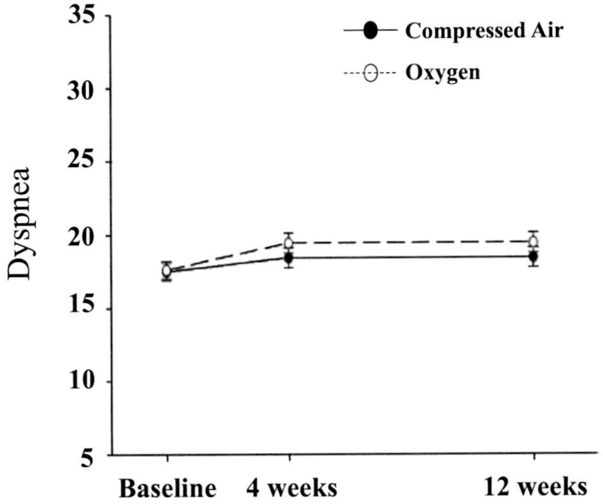

Fig. 11.4 A randomized trial of domiciliary ambulatory oxygen in COPD patients with dyspnea but without resting hypoxemia. Statistically significant but clinically small improvements in dyspnea were observed in the whole study group over the 12 weeks of the study, however, no significant differences in dyspnea score were found between groups receiving air or oxygen (Referred from Ref. [18])

Statistically significant but clinically small improvements in dyspnea and depression were observed in the whole study group over the 12 weeks of the study and resulted from a substantial placebo effect. They concluded that the domiciliary ambulatory oxygen conferred no more benefits than compressed air in terms of dyspnea, quality of life, or function in breathless patients with COPD who do not have severe resting hypoxemia. It has been demonstrated that the inhalation of either oxygen or compressed air induces a relief of breathlessness through the stimulation of nasal receptors by gas flow, however, the precise mechanism is not known [25]. Indeed, in COPD patients with mild hypoxemia at rest, but showing severe desaturation, effectiveness of long-term domiciliary ambulatory oxygen therapy on QOL with more than placebo effect could not be found. However, even though short-term severe hypoxemia has been demonstrated to aggregate systemic inflammation and increase activity of coagulation, the supplemental oxygen prevents exercise-induced oxidative stress in muscle-wasted patients with COPD [26, 27]. Supplemental oxygen during exercise has been recommended in patients in the United States who show mild hypoxemia at rest, but severe desaturation during exercise [28].

11.6 Effects of Supplemental Oxygen on Pulmonary Rehabilitation in Nonhypoxemic COPD at Rest

According to a review on the effectiveness of adding oxygen to exercise training in comparison to exercise training without oxygen supplementation in patients with COPD, both hypoxemic and nonhypoxemic subjects can exercise longer and have less shortness of breath when using oxygen during an exercise-training program [29]. However, few data have demonstrated the effects of oxygen on daily shortness of breath, daily activity, and QOL. Nonoyama et al. [30] undertook a series of individual randomized controlled trials (N-of-1 RCTs) to measure the effect of oxygen on QOL in 27 COPD patients with transient exertional hypoxemia. Oxygen significantly increased exercise capacity in a 5-min walk test. Among the whole group, neither the CRQ nor the St. George's Respiratory Questionnaire showed any statistical or clinical differences between oxygen and placebo. This study does not support the general application of LTOT for patients with COPD who do not meet criteria for LTOT. Furthermore, Spielmanns et al. [31] carried out a 24-week training program with progressively increasing loads and compared the influences of oxygen supplementation by a blinded randomized controlled study. Thirty-six subjects with moderate to severe COPD who were not dependent on LTOT trained under supervision for 24 weeks (3 times/week for 30 min/session) with supplementation of oxygen or compressed air at a flow of 4 L/min. Statistically significant improvements were found in QOL, maximal tolerated load during cycling, peak oxygen uptake, and 6-min walk test after 12 weeks of training, but there were no further benefits of supplemental oxygen.

It has been demonstrated that the addition of noninvasive positive pressure ventilation (NPPV) to an exercise training program in severe COPD (mean PaO_2: 65.4 mmHg at rest under breathing room air) produces greater benefits in exercise tolerance and QOL than after training alone, and suggested that domiciliary NPPV can be used successfully to augment the effects of rehabilitation in severe COPD [32]. Heliox breathing, similar to NPPV, unloads the respiratory muscles and relieves both dyspnea and leg discomfort during exercise [33]. This allows COPD patients to exercise longer prior to exhaustion and enhances the physiological training effect. Despite the current findings, the overall cost of the ventilator setup and the gas mixture makes the use of this therapy cumbersome/impractical and/or too expensive to be incorporated into routine pulmonary rehabilitation programs or training at home.

11.7 HOT for Patients with COPD Showing Severe Hypoxemia Only During Night

COPD patients have been demonstrated to show nocturnal oxygen desaturation (NOD) during sleep, especially during REM sleep, due to hypoventilation and ventilation to perfusion mismatching even though without daytime hypoxemia [34]. Severe NOD can cause cardiac arrhythmias, pulmonary hypertension, and nocturnal death, especially during acute exacerbations. Fletcher et al. have examined the association between pulmonary hemodynamics and NOD in 36 patients with chronic lung disease who had a daytime $PaO_2 > 60$ mmHg, REM sleep-related NOD for greater than 5 min, and the lowest $SpO_2 \leqq 85\,\%$. The patients with NOD showed more hypoxemia and higher Ppa and PVR compared with those in patients with similar degrees of lung disease but without NOD (Ppa: 23.3 ± 4.8 mmHg and PVR: 172.4 ± 53.8 dyn $\times$ s $\times$ cm^{-5} in patients with NOD vs. Ppa: 20.4 ± 4.2 mmHg and PVR: 101.8 ± 27.6 dyn $\times$ s $\times$ cm^{-5} in patients without NOD) [35]. The effects of nocturnal supplemental oxygen on pulmonary hemodynamics for moderate to severe COPD patients with NOD were evaluated in a double-blind, randomized 3-year trial [36]. The subjects were treated with nocturnal oxygen ($n = 19$) or room air ($n = 19$) at 3 L/min, and 13 nondesaturating subjects were followed with no gas therapy. The NOD patients treated with nocturnal supplemental oxygen over 36 months showed a significant downward trend in pulmonary artery pressure (−3.7 mmHg) compared with NOD patients treated with room air (+3.9 mmHg; Fig. 11.5). Mortality was decidedly higher in the desaturating patients compared with nondesaturating subjects, but there was no significant difference between oxygen- and sham-treated desaturating subjects. It was concluded that nocturnal supplemental oxygen used to reverse episodic desaturation in COPD patients with daytime mild hypoxemia has a beneficial effect in reducing pulmonary artery pressure. However, Chaouat et al. [37] have demonstrated that there was no difference in the pulmonary hemodynamics, the rate of patients conducted to daytime oxygen therapy, and survival 2 years following the treatment between the patient groups prescribed nocturnal supplemental oxygen and no oxygen therapy. There are no coincident results. Also, any significant efficacy for QOL and quality of sleep was not obtained [38]. The potential benefits of nocturnal oxygen therapy in patients with mild to moderate daytime hypoxemia remain unclear. Further studies will be needed.

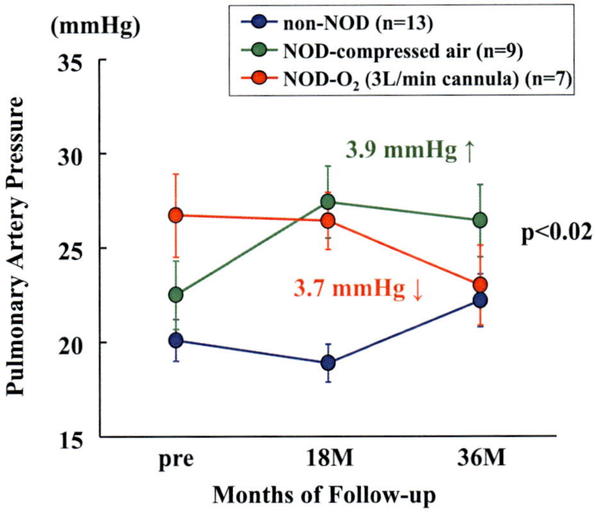

Fig. 11.5 Effect of nocturnal supplemental oxygen on pulmonary artery pressure for moderate to severe COPD patients with nocturnal oxygen desaturation (NOD) and a daytime PaO_2 above 60 mmHg. The NOD patients treated with nocturnal supplemental oxygen (3 L/min) over 36 months showed a significant downward trend in pulmonary artery pressure compared with NOD patients treated with room air (Figure drawn from Ref. [36])

11.8 Oxygen Therapy for Patients with COPD Combined Obstructive Sleep Apnea or Pulmonary Fibrosis

Coexistence of COPD and obstructive sleep apnea (OSA), referred to as overlap syndrome, has been found in 3 % of mild COPD. Overlap patients have worse sleep-related hypoxemia and hypercapnia than patients with COPD or OSA alone [34]. OSA has a similar prevalence in COPD as in a general population of similar age, but oxygen desaturation during sleep is more pronounced when the two conditions coexist. It has also been reported that overlap syndrome showed further increased Ppa and increased rate of all caused death and risk of hospitalization due to exacerbation [39]. Continuous positive airway pressure (CPAP) therapy improves survival and decreases hospitalization [40]. It is important to find the combined OSA by the monitoring SpO_2 during the night. Patients with combined pulmonary fibrosis and emphysema (COPD) have shown severe hypoxemia on effort and poor prognosis although their airflow obstruction is mild [41]. These patients should be prescribed oxygen therapy at an earlier time.

11.9 Introduction of HOT

At the time of introduction of HOT, the PaO_2, $PaCO_2$, and pH should be confirmed, and the presence of hypoxemia also be evaluated not only at rest but also during exercise and sleep. PaO_2 has to maintain a PaO_2 over 60–65 mmHg, and may be better to keep 70–75 mmHg [42]. Concerning inhalational time, 18 h or more a day are desirable. Cancellation of more than 3 h has been reported to worsen pulmonary hypertension [43]. The oxygen flow up to 3 L/min rarely causes an increase in $PaCO_2$ becoming the problem clinically, but it is necessary to confirm it by arterial blood gas analysis. As for high $PaCO_2$ in itself, it does not become taboo for HOT, and it has been reported that patients having a high $PaCO_2$ showed a more beneficial effect on survival [3]. However, for those patients who show their $PaCO_2$ is 55 mmHg or over at rest or lower than 55 mmHg with severe hypoxemia during the night due to hypoventilation during sleep, or those patients who show frequent exacerbation-accompanied hypercapnia, NPPV should be considered to be used together with HOT [44].

11.10 Apparatus and Device Suppling Oxygen

Among oxygen supply devices including an oxygen concentrator, liquid oxygen, and portable oxygen cylinder, more than 90 % of the patients prescribed HOT in Japan use an oxygen concentrator at home and a portable cylinder attached to an oxygen saver, which can be used along with an inhale effort, when going out. When using a portable cylinder attached oxygen saver, it is necessary to confirm whether the device operates normally and check oxygenation during a walk, because the oxygenation varies according to the device and the oxygen supply through the demand valve does not always result in the same effect as the oxygen supply at consecutive flow especially during a walk or if the inhale effort is weak [45]. A portable oxygen concentrator has been developed and provided. However, the style of use of the concentrator is different depending on whether the oxygen supplied is only through an oxygen saver or not only through a saver but also by consecutive flows without a saver; that is, if the concentrator supplies oxygen only through a saver, it cannot be used during sleep. Also, when the portable oxygen concentrator is used, SpO_2 should be monitored using a pulse oximeter because there is a possibility that oxygenation is different in the supplied oxygen concentration between a portable concentrator and a concentrator at home, and the fitness of the patient who will need to manage a battery and possible problems when going out should be carefully considered [46].

11.11 Education and Guidance for HOT

HOT is introduced using a check list and critical path for safety and certainty. HOT will be introduced both in a stable state and at the time of discharge after the patient is restored from exacerbation. In the latter case, it is necessary to confirm that hypoxemia lasts after discharge and is still present in a stable state. At the time of prescription of HOT, we explain to patients and their families the need for HOT and educate them in the directions for use. In other words, we explain and guide how to use the oxygen supply apparatus safely, the observance of the prescribed oxygen flow, the management and maintenance of the apparatus, communication for a disaster and emergency, concerns about daily life, the prevention and communication of the exacerbation, the use of the welfare system, and medical expenses. Those patients showing poor adherence have been shown that the increased rate of severe exacerbation requires hospitalization and increases medical expenses [47]. Also, it has been demonstrated that patients who show good adherence to HOT, increase daily activity, and continuously inhale oxygen during walking and exercise show better prognosis [4]. Therefore, it may lead to prognosis improvement as well as the improvement of QOL that a patient will find it easy to go out thanks to the development and spread of the new more compact and easier to carry oxygen supply apparatus.

Smoking cessation is essential and becomes the premise in starting treatment in patients with COPD. Particularly, we have to confirm the achievement of smoking cessation when oxygen therapy is prescribed. Actually, 24 % of the dangerous matters reported from oxygen-supply companies are smoking during oxygen inhalation, and it is necessary to teach that smoking together with the inhalation of oxygen induces a burn and fire because oxygen promotes combustion. It usually may be enough to monitor daily oxygen therapy by the check of SpO_2, but we have to examine the analysis of arterial blood gas including pH and PCO_2 as needed especially in the patients having type 2 respiratory failure with a high $PaCO_2$. It is important in continuation of HOT to build up a medical network including the close cooperation among the oxygen provider, the patient together with the family, the visiting nurse, and the family doctor, and to provide utmost continuous care including pulmonary rehabilitation, which can reduce the risk of exacerbation and hospitalization and may improve prognosis [48].

The instruction of preparation for a disaster is very important. In patients using an oxygen concentrator with lower than 2 L/min at home, stoppage of the oxygen supply of around two hours is not a problem, but we should grasp the state of each patient and instruct him or her in an appropriate communication. We must instruct the patients to change from the oxygen concentrator to an oxygen cylinder calmly without falling into a panic at the time of the blackout, and teach patients how to handle the oxygen apparatus and explain the importance of handling by the patient himself at any time. In addition, we have to explain the communication of the oxygen supplier to a patient at the disaster because cooperation with the provider who supplies the oxygen is indispensable.

11.12 When Traveling by Airplane

In the patient who shows her PaO_2 at rest less than 70 mmHg, hypoxemia may worsen during long-time movement in a plane due to the hypobaric environment equivalent to 2000 m above sea level. When the PaO_2 under breathing room air at sea level are less than 50 mmHg, or $PaCO_2$ are more than 50 mmHg, movement by plane is a relative taboo [49]. It is also recommended that the oxygen flow needs to increase by 1–2 L/m during a flight for the patient prescribed HOT.

11.13 Conclusion (Future Problems for HOT)

The recommendations for HOT are based on the two randomized non-placebo-controlled trials containing fewer than 300 patients and conducted over 30 years ago. The indications for HOT based on the two studies may not necessarily be representative of today's COPD patients, many of whom are older and have more comorbidity. It would seem important to clarify the true impact of HOT on all-cause mortality in those patients who are currently receiving it, many of whom are elderly with multiple comorbidities. Even though short-time hypoxemia, severe hypoxemia may be worth for health. Further studies should be continued about an application of HOT for those patients with easily induced tissue hypoxemia such as cardiovascular disease and cerebrovascular disease and showing severe desaturation on exertion or during exercise, and/or nocturnal hypoxemia although mild hypoxemia more than 60 mmHg at rest and daytime. Also, we have to verify the efficacy of supplemental oxygen on severe breathlessness and on exercise training in the patients with exercise-induced hypoxemia or nonhypoxemia. The appearance, portability, and uses will be different with the evolution of the oxygen supply device. For example, if a portable oxygen concentrator is downsized and lightweight, and able to supply oxygen at more than 3 L/min flow rate consecutively, furthermore, its battery is lightweight, small size, and lasts for longer than 12 h, ADL and the QOL may be improved. The adaptation for HOT will change if it becomes so. Further examination will be necessary in the future.

References

1. Japanese White Paper on Home Respiratory Care. The Japanese respiratory society and the respiratory failure research group from the Ministry of Health, Labour, and Welfare. Tokyo: Medical Tribune Co. Ltd; 2010.
2. Medical Research Council Working Party. Report of long term domiciliary oxygen therapy in chronic hypoxic cor pulmonale complicating chronic bronchitis and emphysema. Lancet. 1981;1:681–6.
3. Oxygen Therapy Trial Group. Continuous or nocturnal oxygen therapy in hypoxemic chronic obstructive lung disease: a clinical trial. Ann Intern Med. 1980;93:391–8.
4. Petty TL, Bliss PL. Ambulatory oxygen therapy, exercise, and survival with advanced chronic obstructive pulmonary disease (the Nocturnal Oxygen Therapy Trial revisited). Respir Care. 2000;45:204–11.
5. Kira S, Aiba M, Suzuki T, Ishihara T, Takahashi H, Hasunuma K, et al. Improvement of prognosis in patients with chronic respiratory failure using home oxygen therapy. In: Kira S, Petty TL, editors. Progress in domiciliary respiratory care. Amsterdam: Elsevier Science; 1994. p. 337–44.
6. Miyamoto K, Aida A, Nishimura M, Aiba M, Kira S, Kawakami Y, et al. Gender effect on prognosis of patients receiving long-term home oxygen therapy. The Respiratory Failure Research Group in Japan. Am J Respir Crit Care Med. 1995;152:972–6.
7. Ekstrom M, Franklin KA, Strom KE. Increased relative mortality in women with severe oxygen-dependent COPD. Chest. 2010;137:31–6.
8. Fujimoto K, Matsuzawa Y, Yamaguchi S, Koizumi T, Kubo K. Benefits of oxygen on exercise performance and pulmonary hemodynamics in COPD with mild hypoxemia. Chest. 2002;122:457–63.
9. Cooper CB, Waterhouse J, Howardt P. Twelve year clinical study of patients with hypoxic cor pulmonale given long term domiciliary oxygen therapy. Thorax. 1987;42:105–10.
10. Zieliriski J, Tobiasz M, Hawrylkiewicz I, Sliwinski P, Palasiewicz G. Effects of long-term oxygen therapy on pulmonary hemodynamics in COPD patients: a 6-year prospective study. Chest. 1998;113:65–70.
11. Heaton RK, Grant L, McSweeny AJ, Adams KM, Petty TL. Psychologic effects of continuous and nocturnal oxygen therapy in hypoxemic chronic obstructive pulmonary disease. Arch Intern Med. 1983;143:1941–7.
12. Okubadejo AA, O'Shea L, Jones PW, Wedzicha JA. Home assessment of activities of daily living in patients with severe chronic obstructive pulmonary disease on long-term oxygen therapy. Eur Respir J. 1997;10:1572–5.
13. Eaton T, Lewis C, Young P, Kennedy Y, Garrett JE, Kolbe J. Long-term oxygen therapy improves health-related quality of life. Respir Med. 2004;98:285–93.

14. Vestbo J, Hurd SS, Agustí AG, Jones PW, Vogelmeier C, Anzueto A, et al. Global strategy for the diagnosis, management, and prevention of chronic obstructive pulmonary disease: GOLD executive summary. Am J Respir Crit Care Med. 2013;187:347–65.
15. Celli BR, MacNee W, ATS/ERS Task Force. Standards for the diagnosis and treatment of patients with COPD: a summary of the ATS/ERS position paper. Eur Respir J. 2004;23:932–46.
16. McDonald CF, Crockett AJ, Young AH. Adult domiciliary oxygen therapy. Position statement of the Thoracic Society of Australia and New Zealand. Med J Aust. 2005;182:621–6.
17. Górecka D, Gorzelak K, Sliwiński P, Tobiasz M, Zieliński J. Effect of long-term oxygen therapy on survival in patients with chronic obstructive pulmonary disease with moderate hypoxaemia. Thorax. 1997;52:674–9.
18. Moore RP, Berlowitz DJ, Denehy L, Pretto JJ, Brazzale DJ, Sharpe K, et al. A randomised trial of domiciliary, ambulatory oxygen in patients with COPD and dyspnoea but without resting hypoxaemia. Thorax. 2011;66:32–7.
19. Horsfield K, Segel N, Bishop JM. The pulmonary circulation in chronic bronchitis at rest and during exercise breathing air and 80 per cent oxygen. Clin Sci. 1968;34:473–83.
20. Bradley JM, O'Neill B. Short-term ambulatory oxygen for chronic obstructive pulmonary disease. Cochrane Database Syst Rev 2005; CD004356.
21. O'Donnell DE, Laveneziana P. The clinical importance of dynamic lung hyperinflation in COPD. COPD. 2006;3:219–32.
22. Casanova C, Cote C, Martin JM, Pinto-Plata V, de Torres JP, Aguirre-Jaíme A, et al. Distance and oxygen desaturation during the 6-min walk test as predictors of long-term mortality in patients with COPD. Chest. 2008;134:746–52.
23. Garcia-Talavera I, Tauroni A, Trujillo JL, Pitti R, Eiroa L, Aguirre-Jaime A, et al. Time to desaturation less than one minute predicts the need for long-term home oxygen therapy. Respir Care. 2011;56:1812–7.
24. Eaton T, Garrett JE, Young P, Fergusson W, Kolbe J, Rudkin S, et al. Ambulatory oxygen improves quality of life of COPD patients: a randomised controlled study. Eur Respir J. 2002;20:306–12.
25. Liss HP, Grant BJ. The effect of nasal flow on breathlessness in patients with chronic obstructive pulmonary disease. Am Rev Respir Dis. 1988;137:1285–8.
26. Sabit R, Thomas P, Shale DJ, Collins P, Linnane SJ. The effects of hypoxia on markers of coagulation and systemic inflammation in patients with COPD. Chest. 2010;138:47–51.
27. van Helvoort HA, Heijdra YF, Heunks LM, Meijer PL, Ruitenbeek W, Thijs HM, et al. Supplemental oxygen prevents exercise-induced oxidative stress in muscle-wasted patients with chronic obstructive pulmonary disease. Am J Respir Crit Care Med. 2006;173:1122–9.
28. Tarpy SP, Celli BR. Long-term oxygen therapy. N Engl J Med. 1995;333:710–4.
29. Nonoyama M, Brooks D, Lacasse Y, Guyatt GH, Goldstein R. Oxygen therapy during exercise training in chronic obstructive pulmonary disease (Review) Cochrane Database Syst Rev 2007: CD005372.
30. Nonoyama ML, Brooks D, Guyatt GH, Goldstein RS. Effect of oxygen on health quality of life in patients with chronic obstructive pulmonary disease with transient exertional hypoxemia. Am J Respir Crit Care Med. 2007;176:343–9.
31. Spielmanns M, Fuchs-Bergsma C, Winkler A, Fox G, Krüger S, Baum K. Effects of oxygen supply during training on subjects with COPD who are normoxemic at rest and during exercise: a blinded randomized controlled trial. Respir Care. 2015;60:540–8.
32. Garrod R, Mikelsons C, Paul EA, Wedzicha JA. Randomized controlled trial of domiciliary noninvasive positive pressure ventilation and physical training in severe chronic obstructive pulmonary disease. Am J Respir Crit Care Med. 2000;162:1335–41.
33. Palange P, Valli G, Onorati P, Antonucci R, Paoletti P, Rosato A, et al. Effect of heliox on lung dynamic hyperinflation, dyspnea, and exercise endurance capacity in COPD patients. J Appl Physiol. 2004;97:1637–42.

34. McNicholas WT, Verbraecken J, Marin JM. Sleep disorders in COPD: the forgotten dimension. Eur Respir Rev. 2013;22:365–75.
35. Fletcher EC, Luckett RA, Miller T, Costarangos C, Kutka N, Fletcher JG. Pulmonary vascular hemodynamics in chronic lung disease patients with and without oxyhemoglobin desaturation during sleep. Chest. 1989;95:757–64.
36. Fletcher EC, Luckett RA, Goodnight-White S, Miller CC, Qian W, Costarangos-Galarza C. A double-blind trial of nocturnal supplemental oxygen for sleep desaturation in patients with chronic obstructive pulmonary disease and a daytime PaO_2 above 60 mmHg. Am Rev Respir Dis. 1992;145:1070–6.
37. Chaouat A, Weitzenblum E, Kessler R, Charpentier C, Enrhart M, Schott R, et al. A randomized trial of nocturnal oxygen therapy in chronic obstructive pulmonary disease patients. Eur Respir J. 1999;14:1002–8.
38. Lewis CA, Fergusson W, Eaton T, Zeng I, Kolbe J. Isolated nocturnal desaturation in COPD: prevalence and impact on quality of life and sleep. Thorax. 2009;64:133–8.
39. Chaouat A, Weitzenblum E, Krieger J, Ifoundza T, Oswald M, Kessler R. Association of chronic obstructive pulmonary disease and sleep apnea syndrome. Am J Respir Crit Care Med. 1995;151:82–6.
40. Marin JM, Soriano JB, Carrizo SJ, Boldova A, Celli BR. Outcomes in patients with chronic obstructive pulmonary disease and obstructive sleep apnea. The overlap syndrome. Am J Respir Crit Care Med. 2010;182:325–31.
41. Cottin V, Nunes H, Brillet P-Y, Delaval P, Devouassoux G. I. Tillie-Leblond I, et al. Combined pulmonary fibrosis and emphysema: a distinct underrecognised entity. Eur Respir J. 2005;26:586–93.
42. Weitzenblum E, Chaouat A, Kessler R. Long-term oxygen therapy in stable COPD. In: Similowski T, Whitelaw WA, Derenne J, editors. Clinical management of chronic obstructive pulmonary disease. New York: Marcel Dekker; 2002. p. 781–812.
43. Selinger SR, Kennedy TP, Buescher P, Terry P, Parham W, Gofreed D, et al. Effects of removing oxygen from patients with chronic obstructive pulmonary disease. Am Rev Respir Dis. 1987;136:85–91.
44. Köhnlein T, Windisch W, Köhler D, Drabik A, Geiseler J, Hartl S, et al. Non-invasive positive pressure ventilation for the treatment of severe stable chronic obstructive pulmonary disease: a prospective, multicenter, randomized, controlled clinical trial. Lancet Respir Med. 2014;2:698–705.
45. Palwai A, Skowronski M, Coreno A, Drummond C, McFadden Jr ER. Critical comparisons of the clinical performance of oxygen-conserving devices. Am J Respir Crit Care Med. 2010;181:1061–71.
46. Lobato SD, Alises SM. Mobility profiles of patients with home oxygen therapy. Arch Bronconeumol. 2012;48:55–60.
47. Garcia-Aymerich J, Monsó E, Marrades RM, Escarrabill J, Félez MA, Sunyer J, et al. Risk factors for hospitalization for a chronic obstructive pulmonary disease excacerbation EFRAM study. Am J Respir Crit Care Med. 2001;164:1002–7.
48. Rice KL, Dewan N, Bloomfield HE, Grill J, Schult TM, Nelson DB, et al. Disease management program for chronic obstructive pulmonary disease. A randomized controlled trial. Am J Respir Crit Care Med. 2010;182:890–6.
49. Gong Jr H. Air travel and oxygen therapy in cardiopulmonary patients. Chest. 1992;101:1104–13.

Chapter 12
Bronchodilators for COPD: At What Stage Should Therapeutic Intervention Be Initiated?

Takashige Kuraki

Abstract Pharmacologic therapy for COPD is used to reduce symptoms, reduce the frequency and severity of exacerbations, and improve health status and exercise tolerance. Medications that increase the FEV_1 or change other spirometric variables, usually by altering airway smooth muscle tone, are termed bronchodilators, since the improvements in expiratory flow reflect widening of the airways rather than changes in lung elastic recoil. Such medications improve emptying of the lungs, tend to reduce dynamic hyperinflation at rest and during exercise, and improve exercise performance. The extent of these changes, especially in severe and very severe patients, is not easily predictable from the improvement in FEV_1. This chapter will describe some of the information that support the use of mono- or combined bronchodilator therapy in patients with COPD.

Keywords COPD • Bronchodilator

12.1 Introduction: The Physiological Rationale for Using Bronchodilators

Medications that increase the FEV_1 or change other spirometric variables, usually by altering airway smooth muscle tone, are termed bronchodilators, since the improvements in expiratory flow reflect widening of the airways rather than changes in lung elastic recoil. Such medications improve emptying of the lungs, tend to reduce dynamic hyperinflation at rest and during exercise, and improve exercise performance [1].

A schematic description of the innervation of the airways is fundamental for understanding how bronchodilators work and why they have clinical utility. Airway tone is mainly controlled by the vagus nerve, and the parasympathetic nerves

T. Kuraki (✉)
Shimane Prefectural Central Hospital, 4-1-1 Himebara, Izumo-shi, Shimane 693-8555, Japan
e-mail: kuraki@spch.izumo.shimane.jp

H. Nakamura, K. Aoshiba (eds.), *Chronic Obstructive Pulmonary Disease*, Respiratory Disease Series: Diagnostic Tools and Disease Managements,
DOI 10.1007/978-981-10-0839-9_12

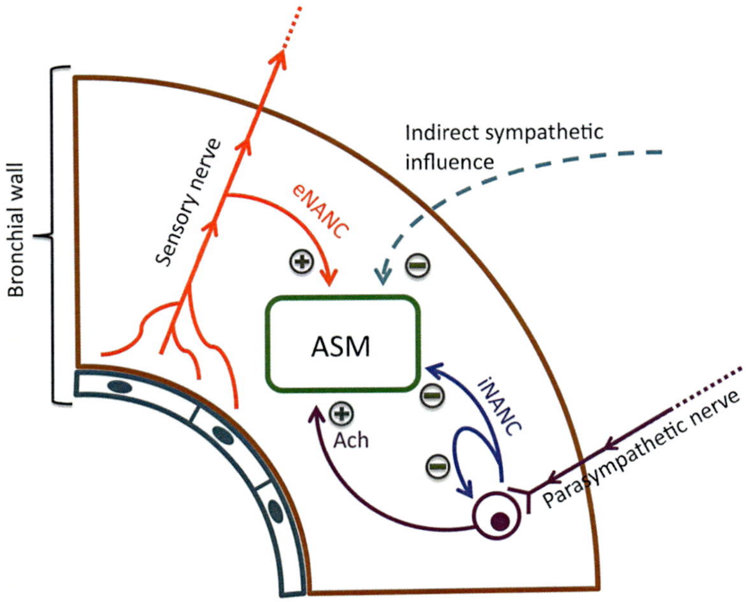

Fig. 12.1 Neural regulation of bronchial tone[2]. *eNANC* excitatory NANC, *Ach* acetylcholine. (Ref : Cazzola M, Pharmacol Rev 2012, 64:450–504.)

carried in the vagus nerve are tonically active, producing a stable, readily reversible baseline tone of the airway smooth muscle (ASM) (Fig. 12.1).

12.1.1 Cholinergic Pathway

Acetylcholine (ACh) is the "classic" neurotransmitter of the parasympathetic nervous system at both the level of ganglionic transmission and the neuroeffector junctions. ACh acts via activation of muscarinic receptors (mAChRs) that belong to the large seven-transmembrane family of G protein-coupled receptors (GPCRs). Five different subtypes of mAChRs have been identified by molecular biological techniques (M_1–M_5), but so far, a sufficient pharmacological and functional characterization has been provided for only four of them (M_1–M_4) [3]. The mAChRs are expressed in almost every cell type of the airway and lung tissue, including airway and vascular smooth muscle, different glandular and surface epithelial cells, endothelial cells, and various inflammatory cells. In humans, M_1 mAChRs seem to be expressed particularly in peripheral lung tissue and in the alveolar wall, but they have not been detected in larger airways, where M_2 and M_3 mAChRs represent the major population of mAChRs. Under "physiological" conditions, the ASM contraction induced by ACh is mediated primarily via the M_3 subtype. M_2 mAChRs couple to adenylyl cyclase via Gi in an inhibitory manner. They functionally oppose the β-AR-mediated increase in cAMP, leading to attenuation of β-AR-induced relaxation of ASM and prevent activation of Ca_2-dependent K (KCa) channels [2, 3].

12.1.2 *Adrenergic Pathway*

β-ARs are present in high concentration in lung tissue, and autoradiographic mapping and in situ hybridization studies show that they are localized to several cell types. β-ARs are subdivided into three types: β_1, β_2, and β_3. They are members of the seven-transmembrane spanning family of GPCRs related to bacteriorhodopsin and are composed of 413 amino acid residues. There is a 65–70 % homology between β_1/ β_3- and β_2-ARs. Binding studies show that approximately 70 % of pulmonary β-ARs are of the β_2-AR subtype. These receptors are localized to ASM (3–4/10^4 per cell), epithelium, vascular smooth muscle, and submucosal glands [4], whereas β1-ARs in the lung are confined to glands and alveoli. There is a uniform distribution of β-ARs on the alveolar wall with a 2:1 ratio of β_1/ β_2-ARs. β_2-AR density increases with increasing airway generation, and high levels are found in the alveolar region. Computed tomography scanning has confirmed that β_2-AR distribution is greater for small rather than large airways. β_2-ARs are also expressed on many proinflammatory and immune cells, including mast cells, macrophages, neutrophils, lymphocytes, eosinophils, epithelial and endothelial cells, and type I and type II alveolar cells [2].

GPCRs are dynamic proteins that switch between an inactive state and an active conformation that can engage G proteins (Fig. 12.2). Persistent activation of a GPCR is achieved through the binding of both an agonist and a G protein at opposite ends of the receptors relative to the lipid bilayer, where the combined binding interactions reduce the energy barriers to the formation of the active state. β_2-ARs are coupled to Gs, where stimulation by a β_2-AR agonist activates adenylyl cyclase and increases cAMP levels. cAMP increases protein kinase A (PKA) activity, which phosphorylates downstream protein modulators. The overall activation of this signal transduction pathway can lead to the inhibition of phosphoinositol hydrolysis, a fall in intracellular Ca_2 levels, and the activation of large-conductance K channels. The hyperpolarization of airway smooth muscle as a result of opening K channels can lead to relaxation of airway smooth muscle. β_2-AR stimulation produces airway relaxation, but prolonged β_2-AR activation leads to a decrease in receptor responsiveness that differs depending on the cell type but is more readily demonstrable in inflammatory cells than ASM [5].

12.1.3 *Non-adrenergic Non-cholinergic Pathway*

Autonomic neural control of ASM tone cannot be fully explained by the functions of the cholinergic and adrenergic nervous systems alone [6]. For example, striking

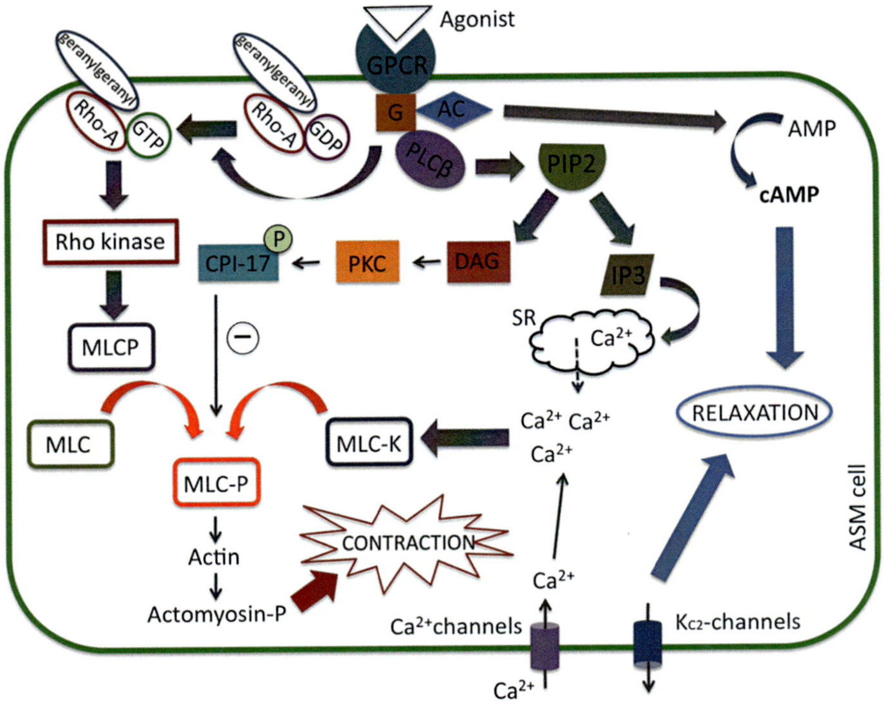

Fig. 12.2 Main intracellular pathways involved in the bronchomotor tone regulation [2]
PLC phospholipase C-, *PIP2* phosphatidylinositol 4,5-bisphosphate, *IP3* inositol 1,4,5-trisphosphate, *DAG* diacylglycerol, *SR* sarcoplasmic reticulum, *MLCK* myosin light-chain kinase, *MLC* myosin light chain, *MLC-P* myosin light-chain phosphorylation, *CPI-17* C kinase-potentiated phosphatase inhibitor, *Rho kinase* Rho-associated serine/threonine kinase, *AC* adenylyl cyclase(Ref : Cazzola M, Pharmacol Rev 2012, 64:450–504.)

changes in ASM tone can be induced even in the presence of an anticholinergic agent (atropine) and a β-AR antagonist (propranolol). There is substantial evidence of contractile and relaxant NANC smooth muscle responses in mammalian airways. In fact, inhibitory NANC (iNANC) innervation is considered the primary neural mechanism mediating ASM relaxation. iNANC relaxation is thought to be generated by a combined effect of vasoactive intestinal peptide (VIP), VIP structure-related peptides (e.g., peptide histidine methionine), and nitric oxide (NO). Indeed, VIP, VIP-like peptides, and NO synthase have been identified in the parasympathetic ganglia and nerve fibers innervating ASM. Furthermore, endogenously released VIP-like and NO-like substances can attenuate ASM contraction induced by ACh. However, the precise anatomical pathways of iNANC innervation of human ASM are not clear. There is also a potent excitatory effect on the ASM involving the "efferent" functions of a specific subtype of bronchopulmonary sensory nerves containing tachykinins (e.g., substance P and neurokinin A) in guinea pig airways, although this is less evident in human airways. When these afferent endings are activated, the impulses trigger the release of tachykinins either locally or propagating antidromically to other peripheral branches via the axonal ramifications. These sensory neuropeptides can activate neurokinin-1 and -2 receptors located on the ASM membrane and produce intense and sustained bronchoconstriction [2, 7].

12.2 Muscarinic Acetylcholine Receptor Antagonists

12.2.1 History

Inhaled mAChR antagonists have been used as treatments for respiratory diseases for centuries. The smoking of plant alkaloids was recommended as a therapy for asthma in the literature of Ayurvedic medicine as early as the seventeenth century. *Atropa belladonna* and *Datura stramonium* are rich in anticholinergic alkaloids such as atropine and stramonium [8]. Unfortunately, atropine, which is a tertiary ammonium compound, is well absorbed into the systemic circulation and penetrates the blood–brain barrier. As a result, it has multiple systemic side effects that limit its clinical usefulness. However, a renewed interest in anticholinergic drugs as therapy for respiratory diseases has been sparked by the development of safe yet effective quaternary anticholinergic compounds (Fig. 12.3). Chemical modifications of the atropine molecule, in particular by making its nitrogen atom pentavalent, have yielded a number of synthetic congeners that are very poorly absorbed from mucosae and cross the blood–brain barrier with difficulty. When given by inhalation, these agents are as effective as atropine at improving lung function but longer acting and much less prone to side effects [9].

12.2.2 Short-Acting Muscarinic Acetylcholine Receptor Antagonists

As well as atropine methonitrate, ipratropium bromide and oxitropium bromide are effective short-acting quaternary anticholinergic drugs that have been used in the treatment of respiratory diseases. Their duration of action is approximately 6–8 h, but compared with SABAs, they have a slower onset of action, although probably a longer duration of action [9].

12.2.2.1 Atropine Methonitrate

Atropine methonitrate, a quaternary ammonium congener of atropine, seems to be a more potent bronchodilator agent than its parent compound, atropine sulfate. In patients with asthma, atropine methonitrate produces a peak bronchodilator effect

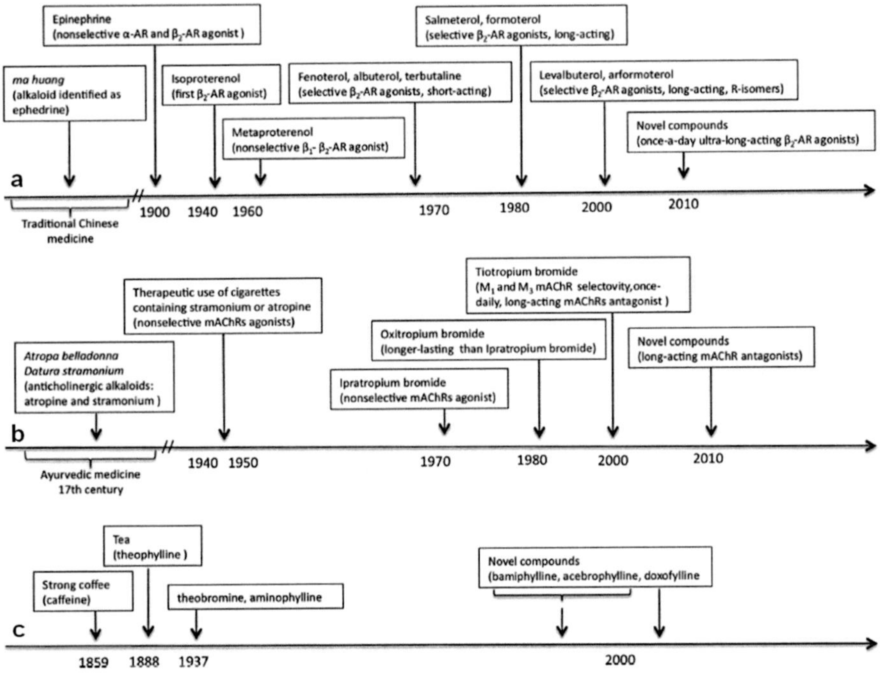

Fig. 12.3 Milestone development of β_2-AR agonists (**a**), antimuscarinics (**b**), and xanthines (**c**) (Ref : Cazzola M, Pharmacol Rev 2012, 64:450–504.) [2]

similar to that of albuterol, both administered in doses that produced close to maximum bronchodilation for the drug concerned, but the effect of atropine is more prolonged, the response being significantly greater at 4 and 6 h than with albuterol [10].

12.2.2.2 Ipratropium Bromide

Ipratropium bromide is unlike atropine; it has low lipid solubility and does not pass the blood–brain barrier. Ipratropium bromide is poorly absorbed by the oral and nasal mucosa, and the swallowed drug is poorly absorbed from the gastrointestinal tract. It is a nonselective antagonist of M_1, M_2, and M_3 mAChRs. Serum ipratropium bromide concentrations are extremely low after inhalation of the drug, peak serum concentrations being achieved at approximately 3 h after administration. The elimination half-life is 3.2–3.8 h, and ipratropium metabolites have little or no anticholinergic activity. Ipratropium bromide starts to act within 15–30 min, but maximal bronchodilation may take up to 90 min in patients with COPD. The duration of action is approximately 6 h, so in comparison with β_2-AR agonists, its broncholytic effect is slower in onset and probably longer in duration.

On the basis of the duration of action, ipratropium bromide is given four times daily, and the maximum number of doses (40 μg) per day should not exceed 12 [11].

12.2.2.3 Oxitropium Bromide

Oxitropium bromide is another quaternary anticholinergic compound but is based on the scopolamine molecule instead of atropine. The peak bronchodilation of oxitropium bromide may take 60–90 min, and its duration is 5–8 h. Oxitropium bromide is considered to have twice the strength of ipratropium bromide per dose. In patients with severe COPD, the FEV_1 and forced vital capacity (FVC) plateau attained at a total cumulative dose of 600 μg of oxitropium bromide was slightly higher than the plateau achieved with 280 μg of ipratropium bromide [12].

12.2.3 Long-Acting Muscarinic Acetylcholine Receptor Antagonists

12.2.3.1 Tiotropium Bromide

Tiotropium bromide is a once-daily, long-acting mAChR antagonist (LAMA) with high potency and kinetic selectivity at the mAChRs. It displays a 6- to 20-fold higher affinity for mAChRs than does ipratropium bromide. Although tiotropium bromide binds to all three mAChRs, it dissociates much faster from the M_2 mAChRs, which results in a more selective antagonist action for M_1 and M_3 mAChR subtypes. Its prolonged pharmacologic activity is the result of its slow dissociation from M_1 and M_3 mAChRs. The half-life of the tiotropium bromide M_3 mAChR complex is approximately 35 h, compared with 0.3 h for ipratropium bromide. The mechanism allowing for the long residency of tiotropium bromide at M_3 mAChRs is not completely known. The increased duration of binding at the M_3 mAChRs results in prolonged improvement in lung function, allowing a once-daily dose compared with the three to four doses per day previously necessary with ipratropium bromide. Tiotropium bromide is rapidly absorbed into the circulation with a peak plasma concentration within 5 min followed by a rapid fall within an hour to a steady state and a terminal half-life of 5–6 days that is independent of dose. The peak onset of bronchodilation with tiotropium bromide occurs between 1 and 3 h with improvements in FEV1 for more than 24 h [13].

12.2.3.2 Glycopyrronium Bromide

Glycopyrronium bromide is a mAChR antagonist that has a dissociation half-life from the human M_3 mAChR that is significantly shorter than tiotropium bromide or aclidinium bromide. In line with this finding, in isolated human bronchi, glycopyrronium bromide elicits a duration of action intermediate between that produced by tiotropium bromide and that of ipratropium bromide. Clinical studies have shown that glycopyrronium bromide has a fast onset of effect that is sustained over 24 h, although another recent study with nebulized glycopyrronium bromide shows that this was probably shorter acting, at least at doses below 50 μg. The safety and efficacy of glycopyrronium bromide have been documented in patients with moderate-to-severe COPD. Glycopyrronium bromide is well tolerated at doses of up to 100 μg in this patient population [14].

12.2.3.3 Aclidinium Bromide

Preclinical studies have demonstrated that aclidinium bromide exhibits M_3/M_2 mAChR kinetic selectivity. This mAChR antagonist dissociates from humanM_3 mAChRs at a rate that was similar to that of ipratropium bromide and 2.6 times faster than that of tiotropium bromide. On the contrary, it dissociates from the same receptors slightly faster than tiotropium bromide and, in line with these findings, is equivalent to ipratropium bromide for speed of onset but with a longer duration. However, in human isolated bronchi, aclidinium bromide has a faster onset and shorter duration of action than tiotropium bromide [15]. Aclidinium bromide has the advantage of rapid hydrolytic inactivation once absorbed into the plasma, thereby enhancing its safety profile.

12.2.3.4 Umeclidinium Bromide

This agent umeclidinium is a novel high-affinity-specific mAChR antagonist. It has similar affinity to the subtypes of muscarinic receptors M_1–M_5. In the airways, it is a potent agent that demonstrates slow functional reversibility at cloned humanM_3 mAChRs and at endogenous mAChR in isolated human bronchus. The competitive and reversible nature of antagonism was shown with human and animal origin receptors and isolated organ preparations. In preclinical in vitro as well as in vivo studies, prevention of methacholine- and acetylcholine-induced bronchoconstrictive effects was dose dependent and lasted longer than 24 h. The clinical relevance of these findings is unknown. The bronchodilation following inhalation of umeclidinium is predominantly a site-specific effect [16].

12.2.4 Novel Long-Acting Muscarinic Acetylcholine Receptor Antagonists

Several other mAChR antagonists are also under development. Unfortunately, the available public information on these bronchodilators is still limited. New agents like CHF 5407, inhaled trospium (ALKS27), and PF-4522971 are under development in 2016 now [2].

12.2.5 Oral Muscarinic Acetylcholine Receptor Antagonists

It is believed that oral anticholinergics are not a treatment option for COPD because of unacceptable side effects [11], whereas inhaled anticholinergics have virtually no systemic absorption. Mepenzolate bromide is one of the oral anticholinergics but has high affinity to M_3 muscarinic acetylcholine receptor and is under redevelopment of COPD.

12.2.6 Side Effects

Anticholinergic drugs are poorly absorbed which limits the troublesome systemic effects seen with atropine. But all of the currently approved inhaled mAChR antagonists have a very wide therapeutic margin and are very well tolerated, in part because they are very poorly absorbed after inhalation. However, if any of these agents makes inadvertent contact with the eye, they can cause papillary dilation.

In older men, who may have prostatic hyperplasia, mAChR antagonists should be used with caution because they can cause urinary retention. Men using both short- and long-acting inhaled mAChR antagonists had a significantly higher risk of acute urinary retention compared with nonusers. Patients with moderate-to-severe renal impairment (creatinine clearance of $<$ 50 ml/min) under treatment with tiotropium bromide should be closely monitored, because tiotropium bromide is predominantly excreted by the kidneys through active secretion.

Paradoxical bronchoconstriction to ipratropium bromide has been reported in humans. It is possible that this results from blockade of prejunctional M_2 mAChRs on airway cholinergic nerves, which normally inhibit ACh release; when the drug is given by nebulizer, however, it is largely explained by the hypotonicity of the nebulizer solution. Paradoxical bronchoconstriction may also occur with other mAChR antagonists.

Concerns have been raised about possible associations of mAChR antagonists with cardiovascular morbidity and mortality. However, the results of the UPLIFT trial and a robust and extensive analysis of more than 19,000 patients participating in placebo-controlled clinical trials with tiotropium bromide indicate that there is no real increased risk for death or cardiovascular morbidity during treatment with this inhaled anticholinergic agent in patients with COPD [13, 17, 18].

12.3 β-Adrenergic Receptor Agonists

12.3.1 History

In traditional Chinese medicine, the botanical ma huang (the plant *Ephedra equisetina*), from which the active material, an alkaloid identified as ephedrine, is extracted, was used for more than 2000 years for the short-term treatment of respiratory symptoms. Beginning at the turn of the last century, the nonselective α-AR and β-AR agonist epinephrine was introduced into clinical practice and administered by the subcutaneous route for the treatment of acute asthma [19]. In the 1940s, the nonselective β-AR agonist isoproterenol was introduced for the treatment of airway disease and became the standard-of-care bronchodilator, although its use was complicated by adverse effects that were due to activation of the β_1-AR in the heart, which elicits tachycardia and predisposes patients to cardiac dysrhythmias. Metaproterenol, a noncatechol resorcinol derivative of isoproterenol, was subsequently developed in the early 1960s. It was an effective bronchodilator when inhaled but also did not discriminate between β_1- and β_2-ARs and thus produced cardiac side effects [20].

The noncatecholamine β_2-AR agonists such as fenoterol, albuterol, and terbutaline differ in their substitutions in the amine group and benzene ring. These structural modifications, conferring resistance to metabolism by COMT, result in a longer half-life and also reduce their potency for β_1-ARs, making them relatively more selective for β_2-ARs (Fig. 12.3). A major limitation of the β_2-AR agonists in use during the 1960s and 1970s was their short duration of action, typically 4 to 6 h. Therefore, the next advance in the development of β_2-AR agonists was the development of the long-acting drugs salmeterol and formoterol, the duration of action of which is approximately 12 h, which made their use for maintenance treatment. A pure *R*-isomer of albuterol, levalbuterol, and the *R*,*R*-enantiomer of formoterol, arformoterol, have been developed. It is claimed that they have a better safety profile than the racemic mixture because they do not have the *S*-enantiomer, which, at least for (*S*)-albuterol, is now known to have unwanted effects in the lung. At present, several once-a-day ultra-long-acting β_2-AR agonists are in different stages of clinical development [2].

12.3.2 Short-Acting Agents

The principal action of β_2-agonists is to relax airway smooth muscle by stimulating β_2-AR, which increases cyclic AMP and produces functional antagonism to bronchoconstriction. The bronchodilator effects of short-acting β_2-agonists usually wear off within 4–6 h. Regular and as-needed use of short-acting β-agonists improve FEV_1 and symptoms. There is little difference in the time course of fenoterol, albuterol, and terbutaline, although there is some evidence that fenoterol might have a slightly longer duration of action. The use of high doses of short-acting β_2-agonists on an as-needed basis in patients already treated with long-acting bronchodilators is not supported by evidence, may be limited by side effects, and cannot be recommended. For single-dose, as-needed use in COPD, there appears to be no advantage in using levalbuterol over conventional bronchodilators [1, 21].

12.3.3 Long-Acting β2-Adrenergic Receptor Agonists

Long-acting inhaled β_2-AR agonists show duration of action of 12 or more hours [22]. The duration of action of β_2-AR agonists in the human bronchus is in the following order: salmeterol >> formoterol > albuterol > terbutaline > fenoterol. Formoterol and salmeterol significantly improve FEV_1 and lung volumes, dyspnea, health-related quality of life, and exacerbation rate, but have no effect on mortality and rate of decline of lung function. A systematic review of trials of salmeterol and formoterol showed a significant reduction in the numbers of patients requiring treatment for exacerbations and the number requiring hospitalization [23, 24]. Salmeterol reduces the rate of hospitalization. Although formoterol and salmeterol are both potent and effective β_2-AR agonists, their different chemical structures confer markedly different pharmacological characteristics.

12.3.3.1 Formoterol

Formoterol is a full agonist of β_2-ARs and has been shown to provide a rapid-onset bronchodilating effect that occurs within minutes after inhalation. A number of studies have shown a comparable clinical effect of formoterol compared with the SABAs albuterol and terbutaline in stable patients with asthma [2]. But an oral formulation of formoterol did not seem to offer a clear advantage to albuterol. In effect, formoterol has a long duration of action when given by inhalation but not when given orally. A dose–response comparison of formoterol in patients with asthma suggested that after inhalation and 50 times more potent after oral administration [25].

12.3.3.2 Salmeterol

Salmeterol is a drug resulting from a specific research program designed to achieve prolonged duration of action by molecular modification of albuterol. Salmeterol is a partial agonist with ~60 and 85 % of the efficacy of isoprenaline, respectively. In contrast to its effects on β_2-ARs, at cardiac β_1-ARs, salmeterol is >10,000-fold weaker than isoprenaline and has a very low efficacy (4 %). The onset of action of salmeterol on ASM is slower than that of other β_2-AR agonists, such as albuterol and formoterol, but it seems to be inherently long acting, in that its effects are independent of concentration as a result of exosite binding, whereas albuterol, fenoterol, and formoterol have shorter durations of action, but this can be prolonged by increasing the concentration of the β_2-AR agonist applied to the tissue [26].

12.3.4 Ultra-Long-Acting β2-Adrenergic Receptor Agonists

A variety of β_2-AR agonists with longer half-lives are currently in development, with the hope of achieving once-daily dosing. These agents include indacaterol, olodaterol, vilanterol, carmoterol, PF-610355, and AZD-3199, the structure of which has not yet been disclosed.

12.3.4.1 Indacaterol

Indacaterol is the first ultra-long-acting β_2-agonist approved for the treatment of COPD that allows for once-daily administration. It is rapidly acting, with an onset of action in 5 min, like salbutamol and formoterol but with a sustained bronchodilator effect, that lasts for 24 h, like tiotropium. In long-term clinical studies in patients with moderate-to-severe COPD, once-daily indacaterol improved lung function significantly more than placebo, and improvements were significantly greater than twice-daily formoterol and noninferior to once-daily tiotropium bromide. Indacaterol was well tolerated at all doses and with a good overall safety profile. These findings suggest that indacaterol can be a first choice drug in the treatment of the patient with mild/moderate stable COPD [27].

12.3.4.2 Olodaterol

Olodaterol is a new long-acting β_2-agonist for COPD. Olodaterol statistically significantly improved lung function in people with moderate to very severe COPD compared with placebo over 24 weeks and was not statistically significantly different from formoterol. Although olodaterol appears to improve lung function as well as formoterol, little evidence is available comparing it directly with other LABAs and LAMAs for COPD, particularly in terms of patient-oriented outcomes such as exacerbations, breathlessness, and quality of life. Olodaterol was often coadministered with tiotropium and ICS and only limited data support its use alone [28].

12.3.4.3 Vilanterol

Vilanterol is a potent, selective β_2-AR agonist in human functional cellular assays. Vilanterol produced rapid bronchodilation in patients with COPD that was maintained over 24 h at all doses. After dosing with vilanterol, there were no serious adverse events or withdrawals due to adverse events. Vilanterol in patients with COPD significantly improved FEV_1 in a dose-dependent manner. Clinically relevant treatment differences of >130 ml in mean FEV_1 were observed. Clinical doses of vilanterol were associated with a low incidence of treatment-related side effects. Vilanterol was often co-administered with umeclidinium and ICS, and only limited data support its use alone [29].

12.3.4.4 Carmoterol

Carmoterol has been demonstrated to be a highly potent and selective β_2-AR agonist. Carmoterol has a similar onset of action compared with albuterol and formoterol and a faster onset of action compared with salmeterol. The duration of tracheal smooth muscle relaxation is longer for carmoterol compared with both formoterol and salmeterol. In COPD, a single use of carmoterol had an effect on 24 h trough FEV_1 that was better than that of two uses of salmeterol given 12 h apart. After a 2-week treatment period, once-daily doses of 2 and 4 μg of carmoterol resulted in placebo-adjusted improvements compared with baseline in trough FEV_1 of 94 and 112 ml [30].

12.3.4.5 LAS100977, PF-610355, and AZD-3199

Abediterol (LAS100977), PF-610355, and AZD-3199 are novel, selective, potent, once-daily LABA in development for treatment of asthma and chronic obstructive pulmonary disease.

12.3.5 Intravenous β2-Adrenergic Receptor Agonists

An interesting new option is the development of a β_2-AR agonist to be administered intravenously. Bedoradrine (MN-221) is a novel, highly selective β_2-adrenoceptor agonist under development for the treatment of acute exacerbation of asthma and COPD. A preliminary small trial showed that bedoradrine added to standard therapy for severe acute asthma exacerbations was safe and provided additional clinical benefit [31].

In a small group of patients with COPD, bedoradrine seemed to improve lung function at all dose levels and reached statistical significance at both 500 and 1200 μg compared with placebo [32].

12.3.6 Transdermal β2-Adrenergic Receptor Agonists

Tulobuterol is the first bronchodilator to be available as a transdermal patch. This drug delivery system ensures that the time at which the peak drug concentration in the blood is reached coincides with the morning dip in respiratory function. The use of the patch also prevents excessive increase in blood drug concentrations, thereby reducing the incidence of systemic adverse reactions. But the efficacy and potentials are not fully recognized, and the tulobuterol patch has been used in the limited regions in the world [33].

12.3.7 Side Effects of β2-Adrenergic Receptor Agonists

Stimulation of β_2-AR can produce resting sinus tachycardia and has the potential to precipitate cardiac rhythm disturbances in susceptible patients, although these seem to have remarkably few clinical implications. Exaggerated somatic tremor is troublesome in some older patients treated with higher doses of β_2-agonists, whatever the route of administration, and this limits the dose that can be tolerated. Although hypokalemia can occur, especially when treatment is combined with thiazide diuretics [34], and oxygen consumption can be increased under resting conditions [35], these metabolic effects show tachyphylaxis unlike the bronchodilator actions. Mild falls in PaO_2 can occur after administration of both short- and long-acting β_2-agonists, but the clinical significance of these changes is doubtful. Despite the concerns raised some years ago related to β_2-agonists in the management of asthma, further detailed study has found no association between β_2-agonist use and an accelerated loss of lung function or increased mortality in COPD [1].

12.4 Methylxanthines

12.4.1 History

One of the earliest reports of the efficacy of methylxanthines in asthma was published in 1859, where Henry Hyde Salter, himself an asthmatic, described his experience that "one of the commonest and best reputed remedies of asthma… is strong coffee." The first analysis of a xanthine derivative extracted from tea leaves was accomplished by Kossel, who was able to extract not only caffeine but also another xanthine derivative, a dimethylxanthine. The name theophylline was then applied to a compound that has two methyl groups (1,3-dimethylxanthine) (Fig. 12.3). Until 1930, xanthine derivatives were used in clinical practice only because of their diuretic and cardiotonic properties. Years later, a combination of theophylline and aminophylline was used intravenously as an effective bronchodilator in acute asthma. Since then, several other xanthines have been synthesized and are used clinically in various parts of the world [2].

12.4.2 Aminophylline

Aminophylline is the ethylenediamine salt of theophylline with higher solubility at a neutral pH. In vivo intravenous aminophylline has an acute bronchodilator effect in patients with asthma that is most likely to be due to a relaxant effect on ASM. Aminophylline also increases diaphragmatic contractility and reverses diaphragm fatigue. However, side effects such as nausea and vomiting are common, and the benefit/risk ratio is unknown. Aminophylline is also widely used for the treatment of acute exacerbations of COPD despite a lack of evidence to support this practice. It remains possible that aminophylline confers a small but clinically significant benefit when added to standard therapy. However, it was unable to find evidence for any clinically important additional effect of aminophylline treatment when used with high-dose nebulized bronchodilators and oral corticosteroids in patients with nonacidotic COPD exacerbations [36].

12.4.3 Theophylline

Theophylline, the most commonly used methylxanthine, is metabolized by cytochrome P450 mixed-function oxidases. Clearance of the drug declines with age. Many other physiological variables and drugs modify theophylline metabolism. Changes in inspiratory muscle function have been reported in patients treated with theophylline, but whether this reflects changes in spirometry or a primary effect on the muscle is not clear. Despite its extensive use in the treatment of respiratory disease, the precise molecular actions of theophylline have not been fully elucidated. Its efficacy in the treatment of patients with COPD or asthma has traditionally been attributed to nonselective phosphodiesterase (PDE) inhibition, resulting in an increase in cAMP by inhibition of PDE_3 and PDE_4 and an increase in cGMP by inhibition of PDE_5. All studies that have shown efficacy of theophylline in COPD were performed with slow-release preparations.

Theophylline is less effective and less well tolerated than inhaled long-acting bronchodilators and is not recommended if those drugs are available and affordable. However, there is evidence for a modest bronchodilator effect compared with placebo in stable COPD. There is also some evidence of symptomatic benefit compared to placebo. Addition of theophylline to salmeterol produced a greater improvement in FEV_1 and breathlessness than salmeterol alone. Low-dose theophylline reduces exacerbations but does not improve post-bronchodilator lung function [37, 38].

Theophylline can also act as a respiratory stimulant. Moreover, theophylline is able to improve diaphragmatic contractility and has anti-inflammatory properties. There is good evidence for inhibitory effects of theophylline on airway inflammation in patients with asthma and COPD, and these effects are seen at plasma concentrations below 10 mg/l [39].

12.4.4 Novel Xanthine

The positive clinical effects of theophylline in airway disease, combined with its advantageous oral bioavailability, has spurred the development of other xanthines, such as bamifylline, acebrophylline, and doxofylline, for the treatment of respiratory disease, with the anticipation that such drugs would have greater efficacy than theophylline but with an improved side effect profile.

12.4.5 Side Effects

Toxicity is dose related, a particular problem with the xanthine derivatives because their therapeutic ratio is small and most of the benefit occurs only when near-toxic doses are given. Methylxanthines are nonspecific inhibitors of all phosphodiesterase enzyme subsets, which explains their wide range of toxic effects. Problems include the development of atrial and ventricular arrhythmias (which can prove fatal) and grand mal convulsions (which can occur irrespective of prior epileptic history). Other side effects include headaches, insomnia, nausea, and heartburn, and these may occur within the therapeutic range of serum theophylline. These medications also have significant interactions with commonly used medications such as digitalis, Coumadin, etc. Unlike the other bronchodilator classes, xanthine derivatives may involve a risk of overdose (either intentional or accidental) [1].

12.5 Novel Classes of Bronchodilators

Novel classes of bronchodilators have proved difficult to develop, but there is still a continued interest in generating new classes of bronchodilators that act via emerging targets, particularly given the recent concerns over the selective phosphodiesterase inhibitors.

There are some pathways to release the ASM constriction like K channel openers, VIP analogs, Rho kinase inhibitors, neuropeptides, and NO donors (Fig. 12.2).

12.5.1 *Selective Phosphodiesterase Inhibitors*

The principal action of selective phosphodiesterase-4 inhibitors is to reduce inflammation by inhibiting of the breakdown of intracellular cyclic AMP. It is a once-daily oral medication with no direct bronchodilator activity, although it has been shown to improve FEV_1 in patients treated with salmeterol or tiotropium [40, 41].

Roflumilast reduces moderate and severe exacerbations treated with corticosteroids by 15–20 % in patients with chronic bronchitis, severe to very severe COPD, and a history of exacerbations. The effects on lung function are also seen when roflumilast is added to long-acting bronchodilators. There are no direct comparisons or add-on studies of roflumilast and inhaled corticosteroids. Phosphodiesterase-4 inhibitors should always be used in combination with at least one long-acting bronchodilator.

As an alternative to oral administration, a number of groups are now investigating the topical application of PDE4 inhibitors as a possible way to improve their efficacy in the treatment of inflammatory airway diseases while minimizing side effects. A non-emetic mixed PDE3/PDE4 has already successfully undergone a number of phase 2 clinical trials in patients with either COPD or asthma. And there are also some recent pilot data showing that PDE5 inhibitors such as sildenafil can have bronchodilator activities.

12.5.2 *Other Types of Bronchodilators*

12.5.2.1 K_ Channel Openers

In ASM cells, K channels, such as large-conductance, voltage-dependent Ca_2-activated K channels (K_{Ca}), or the ATP-dependent K potassium channels (K_{ATP}), play an important role in modulating contractile activity. Activation of these channels will cause cell hyperpolarization that should oppose Ca_2 entry through voltage-dependent Ca_2 channels, leading to smooth muscle relaxation. Consequently, K channel modulators may be of value in the treatment of chronic airway disorders. However, K_{ATP} openers, although effective in relaxing human airways in vitro, are not effective in treating asthma or COPD because they are more potent as vasodilators, which limits the dose that can be administered safely [42].

12.5.2.2 Vasoactive Intestinal Peptide Analogs

VIP, one of the major peptide transmitters in the central and peripheral nervous systems, is abundantly present in the normal human lung, and VIP-immunoreactive nerves are found in the smooth muscle layer and glands of the airway and within the walls of pulmonary and bronchial vessels. The bronchodilatory effect of VIP in human bronchi is almost 100 times more potent than adrenergic dilation induced by isoproterenol. VIP is subject to degeneration by proteases present in the lung lining fluid [43]. As a consequence, several peptidase-resistant VIP analogs have been developed.

12.5.2.3 Rho Kinase Inhibitors

There is now substantial evidence that Rho kinase (RhoK) is involved in bronchoconstriction [44]. RhoK can modulate smooth muscle contraction by multiple mechanisms. Considering that Rho/RhoK signaling is thought to be involved in various processes that contribute to chronic airway diseases, the use of RhoK inhibitors in asthma and COPD therapy clearly holds promise. Inhibition of RhoK reduces contractile responses induced by spasmogens. Indeed, the RhoK inhibitor (Y-27632) has been shown to relax human isolated bronchial preparations. Several analogs of Y-27632 exist that have similarly high inhibitory constants for RhoK and similar smooth muscle relaxant properties.

12.5.2.4 Brain Natriuretic Peptide and Analogs

It is well known that the guanylyl cyclase/cGMP second messenger system has a parallel role to the adenylyl cyclase/cAMP system in ASM, regulating its contractile and proliferative functions. Therefore, it is not surprising that agents activating this signaling pathway bronchodilate in vivo and relax ASM in vitro [45]. Particulate guanylyl cyclases act as plasma membrane receptors for natriuretic and related peptides. Some of them serve as receptors for the natriuretic peptides, a family of peptides that includes atrial natriuretic peptide (ANP), brain natriuretic peptide (BNP), and C-type natriuretic peptide, three peptides known to play important roles in renal and cardiovascular physiology. There is evidence that ANP relaxes human ASM in vitro. Moreover, in humans, exogenous ANP reverses airway hyperresponsiveness when given intravenously or by inhalation in high doses.

12.5.2.5 Nitric Oxide Donors

Exogenous NO has the ability to exert bronchodilatory effects in patients with bronchial asthma [46], and NO has been used in the treatment of preterm children to improve lung capacity. The augmented availability of NO in the lungs may represent a plausible approach for the treatment of asthma and COPD. Nitrates, NO, and NO donors relax ASM in vitro and in guinea pigs and humans, and inhaled NO exerts bronchodilatory effects against methacholine-induced bronchoconstriction in vivo. Studies in bronchial and tracheal smooth muscle have shown that a major target of NO is the enzyme soluble guanylyl cyclase, although NO is also a very active agonist at inducing vascular smooth muscle relaxation. There is therefore a need for suitable NO donors that have minimal effects on the vasculature. The main prototypes of NO donors traditionally used, such as sodium nitroprusside and nitroglycerine, have several well-known adverse effects, such as rapid tachycardia, high toxicity, and rapid induction of tolerance. Likewise, sydnonimines, another well-known class of NO donor drugs, have a characteristically low therapeutic index (because of cyanide toxicity).

At present, a number of groups are designing and synthesizing various chemical compounds capable of modulating NO metabolism for therapeutic purposes that also possess an improved therapeutic index [47]. Specifically, various new classes of NO donors are under intense pharmacological investigation, each characterized by a particular PK and PD profile. The most important obstacle in the field of new NO donor drugs seems to be carefully targeting NO release to lungs at an optimal concentration to achieve a beneficial action and to limit possible adverse effects, particularly on the cardiovascular system.

NO budesonide and ruthenium complex (NO_3) are novel compounds, currently in development for the treatment of chronic respiratory disorders.

12.5.2.6 E-Prostanoid Receptor 4 Agonists

Inhaled prostaglandin E_2 (PGE_2) has been shown to be a bronchodilator in subjects with asthma or COPD. However, PGE_2 itself has the potential to cause the adverse effects of cough and retrosternal burning when inhaled by humans, particularly in subjects with asthma. Moreover, PGE_2 also stimulates other prostaglandin-like receptors having inhibitory and stimulatory activity on the intrinsic tone of the airway smooth muscle. PGE_2 acts predominantly via specific E-prostanoid (EP) receptors.

Whereas it has been established that PGE_2-induced sensory nerve activation and cough are mediated via the EP_3 receptor [48], the EP_4 receptor seems to be the predominant receptor responsible for PGE_2-induced relaxation of human ASM in vitro. Thus, highly potent EP_4 subtype-selective receptor agonists have been suggested to have therapeutic potential without side effects [49].

12.5.2.7 Bitter Taste Receptor Agonists

Bitter taste receptors work as chemoreceptors that interact with taste stimuli to initiate an afferent signal to the brain, where it becomes taste perception. Stimulation of the taste 2 receptors is responsible for the bitter taste. These receptors were recently found on airway smooth muscle. When activated, they caused relaxation through a calcium-dependent mechanism. Agonists to these receptors may make up a new class of useful direct bronchodilators for treating obstructive lung disease, but because they are members of the G protein-coupled receptor superfamily, they may undergo desensitization.

Saccharin, chloroquine, denatonium, aristolochic acid, strychnine, quinine, colchicine, and yohimbine were used in the preclinical studies. Aristolochic acid, strychnine, and yohimbine are probably too toxic to be considered for human use. Perhaps it is worth considering developing an inhalation preparation of quinine for testing in humans with asthma [50].

12.6 Combination Therapy

12.6.1 Pharmacologic Rationale for Combination

GOLD guidelines recommend combination therapy involving two long-acting bronchodilators with differing modes of action in patients whose COPD is not sufficiently controlled with monotherapy (Fig. 12.4). In fact, it seems reasonable to postulate that targeting bronchoconstriction through two distinct mechanisms should maximize the bronchodilator response and help to overcome inter- and intrapatient variability in bronchomotor tone associated with airway obstruction [51]. Moreover, combining two or more classes of molecules allows the use of lower doses to achieve the same efficacy while decreasing adverse effects. Combination therapy with a LABA and an ICS is considered an important approach for treating patients suffering from asthma and patients with severe COPD who have frequent exacerbations [52]. In addition, combination therapy with a LAMA and an ICS seems to be intriguing, although the clinical effects of such combination are largely unknown.

12.6.2 Combining β2-Adrenergic Receptor Agonists and Muscarinic Acetylcholine Receptor Antagonists

12.6.2.1 Pharmacologic Rationale

Airway tone is regulated by both the parasympathetic and sympathetic nervous systems. The complete nature of interactions between the two physiological systems is not yet fully understood, but there is enough evidence to suggest that combining β_2-AR agonists and mAChR antagonists is pharmacologically reasonable for two reasons. First, the addition of a β_2-AR agonist decreases the release of ACh through the modulation of cholinergic neurotransmission by prejunctional β_2-ARs and thereby amplifies the bronchial smooth muscle relaxation induced by the mAChR antagonist. Second, the addition of a mAChR antagonist can reduce bronchoconstrictor effects of ACh, the release of which has been modified by the β_2-AR agonist, and thereby amplify the bronchodilation elicited by the β_2-AR agonist through the direct stimulation of smooth muscle β_2-ARs [53]. Another possibility is the fact that the mAChR antagonist and not the β_2-AR agonist can

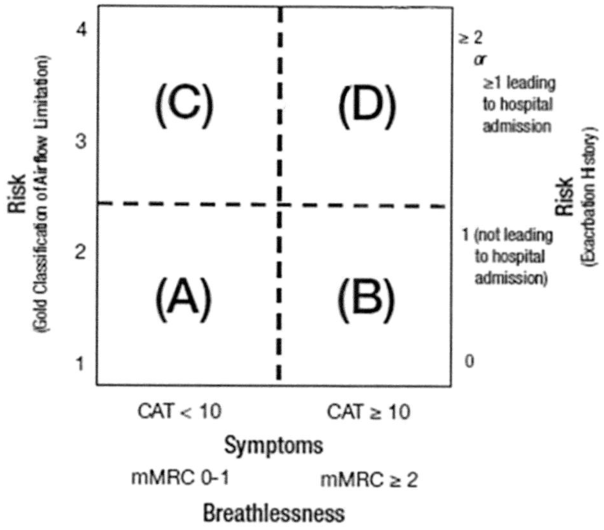

Patient Category	Characteristics	Spirometric Classification	Exacerbations per year	CAT	mMRC
A	Low Risk, Less Symptoms	GOLD 1-2	≤1	< 10	0-1
B	Low Risk, More Symptoms	GOLD 1-2	≤1	≥ 10	≥ 2
C	High Risk, Less Symptoms	GOLD 3-4	≥ 2	< 10	0-1
D	High Risk, More Symptoms	GOLD 3-4	≥ 2	≥ 10	≥ 2

Fig. 12.4 Model of symptom/risk of evaluation of COPD [1]
(From the Global Strategy for Diagnosis, Management, and Prevention of COPD 2016, Global Initiative for Chronic Obstructive Lung Disease (GOLD), http://www.goldcopd.org
COPD chronic obstructive lung disease, *GOLD* Global Initiative for Chronic Obstructive Lung Disease, *mMRC* modified Medical Research Council, *CAT* COPD Assessment Test)

suppress mucus/fluid secretions; hence, surface tension changes that would normally collapse the airways are less likely to occur [54].

12.6.2.2 Clinical Use

Fixed combinations of LABA/LAMA appeared to show a greater degree of improvement in trough FEV_1 when compared with the respective single components. Analysis of synergism on clinical indices including quality of life, exacerbation rates, and disease progression was not possible because dose–response relationships for the single-component drugs were not available, but carefully designed and sufficiently powered studies could help evaluate these missing important efficacy data. Therefore, while FEV_1 may be a relatively poor predicator of improvements in symptom scores, either the dose–response relationship for these phenomena is different or more sensitive measures of small airway caliber (e.g., forced oscillatory techniques) might offer greater predictability. It is therefore likely that the combination therapy provides a complimentary coverage of airway smooth muscle relaxation with a suppression of mucus secretions which benefits the patient provided this is not at the expense of more adverse effects [55]. It remains to be seen whether any purported synergy would allow a dose reduction of both component drugs while still affording clinical meaningful bronchodilation over a 24 h period.

Umeclidinium/vilanterol, glycopyrrolate/indacaterol, and aclidinium/formoterol (available in Canada) are dry-powder inhalers. Tiotropium/olodaterol is a soft mist inhaler. LABA/LAMA combination seems to play an important role in maximizing bronchodilation studies to date indicating that combining different classes of bronchodilators results in significantly greater improvements in lung function and other outcomes compared with individual drugs used alone and that these combinations are well tolerated in patients with moderate-to-severe COPD [56, 57].

12.6.3 Combining β2-Adrenergic Receptor Agonists and Inhaled Corticosteroids

The addition of LABA therapy with ICS has been suggested to improve the efficacy of ICS effects, and a number of molecular interactions between corticosteroids and β_2-ARs have been described [58].

The LABA/ICS combination is now increasingly recommended in patients with COPD because the addition of LABA to ICS provides additional benefits. Several large-scale studies in patients with moderate-to-severe COPD have demonstrated that treatment with salmeterol/fluticasone and formoterol/budesonide leads to significantly greater improvements in lung function, exacerbations, health status, and breathlessness compared with placebo or monotherapy with the component drugs. Compared with placebo, the LABA/ICS combination therapy leads to a significant reduction of a quarter in exacerbation rates. Compared with monocomponent ICS therapy, the LABA/ICS combination significantly reduces morbidity and mortality in COPD. There is a significant reduction in all-cause mortality with the addition of data from the Towards a Revolution in COPD Health (TORCH) study, although in the TORCH study regular treatment with salmeterol/fluticasone narrowly failed to demonstrate a statistically significant benefit on the reduction in all-cause mortality over 3 years [59]. In addition, in the TORCH study, the LABA/ICS combination reduced the rate of decline in FEV_1 in patients with moderate-to-severe COPD by 16 ml/year compared with placebo. However, this improvement was also observed in the LABA-only and ICS-only groups. Moreover, the superiority of combination inhalers should be viewed against the increased risk of side effects, particularly pneumonia in patients with COPD [60].

A next-generation, the ultra-LABA/ICS combination consisting of vilanterol and fluticasone furoate is another combination, had greater improvements than placebo in trough FEV_1 with a good safety and tolerability profile.

12.6.3.1 Combining Muscarinic Acetylcholine Receptor Antagonists and Inhaled Corticosteroids

Experimental evidence has also suggested an influence of corticosteroids on mAChRs, signifying the potential of a LAMA/ICS combination for the treatment of asthma and COPD.

Very few studies published to date have been designed specifically to evaluate the effect of LAMA and ICS combinations on clinical outcomes, and this is an area that warrants future study. Treatment with tiotropium bromide and budesonide in patients with COPD has led to significant improvements in the quality-of-life status according to SGRQ, measuring both dyspnea and lung function, and a reduction of the number of exacerbations of treatment in patients with COPD and chronic asthma [61].

12.6.4 Triple Combination Therapies

Triple therapy with LAMA plus LABA/ICS has also been investigated, demonstrating benefits over monotherapy on lung function. Additionally, a pilot study of patients with advanced COPD reported that triple therapy combined with pulmonary rehabilitation provided a benefit in terms of lung function. Some reports also suggest that triple therapy can provide additional benefits, such as reduction in exacerbation rate and mortality, although a recent systematic review concluded that further, longer-term studies are required to determine the benefits of tiotropium plus LABA and ICS or the additional benefit of ICS on top of LAMA/LABA combinations [56].

12.6.5 Bifunctional Muscarinic Acetylcholine Receptor Antagonists and β2-Adrenergic Receptor Agonists (MABA)

There is another approach that is the design and development of dual-acting agents that combine both mAChR antagonist and β_2-AR agonist pharmacology in a single molecule [54]. This approach may offer several advantages over combination therapy of two separate drug entities. These include the benefit of delivering a fixed ratio into every region of the lung, reducing the complexity of combination inhalers. These agents are known as dual-acting mAChR antagonist–β_2-AR agonist (MABA) bronchodilators. All MABA compounds disclosed so far have an M_3 mAChR antagonist part and a β_2-AR agonist part connected by a linker, the potential synergistic interaction between a LABA and LAMA. It might not be unreasonable to suggest that MABAs are inherently synergistic in terms of their pharmacological effect on airway caliber. A change from baseline trough FEV_1 was 215 and 277 mL with a once-daily dose of 400 and 800 mg GSK961081. A change that was of a similar magnitude to fixed-dose combinations of LABA/LAMA was shown in this analysis to be synergistic. The selectivity of the β_2-agonist and muscarinic antagonist components of the MABA was assumed to be 1:1; the analysis suggests that a threefold lower dose of the MABA is required to produce an equi-effective response with either component acting alone.

12.7 The Role of Bronchodilators in the Management of COPD

In 2011, we saw a substantial revision of the Global Initiative for Chronic Obstructive Lung Disease (GOLD) guidelines for diagnosis, management, and prevention of COPD, which has recently been updated [1]. Recommendations for treatment are no longer based primarily on categorization ("staging") by spirometric assessment, but on categorization by existing symptoms (using validated modified Medical Research Council and COPD Assessment Test questionnaires) and risk (based on severity of airflow limitation and history of exacerbations). This approach acknowledges the importance of consideration of both short- and long-term outcomes when making treatment decisions (Fig. 12.4). The classes of medications commonly used in treating COPD are shown in Tables 12.1, 12.2, 12.3 and 12.4. The choice within each class depends on the availability of medication and the patient's response. A proposed model for initial pharmacological management of COPD according to the individualized assessment of symptoms and exacerbation risk is shown in Table 12.5 [56].

Group A patients have few symptoms and a low risk of exacerbations. Specific evidence for the effectiveness of pharmacologic treatments is not available for patients with $FEV_1 > 80\,\%$ predicted (GOLD 1). However, for all Group A patients, a short-acting bronchodilator used as needed is recommended as first choice based on its effect on lung function and breathlessness. An alternative choice is a combination of short-acting bronchodilators or the introduction of a long-acting bronchodilator. The evidence for this step-up is weak; few studies of the combination exist, and most trials of therapy with long-acting bronchodilators have been performed in patients with more severe airflow limitation.

Group B patients have more significant symptoms but still a low risk of exacerbations. Long-acting bronchodilators are superior to short-acting bronchodilators

Table 12.1 Formulations and typical doses of COPD medications[a] (anticholinergics)

Drug	Inhaler (μg)	Solution for nebulizer (mg/ml)	Duration of action (hours)
Short acting			
Ipratropium bromide	20, 40 (MDI)	0.25–0.5	6–8
Oxitropium bromide	100 (MDI)	1.5	7–9
Long acting			
Tiotropium	18 (DPI), 5 (SMI)		12
Glycopyrronium bromide	44 (DPI)		24
Aclidinium bromide	322 (DPI)		24
Umeclidinium	62.5 (DPI)		24

MDI metered-dose inhaler, *DPI* dry-powder inhaler, *SMI* soft mist inhaler
[a]Not all formulations are available in all countries; in some countries, other formulations may be available

(taken as needed, or prn) and are therefore recommended. There is no evidence to recommend one class of long-acting bronchodilators over another for initial treatment. In the individual patient, the choice should depend on the patient's perception of symptom relief. For patients with severe breathlessness, the alternative choice is a combination of long-acting bronchodilators. Other possible treatments include short-acting bronchodilators and theophylline, the latter of which can be used if inhaled bronchodilators are unavailable or unaffordable.

Group C patients have few symptoms but a high risk of exacerbations. As first choice, a fixed combination of inhaled corticosteroid/long-acting β_2-agonist or a long-acting anticholinergic is recommended. As an alternative choice, a combination of two long-acting bronchodilators or the combination of inhaled corticosteroid/long-acting anticholinergic can be used. Both long-acting anticholinergic and long-acting β_2-agonist reduce the risk of exacerbations, and although good long-term studies are lacking, this principle of combination treatment seems sound. The recommendation for a combination of inhaled corticosteroid/long-acting anticholinergic is not evidence based, but this lack of evidence seems to be the result of lack of interest from the pharmaceutical industry rather than doubts about the rationale. A phosphodiesterase-4 inhibitor used in combination with at least one long-acting bronchodilator could be considered if the patient has chronic bronchitis. Other possible treatments include short-acting bronchodilators and theophylline if long-acting inhaled bronchodilators are unavailable or unaffordable.

Group D patients have many symptoms and a high risk of exacerbations. The first choice of therapy is inhaled corticosteroid plus long-acting β_2-agonist or long-acting anticholinergic. As second choice, a combination of all three classes of drugs (inhaled corticosteroids/long-acting β_2-agonist/long-acting anticholinergic) is recommended. It is also possible to add a phosphodiesterase-4 inhibitor to the treatment chosen as first choice, provided the patient has chronic bronchitis. A

Table 12.2 Formulations and typical Doses of COPD medications[a] (β2-agonist)

Drug	Inhaler (μg)	Solution for nebulizer (mg/ml)	Oral	Vials for injection (mg)	Patch (transdermal)	Duration of action (hours)
Short acting						
Fenoterol	100–200 (MDI)	1	0.05 % (syrup)			4–6
Levalbuterol	45–90 (MDI)	0.21, 0.42				6–8
Salbutamol (albuterol)	100, 200 (MDI and DPI)	5	5 mg (pill), 0.024 % (syrup)	0.1, 0.5		4–6
Terbutaline	400, 500 (DPI)		2.5, 5 mg (pill)			4–6
Long acting						
Formoterol	4.5–12 (MDI and DPI)	0.01[b]				12
Arformoterol		0.0075				12
Salmeterol	25–50 (MDI and DPI)					12
Ultra-long acting						
Indacaterol	75–300 (DPI)					24
Olodaterol	5 (SMI)					24
Tulobuterol					0.5,1,2 mg	24

MDI metered-dose inhaler, *DPI* dry-powder inhaler, *SMI* soft mist inhaler

[a]Not all formulations are available in all countries; in some countries, other formulations may be available

[b]Formoterol nebulized solution is based on the unit dose vial containing 20 mcg in a volume of 2.0 ml

Table 12.3 Formulations and typical doses of COPD medications[a] (xanthines and PGE4 inhibitors)

Drug	Oral	Vials for injection (mg)	Duration of action (hours)
Methylxanthines			
Aminophylline	200–600 mg (pill)	240	up to 24
Theophylline (SR)	100–600 mg (pill)		up to 24
Phosphodiesterase-4 inhibitors			
Roflumilast	500 mcg (pill)		24

MDI metered-dose inhaler, *DPI* dry-powder inhaler, *SMI* soft mist inhaler

[a]Not all formulations are available in all countries; in some countries, other formulations may be available

Table 12.4 Formulations and typical doses of COPD medications[a]

(Combination of β2-agonist plus anticholinergic in one inhaler)			
Drug	Inhaler (mg)	Solution for nebulizer (mg/ml)	Duration of action (hours)
Short-acting β2-agonist plus anticholinergic			
Fenoterol/ipratropium	200/80 (MDI)	1.25/0.5	6–8
Salbutamol/ipratropium	100/20 (SMI)		6–8
Long-acting β2-agonist plus anticholinergic			
Formoterol/aclidinium	12/340 (DPI)		12
Indacaterol/ glycopyrronium	85/43 (DPI)		24
Olodaterol/tiotropium	5/5 (SMI)		24
Vilanterol/ umeclidinium	25/62.5 (DPI)		24

MDI metered-dose inhaler, *DPI* dry-powder inhaler, *SMI* soft mist inhaler
[a]Not all formulations are available in all countries; in some countries, other formulations may be available

phosphodiesterase-4 inhibitor is effective when added to a long-acting bronchodilator, whereas evidence of its benefit when added to inhaled corticosteroid comes from less valid secondary analyses. Other possible treatments include short-acting bronchodilators and theophylline or carbocisteine, which can be used if long-acting inhaled bronchodilators are unavailable or unaffordable [1].

12.8 Route of Drug Delivery to the Airway

12.8.1 Inhaled Route

Inhalation is the preferred mode of delivery of many drugs with a direct effect on airways, particularly for asthma and COPD. The major advantage of inhalation is the delivery of drugs to the airways in doses that are effective with a much lower risk of systemic side effects. This is particularly important with the use of inhaled corticosteroids (ICS), which largely avoids systemic side effects. In addition, inhaled bronchodilators have a more rapid onset of action than when taken orally (Fig. 12.5).

Table 12.5 GOLD guidelines (2016): initial pharmacological management of COPD[a]

Patient group	Recommended first choice	Alternative choice	Other possible treatments[b]
A	SAMA prn. or SABA prn.	LAMA or LABA or SABA + SAMA	Theophylline
B	LAMA or LABA	LAMA + LABA	SABA and/or SAMA Theophylline
C	ICS + LABA or LAMA	LAMA+ LABA or LAMA + PDE-4 I or LABA + PDE-4 I	SABA and/or SAMA Theophylline
D	ICS + LABA and/or LAMA	ICS + LABA + LAMA or ICS + LABA + PDE-4 I or LAMA + LABA or LAMA + PDE-4 I	Carbocisteine N-acetylcysteine SABA and/or SAMA Theophylline

[a]Medications in each box are mentioned in alphabetical order and therefore not necessarily in order of preference
[b]Medications in this column can be used alone or in combination with other options in the recommended first choice and alternative choice columns
From the Global Strategy for Diagnosis, Management and Prevention of COPD 2016, Global initiative for chronic Obstructive Lung Disease (GOLD), http://www.goldcopd.org
Medications in each box are mentioned in alphabetical order and, therefore, not necessarily in the order of preference
prn as needed, *SABA* short-acting β2-agonist, *LABA* long-acting β2-agonist, *SAMA* short-acting muscarinic antagonist, *LAMA* long-acting muscarinic antagonist, *ICS* inhaled corticosteroid, *PDE4I* phosphodiesterase-4 inhibitor

12.8.1.1 Particle Size

The size of particles for inhalation is of critical importance in determining the size deposition in the respiratory tract. The optimum size for particles to settle in the airways is 2–5 μm mass median aerodynamic diameter (MMAD). Larger particles settle out in the upper airways, whereas smaller particles remain suspended and are therefore exhaled. There is increasing interest in delivering drug particles of ~1 μm MMAD, which is now possible using drugs formulated in hydrofluoroalkane (HFA) propellant and soft mist inhaler as Respimat device [63].

12.8.1.2 Pharmacokinetics

Of the total drug delivered, only 10–50 % enters the lower airways with a conventional pressurized metered-dose inhaler. Drugs are absorbed from the airway lumen and have direct effects on target cells of the airway. Drugs may also be absorbed into the bronchial circulation and then distributed to more peripheral airways.

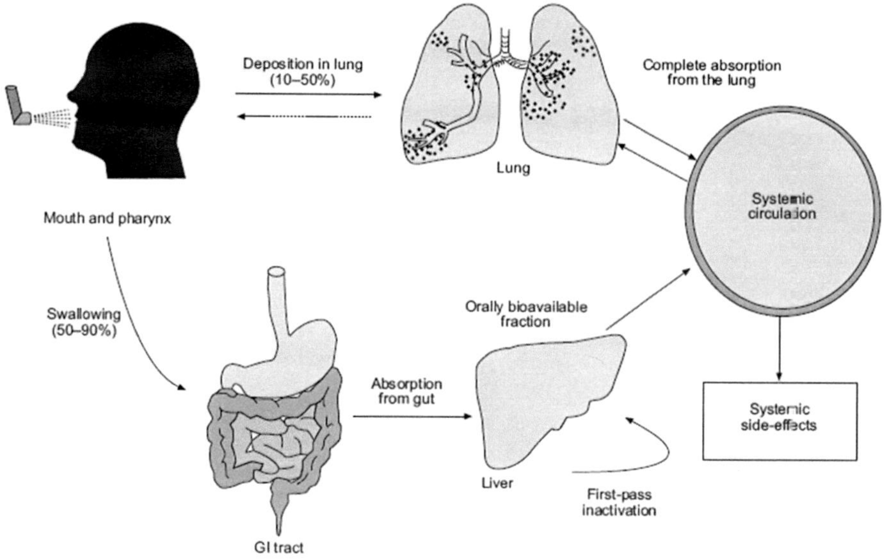

Fig. 12.5 Deposition of inhaled drugs
Inhalation therapy deposits drugs directly, but not exclusively, in the lungs. Distribution between lungs and oropharynx depends mostly on the particle size and the efficiency of the delivery method. Most material will be swallowed and absorbed, entering systemic circulation after undergoing the first-pass effect in the liver. Some drug will also be absorbed into the systemic circulation from the lungs. Use of a large-volume spacer will reduce the amount of drug deposited on the oropharynx, thereby reducing amount swallowed and absorbed from the GI tract, thus limiting systemic effects (From Eur Respir J 2006; 28: 1042–1050)[62]

Drugs with higher molecular weights tend to retain to a greater extent in the airways. Nevertheless, several drugs have greater therapeutic efficacy when given by the inhaled route. More extensive pulmonary distribution of a drug with a smaller MMAD increases alveolar deposition and thus is likely to increase absorption from the lungs into the general circulation resulting in more systemic side effects.

12.8.2 *Oral Route*

Drugs for treatment of pulmonary diseases may also be given orally. The oral dose is much higher than the inhaled dose required to achieve the same effect (typically by a ratio of ~20:1), so that systemic side effects are more common. When there is a choice of inhaled or oral route for a drug, the inhaled route is always preferable, and the oral route should be reserved for the few patients unable to use inhalers. Xanthine is ineffective by the inhaled route; it must be given systemically.

12.8.3 Parenteral Route

The intravenous route should be reserved for delivery of drugs in the severely ill patient who is unable to absorb drugs from the GI tract. Side effects are generally frequent due to the high plasma concentrations.

12.8.4 Transdermal Route

The transdermal route should be reserved for delivery of drugs in the severely ill patient who is unable to use inhalers.

12.9 Conclusion

Bronchodilator medications are central to the symptomatic management of COPD. The principal bronchodilator treatments are anticholinergics, β_2-agonist, and methylxanthines used as monotherapy or in combination. Therapeutic intervention should be initiated on categorization by symptoms and risk.

References

1. Global initiative for chronic Obstructive Lung Disease: Global strategy for the diagnosis, management, and prevention of chronic obstructive pulmonary disease. Revised 2016.
2. Cazzola M, Page CP, Calzetta L, Matera MG. Pharmacology and therapeutics of bronchodilators. Pharmacol Rev. 2012;64:450–504.
3. Racke´ K, Juergens UR, Matthiesen S. Control by cholinergic mechanisms. Eur J Pharmacol. 2006;533:57–68.
4. Carstairs JR, Nimmo AJ, Barnes PJ. Autoradiographic visualization of beta-adrenoceptor subtypes in human lung. Am Rev Respir Dis. 1985;132:541–7.
5. Johnson M. The β-adrenoceptor. Am J Respir Crit Care Med. 1998;158:S146–53.
6. Gu Q, Lee LY. Neural control of airway smooth muscle. In: Laurent GJ, Shapiro SD, editors. Encyclopedia of respiratory medicine. Amsterdam: Elsevier; 2006. p. 138–45.
7. Prakash YS. Airway smooth muscle in airway reactivity and remodeling: what have we learned? Am J Physiol Lung Cell Mol Physiol. 2013;305:L912–33.
8. Miraldi E, Masti A, Ferri S, Barni Comparini I. Distribution of hyoscyamine and scopolamine in *Datura stramonium*. Fitoterapia. 2001;72:644–8.
9. Gross NJ. Anticholinergic agents in asthma and COPD. Eur J Pharmacol. 2006;533:36–9.
10. Pierce RJ, Allen CJ, Campbell AH. A comparative study of atropine methonitrate, salbutamol and their combination in airways obstruction. Thorax. 1979;34:45–50.
11. Scullion JE. The development of anticholinergics in the management of COPD. Int J Chron Obstruct Pulmon Dis. 2007;2:33–40.
12. Hardy JPR, Goggin PL, Graham P. Bronchodilation effect of oxitropium bromide compared with ipratropium bromide (Abstract). Thorax. 1992;48:865.

13. Tashkin DP, Celli B, Senn S, Burkhart D, Kesten S, Menjoge S, Decramer M, UPLIFT Study Investigators. A 4-year trial of tiotropium in chronic obstructive pulmonary disease. N Engl J Med. 2008;359:1543–54.
14. Verkindre C, Fukuchi Y, Fle´male A, Takeda A, Overend T, Prasad N, Dolker M. Sustained 24-h efficacy of NVA237, a once-daily long-acting muscarinic antagonist, in COPD patients. Respir Med. 2010;104:1482–9.
15. Cazzola M. Aclidinium bromide, a novel long-acting muscarinic M3 antagonist for the treatment of COPD. Curr Opin Investig Drugs. 2009;10:482–90.
16. Cahn A, Mehta R, Preece A, Blowers J, Donald A. Safety, tolerability and pharmacokinetics and pharmacodynamics of inhaled once-daily Umeclidinium in healthy adults deficient in CYP2D6 activity: a double-blind, randomized clinical trial. Clin Drug Investig. 2013;33:653–64.
17. Celli B, Decramer M, Leimer I, Vogel U, Kesten S, Tashkin DP. Cardiovascular safety of tiotropium in patients with COPD. Chest. 2010;137:20–30.
18. Singh S, Loke YK, Furberg CD. Inhaled anticholinergics and risk of major adverse cardiovascular events in patients with chronic obstructive pulmonary disease: a systematic review and meta-analysis. JAMA. 2008;300:1439–50.
19. Bullowa JG, Kaplan DM. On the hypodermic use of adrenalin chloride in the treatment of asthmatic attacks. Med News. 1903;83:787–90.
20. Waldeck B. β-adrenoceptor agonists and asthma 100 years of development. Eur J Pharmacol. 2002;445:1–12.
21. Datta D, Vitale A, Lahiri B, ZuWallack R. An evaluation of nebulized levalbuterol in stable COPD. Chest. 2003;124:844–9.
22. Lötvall J. The long and short of β2-agonists. Pulm Pharmacol Ther. 2002;15:497–501.
23. Cazzola M, Matera MG, Santangelo G, Vinciguerra A, Rossi F, D'Amato G. Salmeterol and formoterol in partially reversible severe chronic obstructive pulmonary disease: a dose–response study. Respir Med. 1995;89:357–62.
24. Kew KM, Mavergames C, Walters JA. Long-acting beta2-agonists for chronic obstructive pulmonary disease. Cochrane Database Syst Rev. 2013;10:CD010177.
25. Löfdahl CG, Svedmyr N. Formoterol fumarate, a new β2-adrenoceptor agonist. Allergy. 1989;44:264–71.
26. Johnson M, Butchers PR, Coleman RA, Nials AT, Strong P, Sumner MJ, Vardey CJ, Whelan CJ. The pharmacology of salmeterol. Life Sci. 1993;52:2131–43.
27. Cazzola M, Bardaro F, Stirpe E. The role of indacaterol for chronic obstructive pulmonary disease (COPD). J Thorac Dis. 2013;5:559–66.
28. O'Reilly, J. Chronic obstructive pulmonary disease:olodaterol. NICE: Evidence summary: new medicine Published; 2015.
29. Hanania NA, Feldman G, Zachgo W, Shim JJ, Crim C, Sanford L, Lettis S, Barnhart F, Haumann B. The efficacy and safety of the novel long-acting β2 agonist vilanterol in COPD patients: a randomized placebo-controlled trial. Chest. 2012;2012(142):119–27.
30. Make BJ, Kanniess F, Bateman ED, Linberg SE. Efficacy of 3 different doses of carmoterol, a long-acting β2-agonist in patients with COPD (Abstract). Proc Am Thorac Soc. 2008;5:A961.
31. Nowak R, Iwaki Y, Matsuda K, Johnson K, Dunton AW. Reduced hospital admission and improved pulmonary function following intravenous MN-221 (bedoradrine), a novel, highly selective beta2-adrenergic receptor agonist, adjunctive to standard of care in severe acute exacerbation of asthma (Abstract). Chest. 2010;138:66A.
32. Pearle J, Iwaki Y, Dunton AW, Kitt E, Ruby K. Intravenous MN-221, a novel, highly selective beta2-adrenergic receptor agonist, improves lung function in stable moderate to severe chronic obstructive pulmonary disease patients (Abstract). Chest. 2010;138:487A.
33. Tamura G, Ichinose M, Fukuchi Y, Miyamoto T. Transdermal tulobuterol patch, a long-acting β2-agonist. Allergol Int. 2012;61:219–29.

34. Lipworth BJ, McDevitt DG, Struthers AD. Hypokalemic and ECG sequelae of combined beta-agonist/diuretic therapy. Protection by conventional doses of spironolactone but not triamterene. Chest. 1990;98:811–15.
35. Uren NG, Davies SW, Jordan SL, Lipkin DP. Inhaled bronchodilators increase maximum oxygen consumption in chronic left ventricular failure. Eur Heart J. 1993;14:744–50.
36. Brochard L, Mancebo J, Wysocki M, Lofaso F, Conti G, Rauss A, Simonneau G, Benito S. Gasparetto A, and Lemaire F () Noninvasive ventilation for acute exacerbations of chronic obstructive pulmonary disease. N Engl J Med. 1995;333:817–22.
37. Ram FS, Jones PW, Castro AA, et al. Oral theophylline for chronic obstructive pulmonary disease. Cochrane Database Syst Rev. 2002;4:CD003902.
38. Zhou Y, Wang X, Zeng X, et al. Positive benefits of theophylline in a randomized, double-blind, parallel-group, placebo-controlled study of low-dose, slow-release theophylline in the treatment of COPD for 1 year. Respirology. 2006;11:603–10.
39. Kobayashi M, Nasuhara Y, Betsuyaku T, Shibuya E, Tanino Y, Tanino M, Takamura K, Nagai K, Hosokawa T, Nishimura M. Effect of low-dose theophylline on airway inflammation in COPD. Respirology. 2004;9:249–54.
40. Fabbri LM, Calverley PM, Izquierdo-Alonso JL, et al. Roflumilast in moderate-to-severe chronic obstructive pulmonary disease treated with longacting bronchodilators: two randomised clinical trials. Lancet. 2009;374:695–703.
41. Rabe KF. Update on roflumilast, a phosphodiesterase 4 inhibitor for the treatment of chronic obstructive pulmonary disease. Br J Pharmacol. 2011;163:53–67.
42. Nardi A, Demnitz J, Garcia ML, Polosa R. Potassium channels as drug targets for therapeutic intervention in respiratory diseases. Expert Opin Ther Pat. 2008;18:1361–84.
43. Wu D, Lee D, Sung YK. Prospect of vasoactive intestinal peptide therapy for COPD/PAH and asthma: a review. Respir Res. 2011;12:45.
44. Fernandes LB, Henry PJ, Goldie RG. Rho kinase as a therapeutic target in the treatment of asthma and chronic obstructive pulmonary disease. Ther Adv Respir Dis. 2007;1:25–33.
45. Hamad AM, Range S, Holland E, Knox AJ. Regulation of cGMP by soluble and particulate guanylyl cyclases in cultured human airway smooth muscle. Am J Physiol. 1997;273: L807–13.
46. Högman M, Frostell CG, Hedenström H, Hedenstierna G. Inhalation of nitric oxide modulates adult human bronchial tone. Am Rev Respir Dis. 1993;148:1474–8.
47. Scatena R, Bottoni P, Pontoglio A, Giardina B. Pharmacological modulation of nitric oxide release: new pharmacological perspectives, potential benefits and risks. Curr Med Chem. 2010;17:61–73.
48. Maher SA, Birrell MA, Belvisi MG. Prostaglandin E2 mediates cough via the EP3 receptor: implications for future disease therapy. Am J Respir Crit Care Med. 2009;180:923–8.
49. Buckley J, Birrell MA, Maher SA, Nials AT, Clarke DL, Belvisi MG. EP4 receptor as a new target for bronchodilator therapy. Thorax. 2011;66:1029–35.
50. Doggrell SA. Bitter taste receptors as a target for bronchodilation. Expert Opin Ther Targets. 2011;15:899–902.
51. Cazzola M, Matera MG. The effective treatment of COPD: anticholinergics and what else? Drug Discov Today Ther Strateg. 2006;3:277–86.
52. Chung KF, Caramori G, Adcock IM. Inhaled corticosteroids as combination therapy with β-adrenergic agonists in airways disease: present and future. Eur J Clin Pharmacol. 2009;65:853–71.
53. Cazzola M, Molimard M. The scientific rationale for combining long-acting β2-agonists and muscarinic antagonists in COPD. Pulm Pharmacol Ther. 2010;23:257–67.
54. Cazzola M, Calzetta L, Matera MG. β2-adrenoceptor agonists: current and future direction. Br J Pharmacol. 2011;163:4–17.
55. Spina D. Pharmacology of novel treatments for COPD:are fixed dose combination LABA/LAMA synergistic? Eur Clin Respir J; 2015.

56. Tashkin DP, Ferguson GT. Combination bronchodilator therapy in the management of chronic obstructive pulmonary disease. Respir Res. 2013;14:49–61.
57. Cazzola M, Tashkin DP. Combination of formoterol and tiotropium in the treatment of COPD: effects on lung function. COPD. 2009;6:404–15.
58. Adcock IM, Maneechotesuwan K, Usmani O. Molecular interactions between glucocorticoids and long-acting β2-agonists. J Allergy Clin Immunol. 2002;110:S261–8.
59. Cazzola M, Dahl R. Inhaled combination therapy with long-acting β2-agonists and corticosteroids in stable COPD. Chest. 2004;126:220–37.
60. Calverley PM, Anderson JA, Celli B, Ferguson GT, Jenkins C, Jones PW, Yates JC, Vestbo J, TORCH Investigators. Salmeterol and fluticasone propionate and survival in chronic obstructive pulmonary disease. N Engl J Med. 2007;356:775–89.
61. Choi J, Na J, Kim Y. The effect of tiotropium and inhaled corticosteroid combination therapy in chronic obstructive pulmonary disease (COPD) and chronic obstructive bronchial asthma (COBA) associated with irreversible pulmonary function (Abstract). Am J Respir Crit Care Med. 2007;175:A130.
62. Derendorf H, Nave R, Drollmann A, Cerasoli F, Wurst W. Relevance of pharmacokinetics and pharmacodynamics of inhaled corticosteroids to asthma. Eur Respir J. 2006;28:1042–50.
63. Pitcairn G, Reader S, Pavia D, Newman S. Deposition of corticosteroid aerosol in the human lung by Respimat® Soft Mist™ inhaler compared to deposition by Metered Dose Inhaler or by Turbuhaler® Dry Powder Inhaler. J Aerosol Med. 2005;18:264–72.

Chapter 13
Inhaled Corticosteroids for COPD: Are Inhaled Corticosteroids Required in the Management of COPD?

Masayuki Itoh

Abstract Inhaled corticosteroids (ICSs) strongly suppress airway inflammation and are widely used as the first drugs of choice for the treatment of bronchial asthma. Chronic obstructive pulmonary disease (COPD) is also an inflammatory disease of the airway, but because the type of inflammation in COPD differs from the type of inflammation in asthma and because pathology that diminishes the effectiveness of steroids is postulated in COPD, the therapeutic effect of ICSs in COPD is limited. In fact, there are many negative opinions in regard to the preventive effect of ICSs on the progression of COPD and in regard to their effectiveness in lowering mortality. Although ICS effectiveness in preventing exacerbations and effectiveness in preventing decreased quality of life (QOL) have been reported, it has also been reported that no difference in exacerbation-preventing effect was observed when the results of treatment with ICS/long-acting β agonist (LABA) and long-acting muscarinic antagonist (LAMA) were compared, and that when ICSs were gradually discontinued in COPD patients being treated with ICS/LABA/LAMA, the results showed no increase in exacerbation frequency. When selecting COPD patients for treatment with ICSs, it is necessary to consider not just the benefits of treatment, but overtreatment, increased cost, and risk of pneumonia as well.

Keywords COPD • Inhaled corticosteroids • Exacerbation

13.1 Introduction

According to the Global Initiative for Chronic Obstructive Lung Disease (GOLD) guidelines, combination therapy with a bronchodilator (long-acting muscarinic antagonist [LAMA] or long-acting β agonist [LABA]) and inhaled corticosteroid

M. Itoh (✉)
Department of Respiratory Medicine, Kashiwa Tanaka Hospital, Higashi 65 gaiku 1 Koaota 70-1, Kashiwa, Chiba 277-0803, Japan
e-mail: momo1562002@yahoo.co.jp

H. Nakamura, K. Aoshiba (eds.), *Chronic Obstructive Pulmonary Disease*, Respiratory Disease Series: Diagnostic Tools and Disease Managements,
DOI 10.1007/978-981-10-0839-9_13

(ICS) is indicated in chronic obstructive pulmonary disease (COPD) patients who are GOLD Stage III (forced expiratory volume in 1 s [FEV_1] <50 % predicted normal) or who experience an exacerbation two or more times a year (or who require inpatient treatment for one or more exacerbations a year) [1]. The evidence that served as the basis for these indications consists of the results of large-scale randomized controlled trials (RCTs), including the Inhaled Steroids in Obstructive Lung Disease (ISOLDE) trial and Towards a Revolution in COPD Health (TORCH) trial [2, 3], but there are data analysis issues, the problem of the effectiveness of ICSs not necessarily having been demonstrated in a meta-analysis, etc [4, 5], and adverse effects, including an increased risk of pneumonia, must be taken into consideration when using ICSs. Patients with severe or very severe COPD, who have indications for ICSs according to the guidelines, account for about 20 % of COPD patients; however, there is a survey showing that ICS/LABA is actually being prescribed for 75 % of COPD patients [6], and the high cost and overtreatment with ICSs have become problems [7]. In this chapter, we will explain the effectiveness of ICSs in COPD and the risks and indications.

13.2 Effectiveness of ICSs Against the Airway Inflammation in COPD

Because ICSs strongly inhibit eosinophilic inflammation of the airway, they are widely used as the drugs of first choice for the treatment of bronchial asthma. COPD is also an inflammatory disease of the airway, but the airway inflammation in COPD differs from the eosinophilic inflammation in bronchial asthma, and because neutrophils and macrophages predominate in the inflammation in the stable phase of COPD, the effectiveness of ICSs against the airway inflammation in COPD is limited in comparison with their effectiveness in asthma [8]. However, Confalonieri et al. conducted a detailed study of the effectiveness of ICSs against the airway inflammation in COPD, and the results showed that although the macrophages during induction had increased in number in the COPD patients who had been treated with high-dose (1500 μg/day) beclomethasone dipropionate (BDP) for 2 months or more, there was a significant decrease in the number of neutrophils [9]. Moreover, Llewellyn-Jones et al. reported finding that the neutrophil elastase inhibitory capacity of sputum increased in COPD patients who inhaled fluticasone propionate (FP) 1500 μg/day for 8 weeks and that neutrophil chemotactic activity decreased [10]. In addition, Ozol et al. reported that when they had stable-phase COPD patients inhale budesonide (BUD) for 6 months, the neutrophil fraction and interleukin-8 (IL-8) in their bronchoalveolar lavage fluid (BALF) decreased [11]. Based on the above results, when high doses of ICSs were used, they appeared to have some degree of effectiveness against the neutrophilic airway inflammation in COPD.

According to a meta-analysis that investigated the effectiveness of ICSs against airway inflammation, ICSs increased the number of macrophages in the BALF of COPD patients, but decreased the numbers of cluster of differentiation (CD) 4+ and CD8+ lymphocytes in the airway wall and the numbers of neutrophils and lymphocytes in BALF [12]. Thus, ICSs appeared to also have some degree of inhibitory effect on the lymphocytic inflammation in COPD.

On the other hand, usual steroid effectiveness appears to be decreased in COPD, because histone deacetylase-2 (HDAC2) expression and activity are reduced [13, 14]. After a steroid binds to the glucocorticoid receptor (GR), it enters the nucleus and activates HDAC2, and an anti-inflammatory action called transrepression that inhibits binding of transcription factors such as nuclear factor-kappa B (NF-kB) to the promoter region of pro-inflammatory genes by accelerating histone deacetylation is known to occur, but it appears that because HDAC2 expression and activation are reduced in COPD, the transrepression mechanism of action of steroids is not sufficiently exerted, and their anti-inflammatory effectiveness is weaker [15, 16].

13.3 Clinical Effectiveness of ICSs in COPD

The results of clinical trials of ICSs in COPD are summarized in Table 13.1 [2, 3, 17–65]. FEV_1 values, FEV_1 decline rate, exacerbation frequency, quality of life (QOL), etc. have been assessed as evaluation parameters for the therapeutic effect of ICSs.

13.3.1 Effects of ICSs on Pulmonary Function

Although results of short-term clinical trials showing that ICSs improved FEV_1 have been reported, there have been many reports of long-term large clinical trials showing that ICSs had no preventive effect in relation to FEV_1 or the FEV_1 decline rate (Table 13.1). For example, ICSs had no effect on the FEV_1 decline rate in such long-term, large-scale clinical trials as the European Respiratory Society study on COPD (EUROSCOP), Copenhagen City Lung Study (CCLS), ISOLDE, or Lung Health Study (LHS) [2, 34, 36, 39]. By contrast, in the Groningen Leiden Universities Corticosteroids in Obstructive Lung Disease (GLUCOLD) study, a significant ameliorating effect on the percentage change in FEV_1 was seen in the ICS group (+7.3 mL/year) in comparison with the placebo group (−79 mL/year), and correlations were also seen between slowing of the FEV_1 decline rate and decreases in the numbers of inflammatory cells in the airway [61]. A preventive effect of ICSs on the FEV_1 decline rate was seen in the TORCH trial as well [3], but the possibility of the FEV_1 decline rate in the placebo group having been overestimated because of a dropout case bias was pointed out [66].

Table 13.1 Placebo-controlled trials on the effects of inhaled corticosteroids in COPD

Author/year	Ref	Number of patients	ICS dose (μg/day)	Study duration	Results (FEV1.0, SGRQ, risk of exacerbation, etc)
Robertson et al./1986	[17]	83	BDP 1500	2 weeks	FEV1: →
Weir et al./1990	[18]	127	BDP 1500	2 weeks	FEV1: ↑
Auffarth et al./1991	[19]	24	BUD 1600	8 weeks	FEV1: → PEF: →
Thompson et al./1992	[20]	31	BDP 2000	6 weeks	FEV1: ↑ PEF: →
Kerstjens et al./1992	[21]	182	BDP 800	2.5 years	FEV1:↑
Watson et al./1992	[22]	14	BUD 1200	12 weeks	FEV1: → PEF: → Bronchoconstrictor responsiveness:NS
Wempe et al./1992	[23]	10	BUD 1600	3 weeks	FEV1: → Bronchoconstrictor responsiveness:NS
Weir et al./1993	[24]	105	BDP 1500 or 3000	3 weeks	FEV1: ↑
Weiner et al./1995	[25]	30	BUD 800	6 weeks	FEV1: ↑ (responders to beta2-agonist)
Llewellyn-Jones et al./1996	[10]	17	FP 1500	8 weeks	PEF: →
Renkema et al./1996	[26]	45	BUD 800	2 years	FEV1 decline: NS Frequency and duration of exacerbation: NS
Boothman-Burrell et al./1997	[27]	18	BDP 1000	3 months	FEV1: →
Keatings et al./1997	[28]	13	BUD 1600	2 weeks	FEV1: →
Bourbeau et al./1998	[29]	79	BUD 1600	6 months	FEV1: → 6MWT: → CRQ:NS
Paggiaro et al./1998	[30]	281	FP 1000	6 months	FEV1: ↑ Numbers of exacerbation: NS
Rutgers et al./1998	[31]	44	BUD 1600	6 weeks	FEV1: → PEF: → Symptom score: NS Serum IL-8:↓

(continued)

Table 13.1 (continued)

Author/year	Ref	Number of patients	ICS dose (μg/day)	Study duration	Results (FEV1.0, SGRQ, risk of exacerbation, etc)
Culpitt et al./1999	[32]	25	FP 1000	4 weeks	FEV1: →
					PEF: →
					Symptom score: NS
					Sputum Percentage of neutrophils, IL-8, elastase, MMP-1, MMP-9, SLPI, TIMP-1: NS
Nishimura et al./1999	[33]	30	BDP 3000	4 weeks	FEV1: ↑
Pauwels et al./1999 (EUROSCOP)	[34]	1277	BUD800	3 years	FEV1 decline: NS
Senderovitz et al./1999	[35]	37	BUD 800	6 months	FEV1: →
					Number of exacerbation: NS
Vestbo et al./1999 (CCLS)	[36]	290	BUD 800	3 years	FEV1 decline: NS
					Exacerbation rate: NS
Weiner et al./1999	[37]	168	BUD 800	6 weeks	FEV1: ↑(responders to beta2-agonist)
Weir et al./1999	[38]	98	BDP 2000	2 years	FEV1 decline: NS
					exacerbation rate: NS
Burge et al./2000 (ISOLDE)	[2]	751	FP 1000	3 years	FEV1 decline: NS
					Exacerbation rate: ↓
					Slower decline in respiratory questionnaire score (SGRQ)
Lung Health Study/2000 (LHS)	[39]	1116	Triamcinolone 1200	4.5 years	FEV1 decline: NS
					SF-36: improved
Ferreira et al./2001	[40]	20	BDP 1000	2 weeks	FEV1: →
					Exhaled nitric oxide:↓
Loppow et al./2001	[41]	19	FP 1000	4 weeks	FEV1: →
					Concentration of exhaled nitric oxide, differential cell counts in induced sputum and the number of cells positive for iNOS, levels of LDH, ECP, neutrophil elastase, and IL-8 in sputum supernatants: NS
Mirici et al./2001	[42]	50	BDP 800	12 weeks	FEV1: ↑
					Sputum cell count, proportion of neutrophil: ↓
Hattotuwa et al./2002	[43]	37	FP 1000	3 months	FEV1: →

(continued)

Table 13.1 (continued)

Author/year	Ref	Number of patients	ICS dose (μg/day)	Study duration	Results (FEV1.0, SGRQ, risk of exacerbation, etc)
Mahler et al./2002	[44]	691	FP 1000	24 weeks	FEV1: ↑
					Time to exacerbation: NS
					CRDQ: NS
					CBSQ: NS
Thompson et al./2002	[45]	52	FP 880	3 months	Pre-bronchodilator FEV1: ↑
					Dyspnea score in CRQ: improved
Verhoeven et al./2002	[46]	23	FP 1000	6 months	FEV1 decline: improved
					Bronchoconstrictor responsiveness:→
Calverley et al./2003 (TRISTAN)	[47]	719	FP 1000	1 year	FEV1: ↑
					Exacerbation rate: ↓
					SGRQ: improved
Calverley et al./2003	[48]	513	BUD 800	1 year	FEV1: →
					Time to first exacerbation and number of exacerbation: NS
					SGRQ: improved
Hanania et al./2003	[49]	247	FP 500	24 weeks	FEV1: ↑
					CRDQ:→
Szafranski et al./2003	[50]	403	BUD 800	1 year	FEV1:↑
					Exacerbation rate: NS
					SGRQ: NS
Van Grunsven et al./2003 (DIMCA)	[51]	48	FP 500	2 years	FEV1: ↑(pre- and post-bronchodilator)
					FEV1 decline:NS
					Occurrence of exacerbations: NS
Sin et al./2004	[52]	41	FP 1000	4 weeks	FEV1: →
					CRP: ↓
Yildiz et al./2004	[53]	38	BUD 800	12 weeks	FEV1: →
					SGRQ: improved
Brightling et al./2005	[54]	60	MF 800	2 weeks	CRQ: NS
					FEV1: →
John et al./2005	[55]	22	BDP 800	12 weeks	SGRQ total: NS
					FEV1: →
					PEF: ↑
					IL-10, GM-CSF, IFN-γ, MIP-α from peripheral blood monocyte: NS

(continued)

Table 13.1 (continued)

Author/year	Ref	Number of patients	ICS dose (μg/day)	Study duration	Results (FEV1.0, SGRQ, risk of exacerbation, etc)
Ozol et al./2005	[11]	26	BUD 800	6 months	FEV1: →
					IL-8 levels in BAL: decreased
					Percentages of neutrophils: decreased
GSK, FCO30002/2005	[56]	140	FP 1000	12 weeks	FEV1: →
GSK, FLTA3025/2005	[57]	640	FP 500 or 1000	24 weeks	FEV1: ↑ (FP500)
					CBSQ: NS
					Exacerbation rate: NS
Bourbeau et al./2007	[55]	41	FP 1000	3 months	FEV1: →
					CRQ: NS
Calverley et al./2007 (TORCH)	[3]	3058	FP 1000	3 years	FEV1: ↑
					SGRQ: improved
					Exacerbation rate:↓
					Mortality rate: NS
Calverley et al./2008	[59]	911	MF 800	1 year	FEV1: ↑
					Exacerbations rate:↓
					SGRQ: improved
Sin et al./2008	[60]	289	FP 1000	4 weeks	FEV1: →
					SGRQ: improved
					Number of exacerbations: ↓
					Serum IL-6: NS
					Serum SP-D:↓
Lapperre et al./2009 (GLUCOLD)	[61]	55	FP 1000	30 months	FEV1 decline: improved
					Mucosal CD3+, CD4+, CD8 + cells and mast cells:↓
					Bronchoconstrictor responsiveness: ↓
					CCQ: improved
					Activity score in SGRQ: improved
					MRC dyspnea score: improved
Schermer et al./2009 (COOPT)	[62]	300	FP 1000	3 years	FEV1: →
					CRQ: NS
					Exacerbation rate: NS
Shaker et al./2009	[63]	278	BUD 800	2–4 years	FEV1 decline: NS
					Annual CT change: NS
Guenette et al./2011	[64]	17	FP1000	2 weeks	FEV1: ↑

(continued)

Table 13.1 (continued)

Author/year	Ref	Number of patients	ICS dose (μg/day)	Study duration	Results (FEV1.0, SGRQ, risk of exacerbation, etc)
Tashkin et al./2012	[65]	911	MF 400	26 weeks	FEV1:↑
					Exacerbations rate:↓
					SGRQ: improved

Abbreviations
↑: increased
→: no change
↓: decreased
NS: not significant vs placebo
FP: fluticasone propionate
BUD: budesonide
BDP: beclomethasone dipropionate
MF: mometasone furoate
FEV1: forced expiratory volume in 1 second
PEF: peak expiratory flow
CCQ: Clinical COPD Questionnaire
CRQ: Chronic Respiratory Questionnaire
CRDQ: Chronic Respiratory Disease Questionnaire
CBSQ: Chronic Bronchitis Symptoms Questionnaire
MRC: Medical Research Council
SGRQ: St George's Respiratory Questionnaire
ECP: eosinophil cationic protein
LDH: lactate dehydrogenase
CRP: C-reactive protein
iNOS: inducible nitric oxide synthase
IL: interleukin
GM-CSF: granulocyte-macrophage colony-stimulating factor
IFN-γ: interferon-γ
MIP-1α: macrophage inflammatory protein-1α
SP-D: surfactant protein D
BAL: bronchoalveolar lavage
CT: computed tomography
CCLS: Copenhagen City Lung Study
DIMCA: Detection, Intervention and Monitoring of COPD and Asthma
EUROSCOP: ERS study on COPD
ISOLDE: Inhaled Steroids in Obstructive Lung Disease in Europe
LHS: Lung Health Study
TRISTAN: Trial of Inhaled Steroids and Long-Acting β2 Agonists
TORCH: Towards a Revolution in COPD Health
GLUCOLD: Groningen Leiden Universities Corticosteroids in Obstructive Lung Disease
COOPT: COPD on Primary Care Treatment

In a meta-analysis by van Grunsven et al., it was concluded that an improvement in FEV_1 in response to ICSs had been observed in a 2-year observation period [67]. However, Alsaeedi et al. have stated that the number of RCTs that were suitable for assessment was small and an adequate meta-analysis could not be performed [68]. According to the Cochrane Review, which also analyzed the effectiveness of BDP in improving FEV_1, the number of RCTs that could be assessed was small, and it was impossible to draw a clear conclusion [69]. However, Yang et al. later conducted a meta-analysis of 55 RCTs ($n = 16{,}154$ subjects) and concluded that ICSs had been found to have no preventive effect on the rate of decline in FEV_1 [4].

13.3.2 *Effects of ICSs on QOL*

The QOL of COPD patients has been assessed by means of a variety of questionnaires (Table 13.1), and St George's Respiratory Questionnaire (SGRQ) has recently come into widespread use. The results of the SGRQ in large-scale surveys, including the ISOLDE, Trial of Inhaled Steroids and Long-Acting β2 Agonists (TRISTAN), and TORCH surveys, have shown an ameliorating effect of ICSs on QOL [2, 3, 47, 48, 59, 65]. A similar conclusion was also drawn in a meta-analysis in recent years [4]; however, caution is necessary, because many studies have concluded that ICSs were effective based on statistically significant differences, even though the SGRQ results did not show an improvement of 4 points or more, which is considered significant clinically [70]. Moreover, since the comparisons were not made with the values before using ICSs and the results did not show that ICSs had improved the SGRQ score 4 points or more in comparison with the placebo, the clinical evidence that ICSs improve the QOL of COPD patients can only be said to be scant.

13.3.3 *Exacerbation-Preventing Effect of ICS*

Conflicting results showing that ICSs are effective and ineffective in preventing exacerbations have been published (Table 13.1). A COPD exacerbation-preventing effect of ICSs was shown in ISOLDE, TRISTAN, and TORCH trials [2.3.47]. In the results of meta-analyses, no exacerbation-preventing effect of ICSs was found by van Grunsven et al. [67], whereas Alsaeedi et al. reported a 30 % decrease in exacerbation frequency [68]. In subsequent meta-analyses, Yang et al. concluded that exacerbations had been reduced by ICSs at a rate of one exacerbation in 4 years [4], whereas Agarwal et al. claimed that the exacerbation-preventing effect of ICSs was slight and that the preventive effect of ICSs in previous reports had been exaggerated [5]. Moreover, Ernst et al. pointed out problems in the studies showing that ICSs were effective, i.e., that there were differences between the methods used to diagnose an exacerbation, that intention to treat (ITT) had not been analyzed, that the calculations of the number needed to treat (NNT) were incorrect, etc [71].

13.3.4 Effect of ICSs on the Mortality Rate

A retrospective study by Soriano et al. using the UK General Practice Research Database showed that the hospital admission rate and mortality rate of patients being treated with FP were lower than among patients being treated with just a bronchodilator other than LABA, i.e., with LAMA or short-acting β2 agonist (SABA) [72]. However, no significant differences in mortality rate between the ICS group and placebo group were found in the TORCH trial [3], and a meta-analysis in recent years also reported that ICSs did not affect the COPD mortality rate [4]. Thus, there is little evidence to support ICS effectiveness in reducing the mortality rate.

13.3.5 Effectiveness of Combined Use of an ICS and a Bronchodilator

Clinically, ICSs are being used to treat COPD in combination with bronchodilators, including LABA and LAMA. Szafranski et al. reported that BUD monotherapy did not reduce COPD exacerbations, but that exacerbation frequency declined significantly when BUD was used in combination with formoterol [50], and in the TORCH trial, effectiveness in improving FEV_1 and SGRQ scores in the salmeterol (SAL)/FP combination therapy group was better than in the monotherapy group [3]. Nevertheless, results showing no differences in exacerbation frequency between an ICS/LABA group and a LABA-alone group have also been reported [73], and in the LANTERN trial, which compared ICS/LABA and LABA/LAMA, there were fewer exacerbations in the indacaterol + glycopyrronium (QVA149) group than in the SAL/FP group [74]. Moreover, results of more than one RCT showing greater effectiveness of LABA/LAMA than of ICS/LABA in ameliorating FEV_1 as well have been reported [75, 76]. Furthermore, the results of a meta-analysis also showed that LABA/LAMA was superior to ICS/LABA in relation to ameliorating FEV_1 and its exacerbation-preventing effect, and data showing a lower risk of pneumonia have also been published [77]. According to another meta-analysis, exacerbation-preventing effectiveness was reported to be greatest in a three-drug (tiotropium + BUD/formoterol) combination therapy group [78].

13.4 Effect of Discontinuing ICSs

Various studies have also been conducted on the effects of discontinuing ICSs on COPD. In the COPE study, which compared a group in which FP had been discontinued after 4 months and a group in which it had been continued, the interval before exacerbations was shorter in the group in which FP had been discontinued, and health-related QOL had also decreased [79], and in a study by Choudhury et al., the risk of COPD exacerbations was shown to have increased as a result of discontinuing ICSs [80]. Moreover, in the COPD and Seretide: a Multi-Center Intervention and Characterization (COSMIC) study, which compared a group in which FP had been discontinued after 3 months of treatment with SAL/FP and a group in which it had been continued, the magnitude of the decline in FEV_1 was greater in the group in which it had been discontinued. The difference in moderate-to-severe exacerbation frequency in that study was not significant, but mild exacerbations were more frequent in the group in which FP had been discontinued [81]. O'Brien et al. reported finding that when BDP was discontinued in elderly COPD patients, their FEV_1 decreased, and that shortness of breath evaluated on the Borg scale became severer [82]. Furthermore, in the 5-year observation period in the recent GLUCOLD study as well, when the ICS was discontinued after 30 months of treating patients with moderate-to-severe COPD, worsening of their FEV_1, QOL, and airway hypersensitivity was seen [83].

In contrast to the above results, there have also been results showing that it was possible to safely discontinue ICSs in COPD patients. In the INSTEAD trial, which distributed patients with moderate COPD and no history of exacerbations into a group treated with indacaterol (150 μg once daily) after treatment with SAL/FP (50/500 μg twice daily) for 3 months and an SAL/FP (50/500 μg twice daily) group, no significant differences between the groups in FEV_1, SGRQ scores, or exacerbation frequency were seen 12 weeks later [84]. Moreover, in the OPTIMO trial, which compared an ICS continuation group and ICS discontinuation group of 914 patients (FEV_1 predicted >50 %, exacerbation frequency <2 times/year) being treated with a combination of an ICS and a bronchodilator, no differences were seen between the groups in FEV_1, COPD Assessment Test (CAT) scores, or exacerbation rates 6 months later [85]. Thus, it was possible to discontinue the ICS safely in patients with up to moderate COPD, in which the risk of exacerbation is low. On the other hand, in the 52-week WISDOM trial in which FP was continued or gradually discontinued in FEV_1% predicted <50 %, exacerbation frequency >1/ year COPD patients ($n = 2815$) who were receiving tiotropium (TIO) + SAL + FP triple therapy, no significant difference was seen in exacerbation frequency, but FEV_1 decreased in the group in which FP had been discontinued [86]. Consequently, it appeared to be possible to gradually discontinue ICSs even in patients with severe COPD, who have a high risk of exacerbation, but that their respiratory function might decrease.

13.5 Side Effects of ICSs

Local side effects of ICSs include hoarseness, sore throat, cough, and oral and laryngopharyngeal candidiasis [87], and it is often possible to manage them by gargling after inhalation, changing the type of ICS or device, adjusting the inhalation rate, etc. When prescribing an ICS for COPD patients, it is important to take pneumonia, diabetes, and its systemic effects on bone, etc., into consideration.

13.5.1 Pneumonia

Because bacteria tend to colonize the lower airway of COPD patients, ICSs appear to increase the risk of airway infection [88]. In the TORCH trial, the rate of occurrence of pneumonia was higher in the group receiving drug therapy that included an ICS than in the placebo group [3], and in the INSPIRE trial, the rates of occurrence of pneumonia and candidiasis in the SAL/FP group were about twice as high as in the tiotropium group [89]. In the analysis by Ernst et al., it was found that pneumonia requiring hospitalization increased 70 % when ICSs were used to treat COPD patients, and the risk increased when the dose was 1000 μg or more converted to FP equivalents (relative risk [RR], 2.25; 95 % confidence interval [CI], 2.07–2.44) [90]. The cohort study by Di Santostefano et al. compared the incidence of severe pneumonia among COPD patients who were newly being treated with an ICS or ICS/LABA ($n = 11{,}555$) and a LABA monotherapy group ($n = 6492$), and the results showed that the risk of pneumonia was about 50 % higher among the patients who were newly being treated with an ICS [91]. The increase in pneumonia risk in COPD patients as a result of being treated with an ICS has even been confirmed by meta-analyses [92–94]. Kew et al. calculated a pneumonia risk odds ratios of 1.78 for FP (95 % CI: 1.50–2.12) and 1.62 for BUD (95 %CI: 1.00–2.62) [92]. Treatment with ICSs has also been reported to result in about a twofold increase in the risk of tuberculosis [95].

On the other hand, the risk of pneumonia varies with the type of ICS, and it has been reported to be lower with BUD than with FP [96]. In the PATHOS trial, which retrospectively investigated pneumonia incidence, hospitalization, and mortality rates in a SAL/FP group ($n = 2734$) and BUD/formoterol group ($n = 2734$), the risks of developing and being hospitalized for pneumonia were significantly higher in the SAL/FP group, and pneumonia-related deaths were also more common [97]. In an analysis by Suissa et al., ICSs were associated with a 69 % increase in the rate of occurrence of severe pneumonia (RR 1.69; 95 % CI 1.63–1.75), and the risk associated with SAL/FP was higher than the risk associated with BUD/formoterol [98]. When 6 months had elapsed since the ICS was discontinued, the increased risk of pneumonia was no longer seen. BUD and fluticasone dipropionate (FDP) were also shown to increase the incidence of severe pneumonia in the results of the Cochrane Review, and although there was no significant difference between the two drugs in pneumonia mortality rates, FDP entailed a higher risk of developing mild pneumonia [92]. The reason for the difference in pneumonia risk between BUD and FP has been explained by differences between the drugs in the strength of their immunosuppressant effects and their pharmacokinetic/pharmacodynamic (PK/PD) ratios, but the high 1000 μg FP dosage in many clinical trials seems to be another reason.

13.5.2 Diabetes

No increases in the rate of occurrence of diabetes due to ICSs were seen in the results of the Lung Health Study or EUROSCOP [34, 39], and no increases in the numbers of cases of diabetes were reported as adverse events due to ICSs in the TRISTAN, ISOLDE, or TORCH trials [2, 3, 47]. However, according to the cohort study conducted by Suissa et al. ($n = 388{,}584$), the risk of diabetes was reported to be 34 % higher when an ICS (FP, BDP, BUD, triamcinolone, and flunisolide) was used to treat respiratory disease patients than in the group in which no ICSs were used (95 % CI, 1.17–1.53), and the risk was reported to be particularly higher among the patients who received high dosages, i.e., 1000 μg/day or more converted to FP equivalents [99]. Moreover, based on the results of measuring the blood glucose level of 1698 patients being treated with an ICS (triamcinolone), it was reported that the blood glucose level of the patients who self-reported diabetes increased 1.82 mg/dL for each 100 μg increase in the ICS and that among the diabetes patients who had been prescribed an antiglycemic drug, it increased 2.65 mg/dL [100]. However, O'Byrne et al. analyzed 8 RCTs (BUD, $n = 33{,}496$; non-ICS, $n = 3643$) and stated that the incidence of diabetes/hyperglycemia was 1.3 % in the BUD group and 1.2 % in the non-ICS group and the difference was not significant [101]. In addition, in the cohort study by Flynn et al. (3243 patients treated with an ICS, 1062 patients not treated with an ICS) as well, the hazard ratio (HR) due to ICS was 0.70 (0.43–1.12) for the onset of diabetes and 0.57 (0.24–1.37) for worsening of diabetes, and no effect of the ICS was observed [102]. Moreover, no association was observed between treatment with BDP and the risk of diabetes in the cohort study of elderly subjects ($n = 21{,}645$) conducted by Dendukuri et al. [103]. Based on the above results, the risk of developing diabetes as a result of treatment with an ICS is very small, but caution appears to be necessary in regard to the use of high-dose steroids and patients who have diabetes.

13.5.3 Osteoporosis and Fractures

According to a World Health Organization (WHO) systematic review that investigated the bone effects of ICSs in bronchial asthma and COPD patients, triamcinolone had the greatest adverse effect on bone mineral density (BMD), and was followed by BDP, and then by BUD [104]. In addition, a meta-analysis that investigated the fracture risk associated with ICSs in COPD patients ($n = 17{,}513$) showed that it was increased 21–27 % by ICSs (FP, BUD) and that the risk increased 9 % for each 500 μg increase in dose converted to BDP equivalents [105]. The Nord-Trøndelag Health (HUNT) study, on the other hand, reported a 30 % decrease in female ICS users and 50 % decrease in male ICS users, but that the effects of the ICSs in patients being treated with low to medium doses were slight [106]. By contrast, Yang et al. conducted a meta-analysis in relation to a 3-year or more long-term observations and concluded that ICSs did not have a significant effect on fractures or BMD [4].

13.6 Effectiveness of Combined Use of an ICS and Theophylline

Steroid effectiveness in COPD is attenuated by the decrease in HDAC2, but theophylline is known to have an HDAC2-function-restoring action. For example, it has been reported that when the alveolar macrophages of COPD patients, who have low steroid sensitivity, were exposed to low steroid concentrations, HDAC2 activity and steroid actions were restored. High blood concentrations are needed for theophylline to exert a bronchodilator effect, but low concentrations of around 2 μg/mL appear to be effective in activating HDAC2 [107, 108]. On the other hand, according to a cohort study that assessed 36,492 COPD patients, a significant decrease in frequency of moderate-to-severe exacerbations was observed among the patients treated with an ICS + theophylline in comparison with the patients treated with an ICS + LABA (RR 0.89, 95 % CI 0.87,0.92) [109]. The Theophylline with Inhaled Corticosteroids (TWICS) study, which is checking the effectiveness of ICS and theophylline combination therapy, is currently underway [110].

13.7 Selection of COPD Patients with Indications for ICSs

Steroids have been reported to have a strong therapeutic effect in patients who have a peripheral blood eosinophil count of 2 % or more during a COPD exacerbation [111]. Moreover, because an exacerbation-preventing effect of SAL/FP has been observed in COPD patients with a history of exacerbations if their peripheral blood eosinophil count was 2 % or more in the stable phase, the peripheral blood eosinophil count can serve as a biomarker for selecting patients with ICS indications [112]. By contrast, in COPD complicated by asthma (asthma-COPD overlap syndrome [ACOS]), treatment with ICS/LABA has been found to reduce the risk of hospitalization or death due to COPD in comparison with LABA monotherapy [113]. Moreover, results showing that improvements in sputum eosinophil count and bronchiolar wall thickness on chest computed tomography (CT) scans correlate with improvements in FEV_1 in response to ICSs [114], and correlations between sputum eosinophil counts and steroid responsiveness have also been found [115, 116]. Consequently, some COPD patients, i.e., patients with ACOS, in which COPD is complicated by asthma, and patients with eosinophilic COPD, in which the sputum and peripheral blood eosinophil counts are elevated, appear to have positive indications for ICSs. The characteristics of ACOS are shown in Table 13.2, but treatment with an ICS in combination with bronchodilator is

Table 13.2 Usual features of ACOS

Age of onset	Usually age ≥40 years, but may have had symptoms in childhood or early adulthood
Pattern of respiratory symptoms	Respiratory symptoms including exertional dyspnea are persistent, but variability may be prominent
Lung function	Airflow limitation not fully reversible, but often with current or historical variability
Lung function between symptoms	Persistent airflow limitation
Past history or family history	Frequently a history of doctor-diagnosed asthma (current or previous), allergies and family history of asthma, and/or a history of noxious exposures
Time coarse	Symptoms are partly but significantly reduced by treatment. Progression is usual and treatment needs are high
Chest X-ray	Similar to COPD
Exacerbations	Exacerbation may be more common than in COPD but are reduced by treatment. Comorbidities can contribute to impairment
Airway inflammation	Eosinophils and/or neutrophils in sputum

Adapted from Ref. [117]

Table 13.3 Indicator of a probable response to inhaled corticosteroids in patients with chronic obstructive pulmonary disease

History of asthma or atopy
Onset of respiratory disease prior to the age of 40 years
Cumulative smoking history < 20 pack-years
FEV1 bronchodilator response ≧12 % and ≧400 ml
Normal diffuse capacity
Peripheral blood eosinophilia
Sputum eosinophilia
Not FEV1 <50 % predicted
Not history of frequent exacerbations

Based on [71]

FEV_1 forced expiratory volume in 1 s

strongly recommended for ACOS in the Global Initiative for Asthma (GINA) guideline [117]. Ernst et al. have summarized the characteristics of COPD in which a therapeutic effect of ICSs can be expected in Table 13.3 [71].

13.8 Conclusion

The current GOLD guidelines recommend using an ICS in addition to LABA and LAMA in severe or very severe COPD with recurring exacerbations. The main purpose is to prevent exacerbations, but the exacerbation-preventing effect of ICSs may have been slightly overevaluated in previous reports, and in view of the fact that COPD is a heterogeneous disease, it is necessary to make an effort to search for

COPD phenotypes in which ICSs are of great benefit. At present, ACOS and eosinophilic COPD appear to have positive indications for treatment with ICSs, but further study will be necessary to determine whether the peripheral blood eosinophil count can serve as a biomarker for ICS indications. At the same time, when prescribing ICSs, the fact that the risk of side effects, including pneumonia, increases must also be borne in mind.

References

1. Global Initiative for Chronic Obstructive Lung Disease. Global strategy for the diagnosis, management, and prevention of chronic obstructive pulmonary disease (revised 2011). Global Initiative for Chronic Obstructive Lung Disease, Inc; 2011.
2. Burge PS, Calverley PM, Jones PW, Spencer S, Anderson JA, Maslen TK. Randomised, double blind, placebo controlled study of fluticasone propionate in patients with moderate to severe chronic obstructive pulmonary disease: the ISOLDE trial. BMJ. 2000;320:1297–303.
3. Calverley PM, Anderson JA, Celli B, Ferguson GT, Jenkins C, Jones PW, et al. Salmeterol and fluticasone propionate and survival in chronic obstructive pulmonary disease. N Engl J Med. 2007;356:775–89.
4. Yang IA, Clarke MS, Sim EHA, Fong KM. Inhaled corticosteroids for stable chronic obstructive pulmonary disease (Review). Cochrane Database Syst Rev. 2012;7:CD002991. doi:10.1002/14651858.
5. Agarwal R, Aggarwal AN, Gupta D, Jindal SK. Inhaled corticosteroids vs placebo for preventing COPD exacerbations: a systematic review and metaregression of randomized controlled trials. Chest. 2010;137:318–25. doi:10.1378/chest.09-1305.
6. Mehuys E, Boussery K, Adriaens E, Van Bortel L, De Bolle L, Van Tongelen I, et al. COPD management in primary care: an observational, community pharmacy-based study. Ann Pharmacother. 2010;44:257–66. doi:10.1345/aph.1M481.
7. White P, Thornton H, Pinnock H, Georgopoulou S, Booth HP. Overtreatment of COPD with inhaled corticosteroids—implications for safety and costs: cross-sectional observational study. PLoS One. 2013;8:e75221. doi:10.1371/journal.pone.0075221.
8. Brusselle GG, Joos GF, Bracke KR. New insights into the immunology of chronic obstructive pulmonary disease. Lancet. 2011;378:1015–26. doi:10.1016/S0140-6736(11)60988-4.
9. Confalonieri M, Mainardi E, Della Porta R, Bernorio S, Gandola L, Beghè B, et al. Inhaled corticosteroids reduce neutrophilic bronchial inflammation in patients with chronic obstructive pulmonary disease. Thorax. 1998;53:583–5.
10. Llewellyn-Jones CG, Harris TA, Stockley RA. Effect of fluticasone propionate on sputum of patients with chronic bronchitis and emphysema. Am J Respir Crit Care Med. 1996;153:616–21.
11. Ozol D, Aysan T, Solak ZA, Mogulkoc N, Veral A, Sebik F. The effect of inhaled corticosteroids on bronchoalveolar lavage cells and IL-8 levels in stable COPD patients. Respir Med. 2005;99:1494–500.
12. Jen R, Rennard SI, Sin DD. Effects of inhaled corticosteroids on airway inflammation in chronic obstructive pulmonary disease: a systematic review and meta-analysis. Int J Chron Obstruct Pulmon Dis. 2012;7:587–95. doi:10.2147/COPD.S32765.
13. Ito K, Ito M, Elliott WM, et al. Decreased histone deacetylase activity in chronic obstructive pulmonary disease. N Engl J Med. 2005;352:1967–76.
14. Szulakowski P, Crowther AJ, Jiménez LA, et al. The effect of smoking on the transcriptional regulation of lung inflammation in patients with chronic obstructive pulmonary disease. Am J Respir Crit Care Med. 2006;174:41–50.

15. Barnes PJ. How corticosteroids control inflammation: Quintiles Prize Lecture 2005. Br J Pharmacol. 2006;148:245–54.
16. Barnes PJ, Adcock IM. How do corticosteroids work in asthma? Ann Intern Med. 2003;139:359–70.
17. Robertson AS, Gove RI, Wieland GA, Burge PS. A double-blind comparison of oral prednisolone 40 mg/day with inhaled beclomethasone dipropionate 1500 ug/day in patients with adult onset chronic obstructive airways disease. Eur J Respir Dis Suppl. 1986;146:565–9.
18. Weir DC, Gove RI, Robertson AS, Burge PS. Corticosteroid trials in non-asthmatic chronic airflow obstruction: a comparison of oral prednisolone and inhaled beclomethasone dipropionate. Thorax. 1990;45:112–7.
19. Auffarth B, Postma DS, de Monchy JG, van der Mark TW, Boorsma M, Koëter GH. Effects of inhaled budesonide on spirometric values, reversibility, airway responsiveness, and cough threshold in smokers with chronic obstructive lung disease. Thorax. 1991;46:372–7.
20. Thompson AB, Mueller MB, Heires AJ, Bohling TL, Daughton D, Yancey SW, et al. Aerosolized beclomethasone in chronic bronchitis. Improved pulmonary function and diminished airway inflammation. Am Rev Respir Dis. 1992;146:389–95.
21. Kerstjens HA, Brand PL, Hughes MD, Robinson NJ, Postma DS, Sluiter HJ, et al. A comparison of bronchodilator therapy with or without inhaled corticosteroid therapy for obstructive airways disease. Dutch Chronic Non-Specific Lung Disease Study Group. N Engl J Med. 1992;327:1413–9.
22. Watson A, Lim TK, Joyce H, Pride NB. Failure of inhaled corticosteroids to modify bronchoconstrictor or bronchodilator responsiveness in middle-aged smokers with mild airflow obstruction. Chest. 1992;101:350–5.
23. Wempe JB, Postma DS, Breederveld N, Kort E, van der Mark TW, Koëter GH. Effects of corticosteroids on bronchodilator action in chronic obstructive lung disease. Thorax. 1992;47:616–21.
24. Weir DC, Burge PS. Effects of high dose inhaled beclomethasone dipropionate, 750 micrograms and 1500 micrograms twice daily, and 40 mg per day oral prednisolone on lung function, symptoms, and bronchial hyperresponsiveness in patients with non-asthmatic chronic airflow obstruction. Thorax. 1993;48:309–16.
25. Weiner P, Weiner M, Azgad Y, Zamir D. Inhaled budesonide therapy for patients with stable COPD. Chest. 1995;108:1568–71.
26. Renkema TE, Schouten JP, Koëter GH, Postma DS. Effects of long-term treatment with corticosteroids in COPD. Chest. 1996;109:1156–62.
27. Boothman-Burrell D, Delany SG, Flannery EM, Hancox RJ, Taylor DR. The efficacy of inhaled corticosteroids in the management of non asthmatic chronic airflow obstruction. N Z Med J. 1997;110:370–3.
28. Keatings VM, Jatakanon A, Worsdell YM, Barnes PJ. Effects of inhaled and oral glucocorticoids on inflammatory indices in asthma and COPD. Am J Respir Crit Care Med. 1997;155:542–8.
29. Bourbeau J, Rouleau MY, Boucher S. Randomised controlled trial of inhaled corticosteroids in patients with chronic obstructive pulmonary disease. Thorax. 1998;53:477–82.
30. Paggiaro PL, Dahle R, Bakran I, Frith L, Hollingworth K, Efthimiou J. Multicentre randomised placebo-controlled trial of inhaled fluticasone propionate in patients with chronic obstructive pulmonary disease. International COPD Study Group. Lancet. 1998;351:773–80.
31. Rutgers SR, Koëter GH, van der Mark TW, Postma DS. Short-term treatment with budesonide does not improve hyperresponsiveness to adenosine 5′-monophosphate in COPD. Am J Respir Crit Care Med. 1998;157:880–6.
32. Culpitt SV, Maziak W, Loukidis S, Nightingale JA, Matthews JL, Barnes PJ. Effect of high dose inhaled steroid on cells, cytokines, and proteases in induced sputum in chronic obstructive pulmonary disease. Am J Respir Crit Care Med. 1999;160:1635–9.
33. Nishimura K, Koyama H, Ikeda A, Tsukino M, Hajiro T, Mishima M, et al. The effect of high-dose inhaled beclomethasone dipropionate in patients with stable COPD. Chest. 1999;115:31–7.

34. Pauwels RA, Löfdahl CG, Laitinen LA, Schouten JP, Postma DS, Pride NB, et al. Long-term treatment with inhaled budesonide in persons with mild chronic obstructive pulmonary disease who continue smoking. European Respiratory Society Study on Chronic Obstructive Pulmonary Disease. N Engl J Med. 1999;340:1948–53.
35. Senderovitz T, Vestbo J, Frandsen J, Maltbaek N, Nørgaard M, Nielsen C, et al. Steroid reversibility test followed by inhaled budesonide or placebo in outpatients with stable chronic obstructive pulmonary disease. The Danish Society of Respiratory Medicine. Respir Med. 1999;93:715–8.
36. Vestbo J, Sørensen T, Lange P, Brix A, Torre P, Viskum K. Long-term effect of inhaled budesonide in mild and moderate chronic obstructive pulmonary disease: a randomised controlled trial. Lancet. 1999;353:1819–23.
37. Weiner P, Weiner M, Rabner M, Waizman J, Magadle R, Zamir D. The response to inhaled and oral steroids in patients with stable chronic obstructive pulmonary disease. J Intern Med. 1999;245:83–9.
38. Weir DC, Bale GA, Bright P, Sherwood BP. A double-blind placebo-controlled study of the effect of inhaled beclomethasone dipropionate for 2 years in patients with nonasthmatic chronic obstructive pulmonary disease. Clin Exp Allergy. 1999;29 Suppl 2:125–8.
39. Lung Health Study Research Group. Effect of inhaled triamcinolone on the decline in pulmonary function in chronic obstructive pulmonary disease. N Engl J Med. 2000;343:1902–9.
40. Ferreira IM, Hazari MS, Gutierrez C, Zamel N, Chapman KR. Exhaled nitric oxide and hydrogen peroxide in patients with chronic obstructive pulmonary disease: effects of inhaled beclomethasone. Am J Respir Crit Care Med. 2001;164:1012–5.
41. Loppow D, Schleiss MB, Kanniess F, Taube C, Jörres RA, Magnussen H. In patients with chronic bronchitis a four week trial with inhaled steroids does not attenuate airway inflammation. Respir Med. 2001;95:115–21.
42. Mirici A, Bektas Y, Ozbakis G, Erman Z. Effect of inhaled corticosteroids on respiratory function tests and airway inflammation in stable chronic obstructive pulmonary disease: a randomised, double-blind, Placebo-Controlled Clinical Trial. Clin Drug Invest. 2001;21:835–42.
43. Hattotuwa KL, Gizycki MJ, Ansari TW, Jeffery PK, Barnes NC. The effects of inhaled fluticasone on airway inflammation in chronic obstructive pulmonary disease: a double-blind, placebo-controlled biopsy study. Am J Respir Crit Care Med. 2002;165:1592–6.
44. Mahler DA, Wire P, Horstman D, Chang CN, Yates J, Fischer T, et al. Effectiveness of fluticasone propionate and salmeterol combination delivered via the Diskus device in the treatment of chronic obstructive pulmonary disease. Am J Respir Crit Care Med. 2002;166:1084–91.
45. Thompson WH, Carvalho P, Souza JP, Charan NB. Controlled trial of inhaled fluticasone propionate in moderate to severe COPD. Lung. 2002;180:191–201.
46. Verhoeven GT, Hegmans JP, Mulder PG, Bogaard JM, Hoogsteden HC, Prins JB. Effects of fluticasone propionate in COPD patients with bronchial hyperresponsiveness. Thorax. 2002;57:694–700.
47. Calverley P, Pauwels R, Vestbo J, Jones P, Pride N, Gulsvik A, et al. Combined salmeterol and fluticasone in the treatment of chronic obstructive pulmonary disease: a randomised controlled trial. Lancet. 2003;361(9356):449–56. Erratum in: Lancet. 2003; 361:1660.
48. Calverley PM, Boonsawat W, Cseke Z, Zhong N, Peterson S, Olsson H. Maintenance therapy with budesonide and formoterol in chronic obstructive pulmonary disease. Eur Respir J. 2003;22:912–9.
49. Hanania NA, Darken P, Horstman D, Reisner C, Lee B, Davis S, et al. The efficacy and safety of fluticasone propionate (250 microg)/salmeterol (50 microg) combined in the Diskus inhaler for the treatment of COPD. Chest. 2003;124:834–43.
50. Szafranski W, Cukier A, Ramirez A, Menga G, Sansores R, Nahabedian S, et al. Efficacy and safety of budesonide/formoterol in the management of chronic obstructive pulmonary disease. Eur Respir J. 2003;21:74–81.

51. van Grunsven P, Schermer T, Akkermans R, Albers M, van den Boom G, van Schayck O. Short- and long-term efficacy of fluticasone propionate in subjects with early signs and symptoms of chronic obstructive pulmonary disease. Results of the DIMCA study. Respir Med. 2003;97:1303–12.
52. Sin DD, Lacy P, York E, Man SF. Effects of fluticasone on systemic markers of inflammation in chronic obstructive pulmonary disease. Am J Respir Crit Care Med. 2004;170:760–5.
53. Yildiz F, Basyigit I, Yildirim E, Boyaci H, Ilgazli A. Does addition of inhaled steroid to combined bronchodilator therapy affect health status in patients with COPD? Respirology. 2004;9:352–5.
54. Brightling CE, McKenna S, Hargadon B, Birring S, Green R, Siva R, et al. Sputum eosinophilia and the short term response to inhaled mometasone in chronic obstructive pulmonary disease. Thorax. 2005;60:193–8.
55. John M, Bosse S, Oltmanns U, Schumacher A, Witt C. Effects of inhaled HFA beclomethasone on pulmonary function and symptoms in patients with chronic obstructive pulmonary disease. Respir Med. 2005;99:1418–24.
56. GlaxoSmithKline. A double/blind, randomised, controlled, three parallel group, multicenter study to compare the acute effects of inhaled Flixotide/Salmeterol vs. Decortin/Flixotide/Salmeterol vs. Salmeterol in patients with COPD. 2005. http://www.gsk-clinicalstudyregister.com/study/FCO30002?study_ids=FCO30002#rs. Accessed 9 Dec 2015.
57. GlaxoSmithKline. A randomized, double-blind, parallel-group, comparative trial of inhaled fluticasone propionate 250mcg twice daily, 500mcg twice daily, and placebo twice daily via the DISKUS® inhaler in subjects with chronic obstructive pulmonary disease (COPD). 2005. http://www.gsk-clinicalstudyregister.com/study/FLTA3025?study_ids=FLTA3025#rs. Accessed 9 Dec 2015.
58. Bourbeau J, Christodoulopoulos P, Maltais F, Yamauchi Y, Olivenstein R, Hamid Q. Effect of salmeterol/fluticasone propionate on airway inflammation in COPD: a randomised controlled trial. Thorax. 2007;62:938–43.
59. Calverley PM, Rennard S, Nelson HS, Karpel JP, Abbate EH, Stryszak P, et al. One-year treatment with mometasone furoate in chronic obstructive pulmonary disease. Respir Res. 2008;9:73. doi:10.1186/1465-9921-9-73.
60. Sin DD, Man SF, Marciniuk DD, Ford G, FitzGerald M, Wong E, et al. The effects of fluticasone with or without salmeterol on systemic biomarkers of inflammation in chronic obstructive pulmonary disease. Am J Respir Crit Care Med. 2008;177:1207–14. doi:10.1164/rccm.200709-1356OC.
61. Lapperre TS, Snoeck-Stroband JB, Gosman MM, Jansen DF, van Schadewijk A, Thiadens HA, et al. Effect of fluticasone with and without salmeterol on pulmonary outcomes in chronic obstructive pulmonary disease: a randomized trial. Ann Intern Med. 2009;151:517–27.
62. Schermer T, Chavannes N, Dekhuijzen R, Wouters E, Muris J, Akkermans R, et al. Fluticasone and N-acetylcysteine in primary care patients with COPD or chronic bronchitis. Respir Med. 2009;103:542–51. doi:10.1016/j.rmed.2008.11.003.
63. Shaker SB, Dirksen A, Ulrik CS, Hestad M, Stavngaard T, Laursen LC, et al. The effect of inhaled corticosteroids on the development of emphysema in smokers assessed by annual computed tomography. COPD. 2009;6:104–11. doi:10.1080/15412550902772593.
64. Guenette JA, Raghavan N, Harris-McAllister V, Preston ME, Webb KA, O'Donnell DE. Effect of adjunct fluticasone propionate on airway physiology during rest and exercise in COPD. Respir Med. 2011;105:1836–45. doi:10.1016/j.rmed.2011.08.021.
65. Tashkin DP, Doherty DE, Kerwin E, Matiz-Bueno CE, Knorr B, Shekar T, et al. Efficacy and safety characteristics of mometasone furoate/formoterol fumarate fixed-dose combination in subjects with moderate to very severe COPD: findings from pooled analysis of two randomized, 52-week placebo-controlled trials. Int J Chron Obstruct Pulmon Dis. 2012;7:73–86. doi:10.2147/COPD.S29444.

66. Suissa S. Lung function decline in COPD trials: bias from regression to the mean. Eur Respir J. 2008;32:829–31. doi:10.1183/09031936.00103008.
67. van Grunsven PM, van Schayck CP, Derenne JP, Kerstjens HA, Renkema TE, Postma DS, et al. Long term effects of inhaled corticosteroids in chronic obstructive pulmonary disease: a meta-analysis. Thorax. 1999;54:7–14.
68. Alsaeedi A, Sin DD, McAlister FA. The effects of inhaled corticosteroids in chronic obstructive pulmonary disease: a systematic review of randomized placebo-controlled trials. Am J Med. 2002;113:59–65.
69. De Coster DA, Jones M, Thakrar N. Beclometasone for chronic obstructive pulmonary disease. Cochrane Database Syst Rev. 2013;10:CD009769. doi:10.1002/14651858.
70. Jones PW. Quality of life, symptoms and pulmonary function in asthma: long-term treatment with nedocromil sodium examined in a controlled multicentre trial. Nedocromil Sodium Quality of Life Study Group. Eur Respir J. 1994;7:55–62.
71. Ernst P, Saad N, Suissa S. Inhaled corticosteroids in COPD: the clinical evidence. Eur Respir J. 2015;45(2):525–37. doi:10.1183/09031936.00128914.
72. Soriano JB, Vestbo J, Pride NB, Kiri V, Maden C, Maier WC. Survival in COPD patients after regular use of fluticasone propionate and salmeterol in general practice. Eur Respir J. 2002;20(4):819–25.
73. Rodrigo GJ, Castro-Rodriguez JA, Plaza V. Safety and efficacy of combined long-acting beta-agonists and inhaled corticosteroids vs long-acting beta-agonists monotherapy for stable COPD: a systematic review. Chest. 2009;136:1029–38. doi:10.1378/chest.09-0821.
74. Zhong N, Wang C, Zhou X, Zhang N, Humphries M, Wang L, et al. LANTERN: a randomized study of QVA149 versus salmeterol/fluticasone combination in patients with COPD. Int J Chron Obstruct Pulmon Dis. 2015;10:1015–26. doi:10.2147/COPD.S84436.
75. Vogelmeier CF, Bateman ED, Pallante J, Alagappan VK, D'Andrea P, Chen H, et al. Efficacy and safety of once-daily QVA149 compared with twice-daily salmeterol-fluticasone in patients with chronic obstructive pulmonary disease (ILLUMINATE): a randomised, double-blind, parallel group study. Lancet Respir Med. 2013;1:51–60. doi:10.1016/S2213-2600(12)70052-8.
76. Donohue JF, Worsley S, Zhu CQ, Hardaker L, Church A. Improvements in lung function with umeclidinium/vilanterol versus fluticasone propionate/salmeterol in patients with moderate-to-severe COPD and infrequent exacerbations. Respir Med. 2015;109:870–81. doi:10.1016/j.rmed.2015.04.018.
77. Horita N, Miyazawa N, Tomaru K, Inoue M, Kaneko T. Long-acting muscarinic antagonist + long-acting beta agonist versus long-acting beta agonist + inhaled corticosteroid for COPD: a systematic review and meta-analysis. Respirology. 2015;20:1153–9. doi:10.1111/resp.12603.
78. Tricco AC, Strifler L, Veroniki AA, Yazdi F, Khan PA, Scott A, et al. Comparative safety and effectiveness of long-acting inhaled agents for treating chronic obstructive pulmonary disease: a systematic review and network meta-analysis. BMJ Open. 2015;5:e009183. doi:10.1136/bmjopen-2015-009183.
79. van der Valk P, Monninkhof E, van der Palen J, Zielhuis G, van Herwaarden C. Effect of discontinuation of inhaled corticosteroids in patients with chronic obstructive pulmonary disease: the COPE study. Am J Respir Crit Care Med. 2002;166:1358–63.
80. Choudhury AB, Dawson CM, Kilvington HE, Eldridge S, James WY, Wedzicha JA, et al. Withdrawal of inhaled corticosteroids in people with COPD in primary care: a randomised controlled trial. Respir Res. 2007;8:93.
81. Wouters EF, Postma DS, Fokkens B, Hop WC, Prins J, Kuipers AF, et al. Withdrawal of fluticasone propionate from combined salmeterol/fluticasone treatment in patients with COPD causes immediate and sustained disease deterioration: a randomised controlled trial. Thorax. 2005;60:480–7.
82. O'Brien A, Russo-Magno P, Karki A, Hiranniramol S, Hardin M, Kaszuba M, et al. Effects of withdrawal of inhaled steroids in men with severe irreversible airflow obstruction. Am J Respir Crit Care Med. 2001;164:365–71.

83. Kunz LI, Postma DS, Klooster K, Lapperre TS, Vonk JM, Sont JK, et al. Relapse in FEV1 decline after steroid withdrawal in COPD. Chest. 2015;148:389–96. doi:10.1378/chest.14-3091.
84. Rossi A, van der Molen T, del Olmo R, Papi A, Wehbe L, Quinn M, et al. INSTEAD: a randomised switch trial of indacaterol versus salmeterol/fluticasone in moderate COPD. Eur Respir J. 2014;44:1548–56. doi:10.1183/09031936.00126814.
85. Rossi A, Guerriero M, Corrado A. Withdrawal of inhaled corticosteroids can be safe in COPD patients at low risk of exacerbation: a real-life study on the appropriateness of treatment in moderate COPD patients (OPTIMO). Respir Res. 2014;15:77. doi:10.1186/1465-9921-15-77.
86. Magnussen H, Disse B, Rodriguez-Roisin R, Kirsten A, Watz H, Tetzlaff K, et al. Withdrawal of inhaled glucocorticoids and exacerbations of COPD. N Engl J Med. 2014;371:1285–94. doi:10.1056/NEJMoa1407154.
87. Tattersfield AE, Harrison TW, Hubbard RB, Mortimer K. Safety of inhaled corticosteroids. Proc Am Thorac Soc. 2004;1:171–5.
88. Monsó E, Ruiz J, Rosell A, Manterola J, Fiz J, Morera J, et al. Bacterial infection in chronic obstructive pulmonary disease. A study of stable and exacerbated outpatients using the protected specimen brush. Am J Respir Crit Care Med. 1995;152:1316–20.
89. Wedzicha JA, Calverley PM, Seemungal TA, Hagan G, Ansari Z, Stockley RA. The prevention of chronic obstructive pulmonary disease exacerbations by salmeterol/fluticasone propionate or tiotropium bromide. Am J Respir Crit Care Med. 2008;177:19–26.
90. Ernst P, Gonzalez AV, Brassard P, Suissa S. Inhaled corticosteroid use in chronic obstructive pulmonary disease and the risk of hospitalization for pneumonia. Am J Respir Crit Care Med. 2007;176:162–6.
91. Di Santostefano RL, Sampson T, Le HV, Hinds D, Davis KJ, Bakerly ND. Risk of pneumonia with inhaled corticosteroid versus long-acting bronchodilator regimens in chronic obstructive pulmonary disease: a new-user cohort study. PLoS One. 2014;9:e97149. doi:10.1371/journal.pone.0097149.
92. Kew KM, Seniukovich A. Inhaled steroids and risk of pneumonia for chronic obstructive pulmonary disease. Cochrane Database Syst Rev. 2014;3:CD010115. doi:10.1002/14651858.CD010115.
93. Singh S, Amin AV, Loke YK. Long-term use of inhaled corticosteroids and the risk of pneumonia in chronic obstructive pulmonary disease: a meta-analysis. Arch Intern Med. 2009;169:219–29. doi:10.1001/archinternmed.2008.550.
94. Drummond MB, Dasenbrook EC, Pitz MW, Murphy DJ, Fan E. Inhaled corticosteroids in patients with stable chronic obstructive pulmonary disease: a systematic review and meta-analysis. JAMA. 2008;300:2407–16. doi:10.1001/jama.2008.717.
95. Dong YH, Chang CH, Lin Wu FL, Shen LJ, Calverley PM, Löfdahl CG, et al. Use of inhaled corticosteroids in patients with COPD and the risk of TB and influenza: a systematic review and meta-analysis of randomized controlled trials. Chest. 2014;145:1286–97.
96. Sin DD, Tashkin D, Zhang X, Radner F, Sjöbring U, Thorén A, et al. Budesonide and the risk of pneumonia: a meta-analysis of individual patient data. Lancet. 2009;374:712–9. doi:10.1016/S0140-6736(09)61250-2.
97. Janson C, Larsson K, Lisspers KH, Ställberg B, Stratelis G, Goike H, et al. Pneumonia and pneumonia related mortality in patients with COPD treated with fixed combinations of inhaled corticosteroid and long acting β2 agonist: observational matched cohort study (PATHOS). BMJ. 2013;346:f3306. doi:10.1136/bmj.f3306.
98. Suissa S, Patenaude V, Lapi F, Ernst P. Inhaled corticosteroids in COPD and the risk of serious pneumonia. Thorax. 2013;68:1029–36. doi:10.1136/thoraxjnl-2012-202872.
99. Suissa S, Kezouh A, Ernst P. Inhaled corticosteroids and the risks of diabetes onset and progression. Am J Med. 2010;123:1001–6. doi:10.1016/j.amjmed.2010.06.019.
100. Slatore CG, Bryson CL, Au DH. The association of inhaled corticosteroid use with serum glucose concentration in a large cohort. Am J Med. 2009;122:472–8. doi:10.1016/j.amjmed.2008.09.048.

101. O'Byrne PM, Rennard S, Gerstein H, Radner F, Peterson S, Lindberg B, et al. Risk of new onset diabetes mellitus in patients with asthma or COPD taking inhaled corticosteroids. Respir Med. 2012;106:1487–93. doi:10.1016/j.rmed.2012.07.011.
102. Flynn RW, MacDonald TM, Hapca A, MacKenzie IS, Schembri S. Quantifying the real life risk profile of inhaled corticosteroids in COPD by record linkage analysis. Respir Res. 2014;15:141. doi:10.1186/s12931-014-0141-y.
103. Dendukuri N, Blais L, LeLorier J. Inhaled corticosteroids and the risk of diabetes among the elderly. Br J Clin Pharmacol. 2002;54:59–64.
104. Richy F, Bousquet J, Ehrlich GE, Meunier PJ, Israel E, Morii H. Inhaled corticosteroids effects on bone in asthmatic and COPD patients: a quantitative systematic review. Osteoporos Int. 2003;14:179–90.
105. Loke YK, Cavallazzi R, Singh S. Risk of fractures with inhaled corticosteroids in COPD: systematic review and meta-analysis of randomised controlled trials and observational studies. Thorax. 2011;66:699–708. doi:10.1136/thx.2011.160028.
106. Langhammer A, Forsmo S, Lilleeng S, Johnsen R, Bjermer L. Effect of inhaled corticosteroids on forearm bone mineral density: the HUNT study. Norway Respir Med. 2007;101:1744–52.
107. Ford PA, Durham AL, Russell RE, Gordon F, Adcock IM, Barnes PJ. Treatment effects of low-dose theophylline combined with an inhaled corticosteroid in COPD. Chest. 2010;137:1338–44. doi:10.1378/chest.09-2363.
108. Cosio BG, Iglesias A, Rios A, Noguera A, Sala E, Ito K, et al. Low-dose theophylline enhances the anti-inflammatory effects of steroids during exacerbations of COPD. Thorax. 2009;64:424–9. doi:10.1136/thx.2008.103432.
109. Cyr MC, Beauchesne MF, Lemière C, Blais L. Effect of theophylline on the rate of moderate to severe exacerbations among patients with chronic obstructive pulmonary disease. Br J Clin Pharmacol. 2008;65:40–50.
110. Devereux G, Cotton S, Barnes P, Briggs A, Burns G, Chaudhuri R, et al. Use of low-dose oral theophylline as an adjunct to inhaled corticosteroids in preventing exacerbations of chronic obstructive pulmonary disease: study protocol for a randomised controlled trial. Trials. 2015;16:267. doi:10.1186/s13063-015-0782-2.
111. Bafadhel M, McKenna S, Terry S, Mistry V, Pancholi M, Venge P, et al. Blood eosinophils to direct corticosteroid treatment of exacerbations of chronic obstructive pulmonary disease: a randomized placebo-controlled trial. Am J Respir Crit Care Med. 2012;186:48–55. doi:10.1164/rccm.201108-1553OC.
112. Pavord ID, Lettis S, Locantore N, Pascoe S, Jones PW, Wedzicha JA, et al. Blood eosinophils and inhaled corticosteroid/long-acting β-2 agonist efficacy in COPD. Thorax. 2015. pii: thoraxjnl-2015-207021. doi: 10.1136/thoraxjnl-2015-207021.
113. Gershon AS, Campitelli MA, Croxford R, Stanbrook MB, To T, Upshur R, et al. Combination long-acting β-agonists and inhaled corticosteroids compared with long-acting β-agonists alone in older adults with chronic obstructive pulmonary disease. JAMA. 2014;312:1114–21. doi:10.1001/jama.2014.11432.
114. Kitaguchi Y, Komatsu Y, Fujimoto K, Hanaoka M, Kubo K. Sputum eosinophilia can predict responsiveness to inhaled corticosteroid treatment in patients with overlap syndrome of COPD and asthma. Int J Chron Obstruct Pulmon Dis. 2012;7:283–9. doi:10.2147/COPD.S30651.
115. Brightling CE, Monteiro W, Ward R, Parker D, Morgan MD, Wardlaw AJ, et al. Sputum eosinophilia and short-term response to prednisolone in chronic obstructive pulmonary disease: a randomised controlled trial. Lancet. 2000;356:1480–5.
116. Pizzichini E, Pizzichini MM, Gibson P, Parameswaran K, Gleich GJ, Berman L, et al. Sputum eosinophilia predicts benefit from prednisone in smokers with chronic obstructive bronchitis. Am J Respir Crit Care Med. 1998;158:1511–7.
117. Global Initiative for Asthma. Global strategy for asthma management and prevention: online appendix. 2015. http://www.ginasthma.org/local/uploads/files/GINA_Appendix_2015_May19.pdf.

Chapter 14
New Anti-inflammatory Drugs for COPD: Is There a Possibility of Developing Drugs That Can Fundamentally Suppress Inflammation?

Yasuhiro Yamauchi and Takahide Nagase

Abstract Chronic obstructive pulmonary disease (COPD) is characterized by persistent airflow limitation that is usually progressive and associated with chronic inflammation of the peripheral airways and lung parenchyma. The current therapeutic strategy for COPD consists mainly of the use of bronchodilators, such as long-acting muscarinic antagonists and long-acting beta stimulants. They reduce respiratory symptoms and exacerbations, but do not reduce airway inflammation or prevent disease progression. We have no effective treatments for suppressing airway inflammation in COPD. There are, however, several candidates as anti-inflammatory drugs that would fundamentally suppress airway inflammation in COPD and might prevent progression of COPD. This chapter discusses some of the most promising new therapeutic drugs that have been discovered and describes the status of development of anti-inflammatory drugs in the field of COPD.

Keywords Airway inflammation • Phosphodiesterase inhibitors • Kinase inhibitors • Corticosteroid resistance

14.1 Introduction

Chronic obstructive pulmonary disease (COPD) is characterized by persistent airflow limitation that is usually progressive and associated with chronic inflammation of the peripheral airways and lung parenchyma [1]. This chronic airway inflammation is caused mainly by inhaled noxious particles from smoke and other sources, including outdoor, occupational, and indoor pollution. It results in the narrowing of the small airways and parenchymal destruction and persists through unknown mechanisms, even after long-term smoking cessation. In addition, the persistent airway inflammation may move into systemic inflammation in patients

Y. Yamauchi (✉) • T. Nagase
Department of Respiratory Medicine, Graduate School of Medicine, The University of Tokyo, 7-3-1, Hongo, Bunkyo-ku, Tokyo 113-8655, Japan
e-mail: YAMAUCHIY-INT@h.u-tokyo.ac.jp

H. Nakamura, K. Aoshiba (eds.), *Chronic Obstructive Pulmonary Disease*, Respiratory Disease Series: Diagnostic Tools and Disease Managements, DOI 10.1007/978-981-10-0839-9_14

with COPD. The systemic inflammatory response can cause systemic comorbidities such as cardiovascular and metabolic diseases, which are increasingly recognized as having major impacts on survival in patients with COPD [1].

Chronic inflammation is considered to be related to disease progression and mortality in COPD and should be regulated by treatment. However, current treatments recommended by the guidelines for COPD are mainly bronchodilators to reduce respiratory symptoms and exacerbations. Anti-inflammatory treatment with corticosteroids is not sufficient to suppress the inflammation and disease progression or improve survival [2]. As of this writing, there are no effective and safe drugs for suppressing chronic airway inflammation in COPD [3].

14.2 Inflammation in COPD

Chronic persistent inflammation exists throughout the airways and lung parenchyma in COPD. The airway inflammation consists mainly of increased numbers of T lymphocytes, including CD8 and CD4 cells, B lymphocytes, macrophages, and polymorphonuclear neutrophils [4–7]. These increased numbers of inflammatory cells are associated with the severity of COPD [5].

Many inflammatory mediators are involved in the persistent inflammatory process of COPD. Inhaled noxious particles and oxidative stress due to smoke and air pollution induce airway inflammation by causing release of various cytokines and chemokines, such as tumor necrosis factor-α (TNF-α), CXCL8/interleukin 8 (IL-8), granulocyte-macrophage colony-stimulating factor (GM-CSF), and interferon-inducible protein 10 (CXCL10), from epithelial cells and macrophages [8]. Those mediators recruit inflammatory cells into the airway causing airway inflammation. These inflammatory responses are activated and maintained by autonomous mechanisms, even long after smoking cessation. Moreover, several intracellular signaling pathways, including the mitogen-activated protein kinase (MAPK) pathway, phosphoinositide 3-kinase (PI3K) pathway, and Janus kinase/signal transducers and activators of transcription (JAK/STAT) pathway, and inflammatory transcriptional factors such as nuclear factor-kB (NF-kB) are activated in COPD by various stimuli. Thus, we need to find alternative anti-inflammatory therapies to regulate the persistent airway inflammation in COPD.

14.3 Anti-inflammatory Therapies

14.3.1 Phosphodiesterase Inhibitors

Phosphodiesterase (PDE) regulates the concentrations of cyclic adenosine monophosphate (cAMP) in cells and modulates a broad range of cell functions, including airway smooth muscle contractions and release of inflammatory mediators. Theophylline, a well-known bronchodilator having many physiological activities, works as a phosphodiesterase inhibitor but is weak and nonselective. There are several distinct PDE isozymes, and different PDEs are responsible for cyclic nucleotide hydrolysis in different tissues. Among them, PDE type 4 (PDE4), which is called cAMP-specific phosphodiesterase, has been demonstrated to have broad functional roles in many inflammatory cells [9, 10]. PDE4 inhibitors are reported to effectively inhibit chemotaxis, leukocyte activation, and cytokine production [11] and to reduce the numbers of neutrophils and eosinophils in the sputum of patients with COPD [12]. Thus, PDE4 inhibitors are potentially effective therapies for COPD.

One PDE4 inhibitor, roflumilast, reduces airway inflammation in COPD and improves lung function [13, 14]. Further, orally administered roflumilast reduces the frequency of exacerbation in patients with severe airflow limitation, although adverse effects such as diarrhea, weight loss, nausea, and headache occur [15, 16].

In order to reduce the systemic adverse effects of PDE4 inhibitors, several PDE4 inhibitors have been developed as dry powders for inhalation. One inhaled PDE4 inhibitor, UK-500001, was administered to patients with moderate to severe COPD. Although UK-500001 had no adverse effects, it also showed no therapeutic effects on lung function or symptoms [17]. Another inhaled PDE4 inhibitor, GSK256066, showed anti-inflammatory efficacy in an animal model [18], but it did not show any anti-inflammatory effect and did not improve lung function in patients with COPD [19]. A third inhaled PDE inhibitor, CHF6001, was reported to be more potent in inhibiting PDE4 enzymatic activity than roflumilast, UK-500001, and GSK256066. To date, however, clinical efficacy of CHF6001 in COPD has not been demonstrated [20].

In addition to PDE4 inhibitors, a dual PDE3 and PDE4 inhibitor, RPL554, may provide bronchodilating and anti-inflammatory activities, since the PDE3 inhibitor relaxes airway smooth muscle [21]. Inhaled RPL554 showed anti-inflammatory and bronchoprotective activities and was well tolerated. In addition, combined administration of RPL554 and glycopyrronium interacted synergistically in relaxing both human medium and small isolated bronchi, showing strong relaxation and an extended duration of action, indicating that this combination may prove useful in the treatment of COPD [22].

Thus, several PDE4 inhibitors have been developed for treatment of COPD, but further studies will be needed to assess their efficacy and safety with long-term follow-up.

14.3.2 Specific Inflammatory Mediators

Many different inflammatory mediators, including cytokines, chemokines, growth factors, and lipid mediators, are involved in the pathogenesis of COPD. Theoretical therapeutic approaches for treatment of COPD include inhibition of the mediators by using antibodies specific for them, antagonists of their receptors, or inhibitors of signal transduction. Several specific inhibitors of inflammatory mediators are being developed. However, since many different mediators are closely involved in the pathogenesis of COPD, we do not yet know which mediators would be the best therapeutic targets. Clinical trials are needed to determine the efficacy of mediator inhibition.

14.3.2.1 Cytokines

Many cytokines are increased in patients with COPD and play important roles in airway inflammation [23]. Several therapeutic approaches could be taken to block the cytokines' activities, including specific antibodies for the cytokines or their receptors, antagonists of their receptors, and inhibitors of intracellular signaling pathways.

TNF-α

TNF-α appears to play important roles in the pathogenesis of COPD as a primary mediator driving development of the inflammation and emphysema in COPD. TNF-α activates epithelial and smooth muscle cells in the airways to release inflammatory mediators and promote the fibrotic process in airway remodeling. TNF-α levels are increased in the blood and sputum of patients with COPD [24, 25]. However, administration of an anti-TNF-α antibody, infliximab, did not show any clinical efficacy in moderate–severe COPD. Moreover, in spite of the absence of beneficial effects, the risks of lung cancer and pneumonia were increased [26–28].

IL-1β

IL-1β is a pro-inflammatory cytokine and was demonstrated to be increased in COPD, suggesting that it plays a role in the pathogenesis of COPD by amplifying inflammation [29, 30]. However, an IL-1β-specific antibody, canakinumab, was ineffective in treatment of COPD in a recent unpublished clinical trial [31].

IL-6

IL-6 is also assumed to play an important role in the progression of COPD, and its levels are increased in patients with COPD [24]. An anti-IL-6 receptor antibody, tocilizumab, was effective in patients with rheumatoid arthritis refractory to TNF-α inhibitors [32], but no clinical studies have been conducted in patients with COPD.

IL-17

IL-17 promotes neutrophilic inflammation by inducing production of CXCL1 and CXCL8, which are chemoattractants for neutrophils, by airway epithelial cells [33]. IL-17 is increased in patients with COPD [34], implicating it in the pathogenesis of COPD. Antibodies specific for IL-17 and an IL-17 receptor are available for other indications [32, 35, 36], but no clinical trials have examined their efficacy in treating COPD.

GM-CSF

Granulocyte-macrophage colony-stimulating factor (GM-CSF) is a pro-inflammatory cytokine that promotes leukocyte survival and activation and regulates neutrophil function [37]. It has been implicated in the pathogenesis of COPD. A neutralizing GM-CSF antibody was effective in an animal model of cigarette smoke-induced airway inflammation [38], but no clinical studies have tested this for COPD.

In summary, inhibitors of cytokines, particularly those targeting single cytokines, have not yet shown clinical efficacy in treatment of COPD.

14.3.2.2 Chemokines

CXCL8 (IL-8), which is a chemoattractant for neutrophils and monocytes, is thought to be involved in the pathogenesis of COPD. Levels of IL-8 are elevated in the sputum of patients with COPD and correlate with disease severity [25]. IL-8-specific antibody improved dyspnea in patients with COPD but showed no beneficial effects on lung function, health status, or 6-min walking distance [39].

CXCR2 is a receptor for IL-8 and is expressed on neutrophils. Airway neutrophils are believed to be one of the key players in COPD. Treatment with CXCR2 antagonists reduced sputum neutrophils [40], improved lung function and health status, and reduced exacerbation in COPD [41]. However, they decreased blood neutrophil counts and resulted in an unacceptably high percentage of discontinuing patients. This clinical study suggested that an anti-inflammatory effect expressed via the CXCL8/CXCR2 axis might be clinically important.

14.3.3 Kinase Inhibitors

Many inflammatory genes encoding cytokines, chemokines, and proteinases show increased expression in patients with COPD and are regulated by inflammatory transcription factors via various activated pro-inflammatory kinase pathways. Those kinases are believed to play important roles in the airway inflammation in

COPD. Selective kinase inhibitors are now being used to target those kinases as treatments for COPD.

14.3.3.1 p38 MAPK Inhibitors

The p38 MAPK pathway regulates the expression of many inflammatory genes such as CXCL8 and TNF-α that are involved in COPD. Phosphorylated p38 was reported to be increased in alveolar macrophages and alveolar walls from patients with COPD, so the p38 MAPK pathway seems to be involved in the pathogenesis of COPD [42].

Inhibitors of p38 MAPK inhibited TNF-α release from macrophages of patients with COPD [42]. Further, a p38α-selective MAPK inhibitor reduced pulmonary inflammation in mice exposed to cigarette smoke, whereas dexamethasone was ineffective [43], suggesting that p38 MAPK inhibitors may have potential as treatments for COPD.

An oral p38 MAPK inhibitor, losmapimod, was well tolerated and reduced plasma fibrinogen without significant reduction of IL-6, IL-8, or C-reactive protein [44]. Another oral p38 MAPK inhibitor, PH-797804, improved lung function and dyspnea in patients with moderate to severe COPD [45].

Topical administration of p38 MAPK inhibitors may yield stronger anti-inflammatory effects in the airway. An inhaled p38α MAPK antisense oligonucleotide attenuated airway inflammation in a murine asthma model [46], indicating that p38 MAPK inhibitor inhalation may be an effective treatment for inflammatory airway diseases. Several selective inhaled p38 MAPK inhibitors (GSK-610677, AZD-7624, PF-03715455, and RV-568) are undergoing clinical development for COPD [47, 48].

14.3.3.2 PI3K Inhibitors

PI3Ks generate lipid second messengers that regulate various intracellular signaling pathways involved in inflammatory responses in the small airways in COPD [49–51]. Among the PI3K isoforms, PI3Kγ and PI3Kδ are involved in the pathogenesis of inflammation in respiratory disease [50–52].

An aerosolized PI3Kγ/P13Kδ inhibitor, TG100-115, reduced airway inflammation and airway hyperresponsiveness in a murine asthma model and inhibited airway neutrophilic inflammation in smoke-exposed mice [53].

Inhibition of PI3Kδ reversed oxidative stress-induced glucocorticoid insensitivity by restoring histone deacetylase 2 (HDAC-2) activity in smoke-exposed mice [54, 55].

14.3.3.3 JAK/STAT Inhibitors

Several cytokines implicated in COPD signal via the JAK/STAT pathway, and the activated pathway is associated with COPD [56, 57]. Therefore, inhibition of JAK/STAT signaling may have therapeutic potential for inhibiting airway inflammation in COPD. An oral selective inhibitor of JAK, tofacitinib, was reported to be effective in treatment of rheumatoid arthritis [58] and ulcerative colitis [59]. Its clinical efficacy in COPD should be investigated.

14.3.3.4 NF-kB Inhibitors

NF-kB induces expression of many pro-inflammatory mediators, including cytokines and chemokines, in response to inflammation and smoke exposure [60, 61]. NF-kB is activated in macrophages and epithelial cells of patients with COPD [30], and expression of NF-kB in the epithelium is associated with disease severity [62]. Since IkB kinases (IKKs), especially IKK-β, are essential for NF-kB signaling, their inhibition is a promising approach for intervention in COPD. IKK-β inhibitors are now undergoing development for treatment of airway inflammation in COPD.

14.3.4 Restoration of Corticosteroid Function

Corticosteroid resistance in patients with COPD is reported to be associated with reduced activity of HDAC2, which is caused by oxidative stress. Reduced HDAC2 activity leads to enhanced expression of inflammatory genes and increased acetylation of glucocorticoid receptors, which blocks the anti-inflammatory effects of corticosteroids [63]. Conversely, increasing HDAC2 activity would result in restoration of corticosteroid function and lead to anti-inflammatory effects, thus representing a therapeutic strategy for COPD.

Theophylline was reported to increase HDAC2 activity in alveolar macrophages from patients with COPD [55, 64]. In patients with COPD, combination therapy with an inhaled corticosteroid and low-dose theophylline was more effective than corticosteroid alone in reducing airway inflammation and improving lung function, and low-dose theophylline increased HDAC2 activity in peripheral blood monocytes [65].

Several agents, including formoterol and solithromycin, reversed oxidative stress-induced corticosteroid resistance by inhibiting PI3Kδ signaling in peripheral blood monocytes from patients with COPD [66, 67], so these agents are also potentially effective for treatment for COPD.

14.3.5 Pro-resolving Lipid Mediators

It is unknown why the airway inflammation in COPD persists even after smoking cessation. The conventional wisdom has been that resolution of inflammation is a passive process until inflammatory stimuli are removed. In recent years, however, it has been postulated that resolution of inflammation is a bioactive process mediated by several lipid mediators and that balance between pro-inflammatory and pro-resolving pathways maintains normal immune homeostasis [68, 69]. Those lipid mediators include resolvins, protectins, and maresins, which are bioactive products derived from dietary ω-3 and ω-6 polyunsaturated fatty acids and act on distinct receptors. Among those mediators, resolvin D1, which is a derivative of docosahexaenoic acid, has potent anti-inflammatory effects that suppressed pro-inflammatory mediators [70] and reduced emphysema and chronic inflammation in cigarette smoke-exposed mice [69]. In patients with COPD, pro-resolving and metabolic pathways are disrupted in the lung tissue, presumably due to cigarette smoking. Supplementation with specialized pro-resolving lipid mediators is a potentially important therapeutic strategy for COPD [69].

14.4 Conclusion

Controlling the airway inflammation in COPD should be the main goal of treatment for COPD since it would prevent disease progression, something the current anti-inflammatory therapies for COPD fail to do. Numerous agents have been identified that fundamentally suppress airway inflammation, and several drugs are now undergoing development. Among the drugs discussed above, the most promising agents are the inhaled kinase inhibitors, such as p38 MAPK inhibitors and JAK inhibitors, and drugs able to reverse corticosteroid insensitivity by increasing HDAC2 activity, such as inhaled PI3Kδ inhibitors.

References

1. Vestbo J, Hurd SS, Agusti AG, et al. Global strategy for the diagnosis, management, and prevention of chronic obstructive pulmonary disease: GOLD executive summary. Am J Respir Crit Care Med. 2013;187(4):347–65.
2. Barnes PJ. Inhaled corticosteroids in COPD: a controversy. Respiration. 2010;80(2):89–95.
3. Barnes PJ. New anti-inflammatory targets for chronic obstructive pulmonary disease. Nat Rev Drug Discov. 2013;12(7):543–59.
4. Di Stefano A, Capelli A, Lusuardi M, et al. Severity of airflow limitation is associated with severity of airway inflammation in smokers. Am J Respir Crit Care Med. 1998;158(4):1277–85.
5. Hogg JC, Chu F, Utokaparch S, et al. The nature of small-airway obstruction in chronic obstructive pulmonary disease. N Engl J Med. 2004;350(26):2645–53.

6. Saetta M, Baraldo S, Corbino L, et al. CD8 + ve cells in the lungs of smokers with chronic obstructive pulmonary disease. Am J Respir Crit Care Med. 1999;160(2):711–7.
7. Bourbeau J, Christodoulopoulos P, Maltais F, et al. Effect of salmeterol/fluticasone propionate on airway inflammation in COPD: a randomised controlled trial. Thorax. 2007;62(11):938–43.
8. Chung KF, Adcock IM. Multifaceted mechanisms in COPD: inflammation, immunity, and tissue repair and destruction. Eur Respir J. 2008;31(6):1334–56.
9. Torphy TJ, Undem BJ. Phosphodiesterase inhibitors: new opportunities for the treatment of asthma. Thorax. 1991;46(7):512–23.
10. Hatzelmann A, Morcillo EJ, Lungarella G, et al. The preclinical pharmacology of roflumilast–a selective, oral phosphodiesterase 4 inhibitor in development for chronic obstructive pulmonary disease. Pulm Pharmacol Ther. 2010;23(4):235–56.
11. Spina D. PDE4 inhibitors: current status. Br J Pharmacol. 2008;155(3):308–15.
12. Grootendorst DC, Gauw SA, Verhoosel RM, et al. Reduction in sputum neutrophil and eosinophil numbers by the PDE4 inhibitor roflumilast in patients with COPD. Thorax. 2007;62(12):1081–7.
13. Calverley PM, Sanchez-Toril F, McIvor A, et al. Effect of 1-year treatment with roflumilast in severe chronic obstructive pulmonary disease. Am J Respir Crit Care Med. 2007;176 (2):154–61.
14. Fabbri LM, Calverley PM, Izquierdo-Alonso JL, et al. Roflumilast in moderate-to-severe chronic obstructive pulmonary disease treated with longacting bronchodilators: two randomised clinical trials. Lancet. 2009;374(9691):695–703.
15. Calverley PM, Rabe KF, Goehring UM, et al. Roflumilast in symptomatic chronic obstructive pulmonary disease: two randomised clinical trials. Lancet. 2009;374(9691):685–94.
16. Martinez FJ, Calverley PM, Goehring UM, et al. Effect of roflumilast on exacerbations in patients with severe chronic obstructive pulmonary disease uncontrolled by combination therapy (REACT): a multicentre randomised controlled trial. Lancet. 2015;385(9971):857–66.
17. Vestbo J, Tan L, Atkinson G, et al. A controlled trial of 6-weeks' treatment with a novel inhaled phosphodiesterase type-4 inhibitor in COPD. Eur Respir J. 2009;33(5):1039–44.
18. Nials AT, Tralau-Stewart CJ, Gascoigne MH, et al. In vivo characterization of GSK256066, a high-affinity inhaled phosphodiesterase 4 inhibitor. J Pharmacol Exp Ther. 2011;337 (1):137–44.
19. Watz H, Mistry SJ, Lazaar AL, et al. Safety and tolerability of the inhaled phosphodiesterase 4 inhibitor GSK256066 in moderate COPD. Pulm Pharmacol Ther. 2013;26(5):588–95.
20. Moretto N, Caruso P, Bosco R, et al. CHF6001 I: a novel highly potent and selective phosphodiesterase 4 inhibitor with robust anti-inflammatory activity and suitable for topical pulmonary administration. J Pharmacol Exp Ther. 2015;352(3):559–67.
21. Franciosi LG, Diamant Z, Banner KH, et al. Efficacy and safety of RPL554, a dual PDE3 and PDE4 inhibitor, in healthy volunteers and in patients with asthma or chronic obstructive pulmonary disease: findings from four clinical trials. Lancet Respir Med. 2013;1(9):714–27.
22. Calzetta L, Cazzola M, Page CP, et al. Pharmacological characterization of the interaction between the dual phosphodiesterase (PDE) 3/4 inhibitor RPL554 and glycopyrronium on human isolated bronchi and small airways. Pulm Pharmacol Ther. 2015;32:15–23.
23. Barnes PJ. The cytokine network in chronic obstructive pulmonary disease. Am J Respir Cell Mol Biol. 2009;41(6):631–8.
24. Gan WQ, Man SF, Senthilselvan A, et al. Association between chronic obstructive pulmonary disease and systemic inflammation: a systematic review and a meta-analysis. Thorax. 2004;59 (7):574–80.
25. Keatings VM, Collins PD, Scott DM, et al. Differences in interleukin-8 and tumor necrosis factor-alpha in induced sputum from patients with chronic obstructive pulmonary disease or asthma. Am J Respir Crit Care Med. 1996;153(2):530–4.
26. Rennard SI, Fogarty C, Kelsen S, et al. The safety and efficacy of infliximab in moderate to severe chronic obstructive pulmonary disease. Am J Respir Crit Care Med. 2007;175 (9):926–34.

27. Dentener MA, Creutzberg EC, Pennings HJ, et al. Effect of infliximab on local and systemic inflammation in chronic obstructive pulmonary disease: a pilot study. Respiration. 2008;76 (3):275–82.
28. Rennard SI, Flavin SK, Agarwal PK, et al. Long-term safety study of infliximab in moderate-to-severe chronic obstructive pulmonary disease. Respir Med. 2013;107(3):424–32.
29. Bafadhel M, McCormick M, Saha S, et al. Profiling of sputum inflammatory mediators in asthma and chronic obstructive pulmonary disease. Respiration. 2012;83(1):36–44.
30. Caramori G, Adcock IM, Di Stefano A, et al. Cytokine inhibition in the treatment of COPD. Int J Chron Obstr Pulmon Dis. 2014;9:397–412.
31. Novartis. Safety and efficacy of multiple doses of Canakinumab (ACZ885) in chronic obstructive pulmonary disease (COPD) patients. 2014 [cited 2016 January 3rd]. Available from: http://clinicaltrials.gov/show/NCT00581945
32. Strand V, Burmester GR, Ogale S, et al. Improvements in health-related quality of life after treatment with tocilizumab in patients with rheumatoid arthritis refractory to tumour necrosis factor inhibitors: results from the 24-week randomized controlled RADIATE study. Rheumatology (Oxford). 2012;51(10):1860–9.
33. Matsuzaki H, Mikami Y, Makita K, et al. Interleukin-17A and toll-like receptor 3 ligand poly (I:C) synergistically induced neutrophil chemoattractant production by bronchial epithelial cells. PLoS One. 2015;10(10), e0141746.
34. Di Stefano A, Caramori G, Gnemmi I, et al. T helper type 17-related cytokine expression is increased in the bronchial mucosa of stable chronic obstructive pulmonary disease patients. Clin Exp Immunol. 2009;157(2):316–24.
35. Papp KA, Leonardi C, Menter A, et al. Brodalumab, an anti-interleukin-17-receptor antibody for psoriasis. N Engl J Med. 2012;366(13):1181–9.
36. Leonardi C, Matheson R, Zachariae C, et al. Anti-interleukin-17 monoclonal antibody ixekizumab in chronic plaque psoriasis. N Engl J Med. 2012;366(13):1190–9.
37. Saha S, Doe C, Mistry V, et al. Granulocyte-macrophage colony-stimulating factor expression in induced sputum and bronchial mucosa in asthma and COPD. Thorax. 2009;64(8):671–6.
38. Vlahos R, Bozinovski S, Chan SP, et al. Neutralizing granulocyte/macrophage colony-stimulating factor inhibits cigarette smoke-induced lung inflammation. Am J Respir Crit Care Med. 2010;182(1):34–40.
39. Mahler DA, Huang S, Tabrizi M, et al. Efficacy and safety of a monoclonal antibody recognizing interleukin-8 in COPD: a pilot study. Chest. 2004;126(3):926–34.
40. Holz O, Khalilieh S, Ludwig-Sengpiel A, et al. SCH527123, a novel CXCR2 antagonist, inhibits ozone-induced neutrophilia in healthy subjects. Eur Respir J. 2010;35(3):564–70.
41. Rennard SI, Dale DC, Donohue JF, et al. CXCR2 antagonist MK-7123. A phase 2 proof-of-concept trial for chronic obstructive pulmonary disease. Am J Respir Crit Care Med. 2015;191 (9):1001–11.
42. Renda T, Baraldo S, Pelaia G, et al. Increased activation of p38 MAPK in COPD. Eur Respir J. 2008;31(1):62–9.
43. Medicherla S, Reddy M, Ying J, et al. p38alpha-selective MAP kinase inhibitor reduces tumor growth in mouse xenograft models of multiple myeloma. Anticancer Res. 2008;28 (6A):3827–33.
44. Lomas DA, Lipson DA, Miller BE, et al. An oral inhibitor of p38 MAP kinase reduces plasma fibrinogen in patients with chronic obstructive pulmonary disease. J Clin Pharmacol. 2012;52 (3):416–24.
45. MacNee W, Allan RJ, Jones I, et al. Efficacy and safety of the oral p38 inhibitor PH-797804 in chronic obstructive pulmonary disease: a randomised clinical trial. Thorax. 2013;68 (8):738–45.
46. Duan W, Chan JH, McKay K, et al. Inhaled p38alpha mitogen-activated protein kinase antisense oligonucleotide attenuates asthma in mice. Am J Respir Crit Care Med. 2005;171 (6):571–8.

47. Millan DS, Bunnage ME, Burrows JL, et al. Design and synthesis of inhaled p38 inhibitors for the treatment of chronic obstructive pulmonary disease. J Med Chem. 2011;54(22):7797–814.
48. Norman P. Investigational p38 inhibitors for the treatment of chronic obstructive pulmonary disease. Expert Opin Investig Drugs. 2015;24(3):383–92.
49. Marwick JA, Chung KF, Adcock IM. Phosphatidylinositol 3-kinase isoforms as targets in respiratory disease. Ther Adv Respir Dis. 2010;4(1):19–34.
50. Larocca NE, Moreno D, Garmendia JV, et al. Inhibitors of phosphoinositol 3 kinase and NFkappaB for the treatment of chronic obstructive pulmonary disease. Rec Pat Inflamm Allergy Drug Discov. 2011;5(3):178–83.
51. Ito K, Caramori G, Adcock IM. Therapeutic potential of phosphatidylinositol 3-kinase inhibitors in inflammatory respiratory disease. J Pharmacol Exp Ther. 2007;321(1):1–8.
52. Thomas MJ, Smith A, Head DH, et al. Airway inflammation: chemokine-induced neutrophilia and the class I phosphoinositide 3-kinases. Eur J Immunol. 2005;35(4):1283–91.
53. Doukas J, Eide L, Stebbins K, et al. Aerosolized phosphoinositide 3-kinase gamma/delta inhibitor TG100-115 [3-[2,4-diamino-6-(3-hydroxyphenyl)pteridin-7-yl]phenol] as a therapeutic candidate for asthma and chronic obstructive pulmonary disease. J Pharmacol Exp Ther. 2009;328(3):758–65.
54. Marwick JA, Caramori G, Stevenson CS, et al. Inhibition of PI3Kdelta restores glucocorticoid function in smoking-induced airway inflammation in mice. Am J Respir Crit Care Med. 2009;179(7):542–8.
55. To Y, Ito K, Kizawa Y, et al. Targeting phosphoinositide-3-kinase-delta with theophylline reverses corticosteroid insensitivity in chronic obstructive pulmonary disease. Am J Respir Crit Care Med. 2010;182(7):897–904.
56. Bakke PS, Zhu G, Gulsvik A, et al. Candidate genes for COPD in two large data sets. Eur Respir J. 2011;37(2):255–63.
57. Yew-Booth L, Birrell MA, Lau MS, et al. JAK-STAT pathway activation in COPD. Eur Respir J. 2015;46(3):843–5.
58. Fleischmann R, Kremer J, Cush J, et al. Placebo-controlled trial of tofacitinib monotherapy in rheumatoid arthritis. N Engl J Med. 2012;367(6):495–507.
59. Sandborn WJ, Ghosh S, Panes J, et al. Tofacitinib, an oral Janus kinase inhibitor, in active ulcerative colitis. N Engl J Med. 2012;367(7):616–24.
60. Kwak JH, Jung JK, Lee H. Nuclear factor-kappa B inhibitors; a patent review (2006–2010). Exp Opin Ther Pat. 2011;21(12):1897–910.
61. Pasparakis M. Role of NF-kappaB in epithelial biology. Immunol Rev. 2012;246(1):346–58.
62. Di Stefano A, Caramori G, Oates T, et al. Increased expression of nuclear factor-kappaB in bronchial biopsies from smokers and patients with COPD. Eur Respir J. 2002;20(3):556–63.
63. Ito K, Yamamura S, Essilfie-Quaye S, et al. Histone deacetylase 2-mediated deacetylation of the glucocorticoid receptor enables NF-kappaB suppression. J Exp Med. 2006;203(1):7–13.
64. Cosio BG, Tsaprouni L, Ito K, et al. Theophylline restores histone deacetylase activity and steroid responses in COPD macrophages. J Exp Med. 2004;200(5):689–95.
65. Ford PA, Durham AL, Russell RE, et al. Treatment effects of low-dose theophylline combined with an inhaled corticosteroid in COPD. Chest. 2010;137(6):1338–44.
66. Rossios C, To Y, Osoata G, et al. Corticosteroid insensitivity is reversed by formoterol via phosphoinositide-3-kinase inhibition. Br J Pharmacol. 2012;167(4):775–86.
67. Kobayashi Y, Wada H, Rossios C, et al. A novel macrolide/fluoroketolide, solithromycin (CEM-101), reverses corticosteroid insensitivity via phosphoinositide 3-kinase pathway inhibition. Br J Pharmacol. 2013;169(5):1024–34.
68. Serhan CN. Novel lipid mediators and resolution mechanisms in acute inflammation: to resolve or not? Am J Pathol. 2010;177(4):1576–91.
69. Hsiao HM, Thatcher TH, Colas RA, et al. Resolvin D1 reduces emphysema and chronic inflammation. Am J Pathol. 2015;185(12):3189–201.

70. Hsiao HM, Sapinoro RE, Thatcher TH, et al. A novel anti-inflammatory and pro-resolving role for resolvin D1 in acute cigarette smoke-induced lung inflammation. PLoS One. 2013;8(3), e58258.

Chapter 15
Exacerbation of COPD: Why Do Exacerbations of COPD Attract Attention? Are There Any Preventive Methods?

Masamichi Mineshita

Abstract Chronic obstructive pulmonary disease (COPD) exacerbation is defined as an acute event characterized by a worsening of the patient's respiratory symptoms that is beyond the normal day-to-day variations and leads to a change in medication. Since exacerbations are associated with deterioration of quality of life, accelerated rate of decline of lung function, increased mortality, and high socioeconomic costs, the prevention of exacerbations is one of the main targets of maintenance therapy for COPD. Exacerbations are largely a feature of moderate-to-severe COPD, with some COPD patients predisposed to frequent exacerbation phenotype, whose pulmonary functions show rapid deterioration. The most commonly used medications for COPD exacerbations are antibiotics, bronchodilators, and corticosteroids (ABC approach), while appropriate oxygen therapy and ventilator support are widely accepted as two major non-pharmacologic treatments. COPD exacerbations can often be prevented. Conforming to the management strategy for stable COPD patients is essential. Many types of pharmacologic and non-pharmacologic interventions such as long-acting inhaled bronchodilators and corticosteroids, phosphodiesterase inhibitor, and pulmonary rehabilitation program for posthospitalization periods are reported to be effective. Further understanding into the nature of exacerbations, invention of new effective interventions, and investigations to identify suitable combinations for interventions are required to develop more rational, preventive regimes for exacerbation.

Keywords Frequent exacerbation phenotype • ABC approach • Pulmonary rehabilitation • Oxygen therapy • Noninvasive mechanical ventilation

M. Mineshita (✉)
Internal Medicine, Division of Respiratory Medicine, St. Marianna University School of Medicine, 2-16-1, Sugao, Miyamae-ku, Kawasaki-City, Kanagawa, Japan
e-mail: m-mine@marianna-u.ac.jp

H. Nakamura, K. Aoshiba (eds.), *Chronic Obstructive Pulmonary Disease*,
Respiratory Disease Series: Diagnostic Tools and Disease Managements,
DOI 10.1007/978-981-10-0839-9_15

15.1 Introduction

Chronic obstructive pulmonary disease (COPD) exacerbation is defined as an acute event characterized by a worsening of the patient's respiratory symptoms that is beyond the normal day-to-day variations and leads to a change in medication [1]. Fifty to 70 % of exacerbations are caused by respiratory infections, 10 % exacerbations by environmental pollution, and up to 30 % of exacerbations by unknown etiology [2]. These extrinsic and internal stimuli add to the inflammatory load of preexisting airway inflammation in the lower airway of COPD patients, leading to tissue damage and clinical deterioration.

Reported frequency of exacerbations is around 1.0 per year, and this rate tends to increase according to severity of airflow limitation [3–5]. On the other hand, previous studies have shown that a considerable number of exacerbations will not be reported to medical staff [6]. The symptoms of exacerbation vary in severity between patients and by their history of COPD. Therefore, a personalized approach is required to manage exacerbations of the individual patient. Exacerbations are associated with deterioration in quality of life, an accelerated rate of decline for lung function, an increased mortality, and high socioeconomic costs [1, 7, 8]. Therefore, the prevention and management of exacerbations are important issues for the treatment of COPD patients.

In this chapter, we will describe risk factors, diagnosis and assessments, managements, preventions, and the impact exacerbations have on patients with COPD.

15.2 Risk Factors of Exacerbation

Exacerbations are largely a feature of moderate-to-severe COPD. Exacerbation rates in the first year of follow-up were 0.85 per person for patients with stage 2 COPD, 1.34 for patients with stage 3, and 2.00 for patients with stage 4, reported by the evaluation of COPD longitudinally to identify predictive surrogate endpoints (ECLIPSE) study [5]. Although Nishimura et al. reported a much lower exacerbation frequency in a Japanese cohort of COPD patients, exacerbation frequency was higher in subjects with severe airflow limitation [9]. Thus, the progression of flow limitation is thought to be one of the risk factors for exacerbations.

Hurst et al. reported that the single best predictor for exacerbations, across all GOLD stages, was the patient's history of exacerbations. They reported that the frequent exacerbation phenotype appeared to be relatively stable over a period of 3 years, and exacerbation frequency in the first year had a sensitivity of 60 % and a specificity of 83 % for the frequency in the second year [5]. Because exacerbations can produce a permanent reduction in lung function, COPD patients who experience more exacerbations would have a faster decline than those with fewer exacerbations. Therefore, it is accepted that exacerbation frequency tends to be higher in patients with severe airflow limitation.

Hurst et al. also reported that frequent exacerbation phenotype was associated with a history of gastroesophageal reflux diseases (GERD), poorer quality of life, and elevated white cell counts [5]. Terada et al. prospectively studied the clinical significance of GERD symptoms on exacerbation in 82 moderate-to-severe COPD patients. GERD symptoms were evaluated using the frequency scale for the symptoms of GERD (FSSG). They reported that the frequency of exacerbation was significantly associated with the FSSG score [10]. They also reported that the prevalence of abnormal swallowing reflex was significantly higher in subjects with COPD than in the control group and that abnormal swallowing reflex was significantly associated with frequent exacerbations [11]. The combination of GERD and abnormal swallowing reflex might cause bronchopulmonary inflammation and bacterial colonization, which are predisposed to COPD exacerbations.

Although exacerbations negatively affect a patient's quality of life, poor quality of life is reported to associate with readmission after COPD exacerbation. Osman et al. examined whether quality of life scores could predict readmission in 266 COPD patients who were admitted with exacerbation. Quality of life was evaluated using the St George's Respiratory Questionnaire (SGRQ). They revealed that worse SGRQ scores were significantly associated with the readmission of COPD patients over 12 months [12]. Nishimura et al. also reported that impaired health-related quality of life and weight loss were independent risk factors for COPD exacerbations [9].

It has previously been reported that patients with frequent exacerbations had higher median stable sputum levels of IL-6 and IL-8 [13]. Thomsen et al. evaluated the association between elevated levels of inflammatory biomarkers in individuals with stable COPD and an increased risk of exacerbations, using 6574 COPD patients from the Copenhagen City Heart Study and the Copenhagen General Population Study. They revealed that simultaneously elevated levels of CRP, fibrinogen, and leukocyte counts in individuals with COPD were associated with an increased risk of exacerbation, even in those with milder COPD and in those without previous exacerbations [14].

Computed tomography (CT) is becoming an essential tool for evaluating COPD, and studies have been planned to evaluate the association between quantitative CT measures and COPD exacerbation frequency. Han et al. evaluated the association between the percentage of emphysematous lesions and airway wall thickness and the exacerbation frequency using data from participants in the COPD Gene Study. They found that independent of the severity of airflow obstruction, a 5 % increase in total lung emphysema in those with 35 % or greater emphysema is associated with a 1.18-fold increase in exacerbation frequency, and a 1-mm increase in segmental airway wall thickness is associated with a 1.84-fold increase in exacerbation frequency [15]. Pulmonary hypertension is reported to be one of risk factors for death and readmission in patients discharged after a severe COPD exacerbation [16]. In regard to evaluation of pulmonary arterial pressure using CT, the ratio of diameter of the main pulmonary artery to diameter of the ascending aorta (PA:A ratio) correlates with the mean pulmonary arterial pressure [17]. Wells et al. revealed that a PA:A ratio of more than 1 was associated with future exacerbations of COPD, particularly those requiring hospitalization [18].

Environmental pollution, such as high levels of ozone and particulate air pollution, is also important as a risk factor for exacerbation, and previous studies have reported significant associations between inhalable particulate matter with aerodynamic diameters ≤ 10 μm (PM_{10}) and increased COPD hospitalizations and mortality [2, 8]. Recently, Li et al. performed a systematic review and meta-analysis to evaluate the relationship between short-term particulate matter with aerodynamic diameters ≤ 2.5 μm ($PM_{2.5}$) exposure and COPD hospitalizations and mortality and found that a 10-ug/m^3 increase in daily $PM_{2.5}$ was associated with a 3.1 % increase in COPD hospitalizations and a 2.5 % increase in COPD mortality [19].

15.3 Diagnosis and Assessment of Exacerbation

The diagnosis of exacerbation is based on clinical presentation of the patients [1, 20]. COPD exacerbation is an acute clinical worsening of symptoms, such as baseline dyspnea, cough, and sputum production, beyond a normal day-to-day variation and may necessitate a change in regular treatment. The first diagnostic step is based on the patient's medical history. These histories consist of patient symptoms, such as dyspnea, sputum volume and color, severity of COPD, present drug treatment, frequency of exacerbations, and the presence of comorbidities. The second step to assess severity is physical examination. Findings such as the use of accessory respiratory muscles, paradoxical chest wall motion, attenuated or absent breath sounds, central cyanosis, cardiovascular signs (increase in pulse heart rate, heart failure, peripheral edema, hemodynamic instability), and altered mental status are considered signs of a severe exacerbation. Cardiopulmonary diseases, such as pneumonia, pneumothorax, pulmonary embolism, and heart failure, are often associated with COPD and show clinical symptoms indistinguishable from exacerbations. The following standard tests are performed to assess the severity of an exacerbation, diagnose comorbidities, and exclude alternative diagnoses: pulse oximetry, arterial blood gas analysis, routine blood and biochemical tests, Gram stain and culture when sputum is purulent, chest radiography and/or CT, ECG, and cardiac function. According to the effects of exacerbations on the cardiovascular system, Wells et al. reported that the PA:A ratio increases at the time of severe exacerbation, and the PA:A ratio of more than 1 predicts cardiac injury and a more severe hospital course [21].

15.4 Management of Exacerbation

15.4.1 Pharmacologic Treatment

The most commonly used medications for COPD exacerbation are antibiotics, bronchodilators, and corticosteroids (ABC approach), although the routine use of antibiotics in exacerbations remains controversial.

Since 50–70 % of exacerbations reported are caused by respiratory infections including viral infections, it is thought that selected patients whose exacerbations seemed to be caused by or accompanied with bacterial infection will benefit from antibiotic medications. According to GOLD recommendations [1], antibiotics should be given to patients with exacerbations of COPD who have three cardinal symptoms – increase in dyspnea, sputum volume, and sputum purulence; have two of the cardinal symptoms, if increased purulence of sputum is one of the two symptoms; or require mechanical ventilation (invasive or noninvasive).

Lower airway bacterial colonization is common in COPD patients, and the most commonly isolated organisms are *Haemophilus influenzae*, *Streptococcus pneumoniae*, and *Moraxella catarrhalis*. *Pseudomonas aeruginosa* can also be isolated in more advanced diseases, and this airway bacterial prevalence and load are reported to increase at COPD exacerbations [2, 22]. Although the efforts to elucidate the causative organisms are required and important, antibacterial treatment should be started if clinical symptoms, sputum appearance, blood and biochemical tests, and medical history show the possibility of bacterial infection. Soler et al. suggested that a combination of patient-reported sputum purulence and CRP might be a useful guide to initiate antibiotics [23]. The choice of antibiotic is determined by considering commonly isolated organisms and the local bacterial resistance pattern. Although the recommended length of antibiotic therapy is usually 5–10 days, El Moussaoui et al. stated that a short course (less than 5 days) of antibiotic treatment is as effective as the traditionally longer treatment in patients with mild to moderate exacerbations [24].

Short-acting inhaled β2 agonists (SABA) and anticholinergic agents (SAMA) are usually adopted as the main treatment modality for exacerbations. Although there are no trials reported for short-acting bronchodilator agents, they reduce symptoms and improve airflow obstruction in patients with exacerbation. The effects of SABAs are faster than SAMAs; however, there seems to be no difference in bronchodilator effects. Their effects last for 4–6 h, and repeated inhalation is usually required during treatment of exacerbation. Bronchodilator effects are equivalent between metered dose inhalers and nebulizers in patients with exacerbation, although nebulizers with a mouthpiece appear to be more convenient for sicker patients [20]. Methylxanthines are considered a second-line therapy, only to be used in selected cases when there is an insufficient response to short-acting bronchodilators, whereas potentially important adverse events of nausea and vomiting were significantly increased [20, 25].

International guidelines and systematic reviews recommend systemic glucocorticoid therapy in the management of exacerbation. Previous trials have shown that glucocorticoid therapy benefits clinical outcomes, reduces the length of hospital stay, and accelerates recovery of pulmonary function [1, 20, 26]. Leuppi et al. conducted a randomized multicenter trial to investigate whether a 5-day systemic glucocorticoid (40 mg of prednisone) treatment in patients with COPD exacerbation is non-inferior to the conventional 14-day treatment. They found that the 5-day treatment with systemic glucocorticoids was non-inferior to the 14-day treatment with regard to re-exacerbation within 6 months after exacerbation with significantly reduced glucocorticoid exposure [27]. According to their result, GOLD guideline recommends a dose of 40 mg prednisone per day for 5 days, although there are insufficient data to allow firm conclusions concerning the optimal duration of corticosteroid therapy for acute COPD exacerbations [28]. Although there is no guidance regarding how to adjust the optimal dose of steroids, the high-dose steroid (methylprednisolone $>$ 240 mg/day) group is associated with worse outcomes and more frequent adverse effects than lower-dose steroid (methylprednisolone $\leq$ 240 mg/day) group even in critically ill patients with exacerbation [29]. The optimum dose setting of steroids according to disease severity for the treatment of exacerbation remains to be elucidated.

To improve patient's whole-body condition is always critically important. An appropriate fluid balance with the administration of diuretics, nutritional aspects, anticoagulants, and cardiovascular agents is introduced according to the clinical condition of the patient [20].

15.4.2 Non-pharmacologic Treatment

Oxygen therapy and ventilator support are two major non-pharmacologic treatments and are widely accepted in the management of exacerbation. Controlled oxygen therapy is essential for acute respiratory failure during exacerbation. Supplemental oxygen should be titrated to maintain optimal values PaO2 $>$ 60 Torr or SaO2 $>$ 90 %. Especially in hypercapnic respiratory failure, higher inspired oxygen concentration can result in the suppression of respiratory drive, detrimental carbon dioxide retention, and carbon dioxide narcosis. Although pulse oximetry is useful in clinical practice for adjusting oxygen concentration, arterial blood gases should be checked around 30 min later to ensure satisfactory oxygenation without carbon dioxide retention or acidosis. Low-flow devices such as nasal cannula are commonly used in clinical settings, but they are less accurate. Venturi masks (high-flow devices) offer more accurately controlled inspired oxygen concentrations. Recently, high-flow oxygen through nasal cannula, a heated, humidified, and high-flow oxygen delivery system, has been introduced as a treatment modality for acute respiratory failure [30]. Although the benefits of high-flow oxygen for patients with COPD exacerbations were reported [31], sufficient evidence on an indication, contraindication, appropriate condition setting, and patient selection criteria for exacerbation treatment remains to be elucidated.

When the respiratory condition of a patient deteriorates in spite of adequate pharmacological and oxygen therapies, ventilator support is indicated. Mechanical ventilation can be delivered noninvasively (nasal or facial mask) or invasively (tracheal tube or tracheostomy) and assist the patient's respiration by applying positive pressure in accordance with the patient's respiratory timing.

Noninvasive mechanical ventilation (NIV) is widely used in patients hospitalized for acute hypercapnic exacerbations, and the reported success rate was more than 80 %. NIV has been shown to improve arterial blood findings; decrease respiratory rate and work of breathing, severity of breathlessness, and complications such as ventilator-associated pneumonia; and reduce the need for endotracheal intubation, the length of hospital stay, and in-hospital mortality rate [1, 20, 32]. The indications of NIV for GOLD guidelines are respiratory acidosis (arterial pH $\leq$ 7.35 and/or PaCO2 $\geq$ 45 Torr) and severe dyspnea with clinical signs suggestive of respiratory muscle fatigue, increased work of breathing, or both, such as the use of respiratory accessory muscles, paradoxical motion of the abdomen, or retraction of the intercostal spaces. On the other hand, the considered contraindications for NIV are respiratory or cardiac arrest, uncooperative patients, cases with required airway management, severe hemodynamic instability, and facial deformities that interfere NIV setting. Invasive ventilation is indicated when a patient is unsuitable for NIV, or an initial trial of NIV ends in failure. Major risk factors of invasive ventilations are ventilator-acquired pneumonia, barotrauma, and failure to wean to spontaneous breathing. Despite the need for invasive ventilation, acute mortality among COPD patients with respiratory failure is lower than mortality among patients ventilated for non-COPD causes. Esteban et al. investigated the mortality rate in 5183 patients who received mechanical ventilation. The overall mortality rate in 28 days was 30.7 %. On the other hand, the mortality rate of COPD exacerbation in patients who received mechanical ventilation was 22 % [33]. Long-term follow-up after index hospitalization with acute exacerbation revealed that a longer duration of disease, longer time elapsed since the first hospitalization, lower PaO_2, lower albumin level, and lower BMI were main factors related to long-term mortality [34].

Since multidisciplinary pulmonary rehabilitation can improve dyspnea, quality of life, and exercise capacity in stable COPD, the effects of rehabilitation to counteract deleterious consequences of a hospital admission for an acute exacerbation have been studied. Seymour et al. reported that outpatient pulmonary rehabilitation administered shortly after hospitalization for acute exacerbation improved exercise capacity, health status, and reduced frequencies of re-exacerbation that requires hospital admission or attendance in the subsequent 3 months [35]. Pulmonary rehabilitation in the posthospitalization period also reduces healthcare use, readmissions, and mortality, although poor referral and uptake rates for early outpatient rehabilitation following hospitalization are pointed [36, 37]. On the other hand, recent trials showed that an early progressive rehabilitation program started within 48 h of hospital admission for an acute exacerbation did not reduce the risk of subsequent readmission or enhance recovery of physical function [38]. Further research to reveal the optimal duration and intensity of rehabilitation and to investigate the methods to improve patient's acceptability to rehabilitation is required.

15.4.3 Hospital Admission

GOLD guidelines describe the potential indications for hospital admission as follows:

Marked increase in intensity of symptoms
Severe underlying COPD
Onset of new physical signs
Failure of an exacerbation to respond to initial medical management
Presence of serious comorbidities
Frequent exacerbations
Older age
Insufficient home support

Prediction tools, such as the dyspnea, eosinopenia, consolidation, acidemia, and atrial fibrillation (DECAF) scores, are investigated to create appropriate management strategies according to the mortality risk of patients with exacerbation [39]. Although optimized treatment should be established for the individual patient prior to discharge, home support by a family doctor and nurse may permit earlier discharge of patients without increasing readmission rates.

15.5 Prevention of Exacerbation

The prevention of exacerbations is recognized as one of the main targets in maintenance therapy for COPD since exacerbations lead to the deterioration of patient's condition and cause an economic and public health burden. COPD exacerbations can often be prevented by conforming to the management strategy for stable COPD patients. Smoking cessation is very important, and all healthcare providers should strongly enforce measures against active smoking in COPD patients. Annual influenza vaccine is also recommended to reduce the rate and severity of influenza symptoms. Guidelines also recommend pneumococcal vaccination, although a meta-analysis failed to find significant effects of pneumococcal vaccination on morbidity or mortality in patients with COPD [40].

15.5.1 Pharmacologic Prevention

Two classes of long-acting inhaled bronchodilators, long-acting antimuscarinic agents (LAMAs) and long-acting β agonists (LABAs), are key drugs for COPD treatment, and many clinical trials have elucidated the efficacy of these drugs for the prevention of exacerbation.

The UPLIFT trial enrolled 5993 COPD patients to assess the use of tiotropium. This study revealed that tiotropium (LAMA) significantly delayed the time of first exacerbation and first hospitalization. Tiotropium treatment also revealed a 14 % reduction in the mean number of exacerbations [4]. Glycopyrronium bromide, a new LAMA, is reported to have similar effects for the prevention of exacerbations. LABAs, such as salmeterol, formoterol, and indacaterol, also have the preventive effects for exacerbation, although the effectiveness is a little less than LAMAs [4, 41]. Recently, combined inhalers of LABA and LAMA were developed and available for general use. The SPARK study was designed to evaluate the effect of QVA149, once daily fixed-dose combination of indacaterol 110 μg and glycopyrronium 50 μg, on exacerbation in patients with severe-to-very-severe COPD. This study found that QVA149 significantly reduced the rate of moderate-to-severe exacerbations versus glycopyrronium by 12 %, although QVA149 did not significantly reduce exacerbation rates compared with open-label tiotropium. The rate of all (mild, moderate, and severe) exacerbations was significantly reduced by 15 % with QVA149 compared with glycopyrronium and by 14 % compared with tiotropium [42].

LABAs are also combined with inhaled corticosteroid (ICS) and widely used for asthma and COPD management. The TORCH study was planned to reveal the effects of ICS and LABA combination on survival in COPD patients. In this study, 6122 patients were randomized to treatment with fluticasone-salmeterol, fluticasone, salmeterol, or placebo [3]. The annual rate of exacerbations in the combined regimen group (0.85) was significantly lower than the placebo group (1.13), salmeterol (0.97), and fluticasone (0.93). Meta-analysis reports confirmed that ICS and LABA combination inhalers reduce exacerbation compared with placebo and LABA alone. On the other hand, potential increased risks of pneumonia that were associated with ICS-containing therapies are noted [3, 41].

Although combination therapy of ICS, LABA, and LAMA (triple therapy) is applied for COPD patients to improve pulmonary functions and QOL, the benefit of ICS in a regimen including LABA and LAMA on the prevention of exacerbation was not evaluated in an adequately powered study. The WISDOM study was a 12-month, double-blind, parallel-group study that enrolled 2485 COPD patients with a history of exacerbation [43]. During the 6-week run-in period, triple therapy consisted of tiotropium, salmeterol, and fluticasone and was prescribed for all participants. Patients were then randomly assigned to continued triple therapy or withdrawal from ICS over a 12-week period. This study revealed that in patients with severe COPD receiving LABA and LAMA, the risk of moderate or severe exacerbations was similar to those who discontinued ICS. On the other hand, ICS withdrawal caused a greater deterioration in pulmonary function.

To elucidate the abilities of these inhalation drugs, close monitoring of patients' medication adherence and inhalation techniques are required.

The selective phosphodiesterase inhibitor roflumilast is reported to reduce COPD exacerbations in COPD patients with severe airflow limitation, bronchitic symptoms, and a history of exacerbations. The rate of moderate-to-severe exacerbations was 1.14 per patient per year with roflumilast and 1.37 per patient per year with placebo [44]. A recent study revealed that roflumilast reduced exacerbations and hospital admissions in severe COPD patients with chronic bronchitis who were predisposed to frequent and severe exacerbations despite ICS and LABA or triple therapy [45]. The gastrointestinal side effects of roflumilast, such as nausea, diarrhea, and weight loss, were noted and may limit its effectiveness.

Macrolides have airway anti-inflammatory actions in addition to their antibiotic effects, and studies were conducted to elucidate the effects of macrolides on the prevention of exacerbation. Albert et al. performed a randomized trial to investigate the effects of azithromycin in reducing the frequency of exacerbation in 1142 COPD patients with an increased risk of exacerbation [46]. They reported that the frequency of exacerbations was 1.48 exacerbations per patient per year in the azithromycin group, compared with 1.83 per patient per year in the placebo group ($P = 0.01$). However, since there are concerns on antibiotic resistance and potential cardiac toxicity, GOLD guidelines do not describe azithromycin as a preventive option for COPD exacerbations. Uzun et al. stated that maintenance treatment with azithromycin should be considered for use in patients with COPD who have the frequent exacerbator phenotype and are refractory to standard care [47].

Although a Chinese randomized study reported the preventive effects of N-acetylcysteine 600 mg twice daily [48], other trails on the use of mucolytics to prevent COPD exacerbations are contradictory.

Because many COPD patients have cardiovascular comorbidities such as chronic heart failure, the effects of treatment with β-blockers on COPD patients have been investigated. Although deterioration of pulmonary function caused by β-blockers was a concern, Bhatt et al. reported that β-blockers could be tolerated in severe COPD patients and were associated with a significant reduction in exacerbation [49]. Although the effectiveness of β-blockers in decreasing COPD exacerbations should be confirmed in a randomized, placebo-controlled study, cardioprotective effects of β-blockers seem to be helpful, especially in COPD patients with cardiovascular diseases.

15.5.2 Non-pharmacologic Prevention

Several non-pharmacologic interventions have been studied in clinical trials, with the aim of preventing exacerbations. Compared with usual care, pulmonary rehabilitation in the posthospitalization period is safe and significantly reduces readmissions during follow-up, although a recent report failed to reveal the effects of acute phase progressive rehabilitation during hospital admission for exacerbation on risk reduction of the subsequent readmission [8–36]. The early and tailored in-hospital rehabilitation program taking into account of patient's condition might enhance recovery and reduce readmissions for acute exacerbations. Since abnormal swallowing reflex in COPD patients seem to be associated with frequent exacerbations, an intervention for swallowing reflex might be a useful therapeutic strategy for preventing exacerbations [11].

Several randomized control studies reported that the combination of disease education, self-management programs, and action plans in reduction was thought to be effective in reducing exacerbation. However, a randomized trial that compared an educational program, written action plans, and access to a case manager by phone with usual care was terminated early by the data monitoring committee because of excess mortality in the intervention group [50]. Although available data of this study could not explain the excess mortality in the intervention group, the safety of self-management programs and exacerbation action plans require further evaluation before this strategy can be recommended for all patients [41].

15.6 Impact of Exacerbations on COPD Patients

Exacerbations severely impact the health status of COPD patients such as reductions in quality of life and cardiopulmonary functions and increased risk of death.

Quality of life for COPD patients significantly deteriorated during and after exacerbations [51]. Spencer et al. investigated the adverse effects of infective exacerbation on 438 patients with COPD exacerbation [51]. SGRQ scores were obtained at baseline and at 4, 12, and 26 weeks after exacerbation. They revealed that single exacerbations had a large and sustained effect on health status. Although the initial recovery of SGRQ scores was rapid, the recovery period was over 6 months in patients with no further exacerbations. At baseline assessment for exacerbation, SGRQ scores were worse in patients who had a subsequent exacerbation during follow-up.

Exacerbations have negative impacts on pulmonary function. During COPD exacerbations, airway resistance is abruptly increased, and COPD patients with exacerbation show significant airflow obstruction and lung hyperinflation (Fig. 15.1). Although pulmonary functions gradually improve with treatment, around one quarter of exacerbations had incomplete recovery after 35 days [52]. Therefore, repeated exacerbations progressively worsen airflow limitation. Donaldson et al. investigated the correlation between exacerbation frequency and an accelerated decline in pulmonary function. COPD patients with frequent exacerbations show a significantly faster decline in FEV1 and peak expiratory flow than infrequent exacerbators [7]. Exacerbations are also involved in emphysema progression. Tanabe et al. explored the effects of exacerbations on emphysema

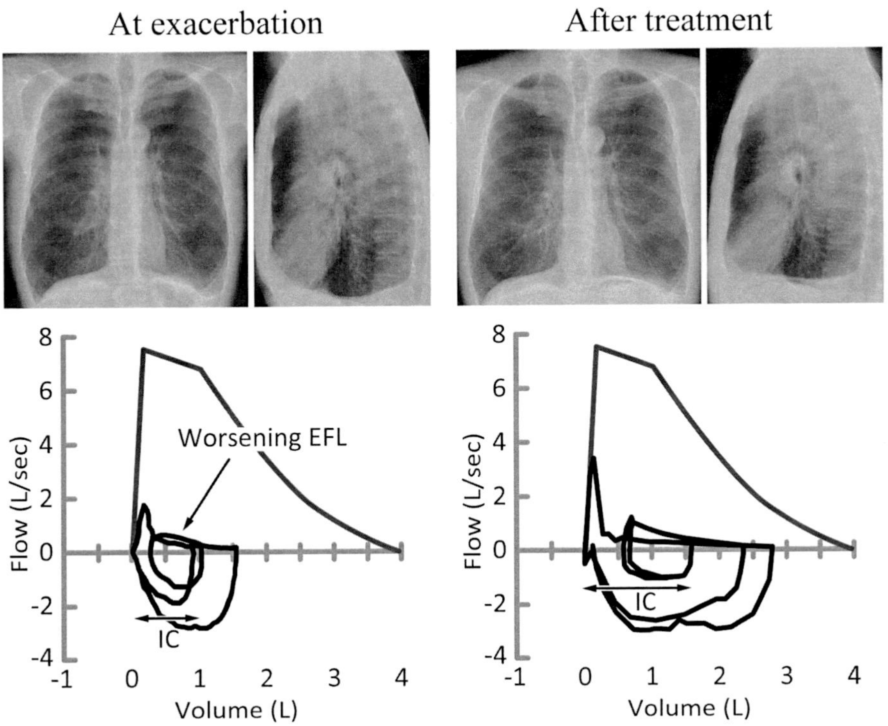

Fig. 15.1 Changes in the level of hyperinflation and pulmonary function during recovery from exacerbation. Chest X-ray films and flow-volume loops from a patient obtained after onset of exacerbation (*left*) and at stable condition after exacerbation (*right*). After exacerbation, there is evidence of worsening expiratory flow limitation (EFL) resulting in hyperinflation on X-ray film. Inspiratory capacity (IC) also decreased. After treatment, an improvement in EFL caused an increase in IC and an improvement in hyperinflation

progression by analyzing CT images for both the percentage of the lung field occupied by low-attenuation areas and fractal analysis using a longitudinal COPD cohort and found that annual changes in CT parameters of emphysema are greater in patients with a history of exacerbation [53].

Exacerbations profoundly affect the cardiovascular system, and this might account for significant morbidity and mortality. Freixa et al. prospectively evaluated 342 moderate-to-severe COPD patients' first admission with exacerbation. Transthoracic echocardiography was performed in clinically stable condition, at least 3 months after discharge. They revealed that cardiac abnormalities, such as right ventricular enlargement and pulmonary hypertension, are highly prevalent in COPD patients at the time of their first severe exacerbation, even in the absence of established cardiac disease or cardiovascular risk factors [54]. CT evaluation seems to be useful to evaluate the adverse effects on the cardiac system caused by exacerbation [18, 21]. Further investigations using novel markers such as the cross-sectional area of small pulmonary vessels are waited [55].

Exacerbations of COPD are associated with high in-hospital and post-discharge mortality. Reported mortality rates vary from 2.5 to 30 % depending upon patient characteristics and the design of the study. A recent investigation from the European Respiratory Society COPD audit that was designed as a prospective, observational, and noninterventional cohort trial found that 10.8 % of those admitted with exacerbated COPD died during the observational period, from admission to 90 days after discharge. In expired patients, 45.7 % died while still in hospital, whereas 54.3 % died during the 90-day post-discharge follow-up. The risk associated with mortality was higher age, the presence of acidotic respiratory failure, subsequent need for ventilator support, and the presence of comorbidity [56]. According to the long-term history and mortality after COPD exacerbations, Suissa et al. conducted an epidemiological study with a cohort of patients at first hospitalization for COPD using healthcare databases. The cohort included 73,106 patients, and during the 17-year follow-up period, 50,580 died with 50 and 75 % mortality at 3.6 and 7.7 years, respectively. They also reported a rapid decline in health status after the second severe exacerbation and high mortality in the weeks following every severe exacerbation. From these results, they stated the importance of delaying the second severe exacerbation and intensifying inpatient treatment of COPD exacerbation to prevent excessive early mortality [57].

15.7 Conclusion

Why does COPD exacerbation attract attention? Are there any preventive methods?

Exacerbations of COPD attract attention because they are associated with the deterioration in quality of life, an accelerated rate of decline for lung function, and increased mortality. Furthermore, high socioeconomic costs on healthcare resources are required to manage COPD exacerbation. Therefore, the prevention of exacerbations is recognized as one of the main targets of maintenance therapy for COPD.

COPD exacerbations are preventable, at least in part. Conforming to the management strategies in stable COPD patients is essential, and many types of pharmacologic and non-pharmacologic interventions are available. However, an optimal combination of these strategies remains to be defined and seems to vary depending upon the characteristics of the patient. Further understanding in the nature of exacerbations, the development of more effective interventions, and investigations to define suitable combinations of these interventions are required to develop rational, preventive regimes for exacerbation.

References

1. The global strategy for the diagnosis, management and prevention of chronic obstructive pulmonary diseases. Updated 2015. Global Initiative for Chronic Obstructive Lung Disease (GOLD). http://www.goldcopd.org. Accessed 9 Dec 2015.
2. Sapey E, Stockley RA. COPD exacerbations. 2: aetiology. Thorax. 2006;61:250–8.
3. Calverley PM, Anderson JA, Celli B, Ferguson GT, Jenkins C, Jones PW, et al. Salmeterol and fluticasone propionate and survival in chronic obstructive pulmonary disease. N Engl J Med. 2007;356:775–89.
4. Tashkin DP, Celli B, Senn S, Burkhart D, Kesten S, Menjoge S, et al. A 4-year trial of tiotropium in chronic obstructive pulmonary disease. N Engl J Med. 2008;359:1543–54.
5. Hurst JR, Vestbo J, Anzueto A, Locantore N, Müllerova H, Tal-Singer R, et al. Susceptibility to exacerbation in chronic obstructive pulmonary disease. N Engl J Med. 2010;363:1128–38.
6. Langsetmo L, Platt RW, Ernst P, Bourbeau J. Underreporting exacerbation of chronic obstructive pulmonary disease in a longitudinal cohort. Am J Respir Crit Care Med. 2008;177:396–401.
7. Donaldson GC, Seemungal TA, Bhowmik A, Wedzicha JA. Relationship between exacerbation frequency and lung function decline in chronic obstructive pulmonary disease. Thorax. 2002;57:847–52.
8. Wedzicha JA, Seemungal TA. COPD exacerbations: defining their cause and prevention. Lancet. 2007;370:786–96.
9. Nishimura M, Makita H, Nagai K, Konno S, Nasuhara Y, Hasegawa M, et al. Annual change in pulmonary function and clinical phenotype in chronic obstructive pulmonary disease. Am J Respir Crit Care Med. 2012;185:44–52.
10. Terada K, Muro S, Sato S, Ohara T, Haruna A, Marumo S, et al. Impact of gastro-oesophageal reflux disease symptoms on COPD exacerbation. Thorax. 2008;63:951–5. doi:10.1136/thx.2007.092858.
11. Terada K, Muro S, Ohara T, Kudo M, Ogawa E, Hoshino Y, et al. Abnormal swallowing reflex and COPD exacerbations. Chest. 2010;137:326–32. doi:10.1378/chest.09-0482.
12. Osman IM, Godden DJ, Friend JA, Legge JS, Douglas JG. Quality of life and hospital re-admission in patients with chronic obstructive pulmonary disease. Thorax. 1997;52:67–71.
13. Bhowmik A, Seemungal TA, Sapsford RJ, Wedzicha JA. Relation of sputum inflammatory markers to symptoms and lung function changes in COPD exacerbations. Thorax. 2000;55:114–20.
14. Thomsen M, Ingebrigtsen TS, Marott JL, Dahl M, Lange P, Vestbo J, et al. Inflammatory biomarkers and exacerbations in chronic obstructive pulmonary disease. JAMA. 2013;309:2353–61. doi:10.1001/jama.2013.5732.
15. Han MK, Kazerooni EA, Lynch DA, Liu LX, Murray S, Curtis JL, et al. Chronic obstructive pulmonary disease exacerbations in the COPDGene study: associated radiologic phenotypes. Radiology. 2011;261:274–82. doi:10.1148/radiol.11110173.
16. McGhan R, Radcliff T, Fish R, Sutherland ER, Welsh C, Make B. Predictors of rehospitalization and death after a severe exacerbation of COPD. Chest. 2007;132:1748–55.
17. Devaraj A, Wells AU, Meister MG, Corte TJ, Wort SJ, Hansell DM. Detection of pulmonary hypertension with multidetector CT and echocardiography alone and in combination. Radiology. 2010;254:609–16. doi:10.1148/radiol.09090548.
18. Wells JM, Washko GR, Han MK, Abbas N, Nath H, Mamary AJ, et al. Pulmonary arterial enlargement and acute exacerbations of COPD. N Engl J Med. 2012;367:913–21. doi:10.1056/NEJMoa1203830.
19. Li MH, Fan LC, Mao B, Yang JW, Choi AM, Cao WJ, et al. Short term exposure to ambient fine particulate matter (PM2.5) increases hospitalizations and mortality of chronic obstructive pulmonary disease: a systematic review and meta-analysis. Chest. 2015 Jun 25. doi: 10.1378/chest.15-0513.
20. Rodríguez-Roisin R. COPD exacerbations.5: management. Thorax. 2006;61:535–44.

21. Wells JM, Morrison JB, Bhatt SP, Nath H, Dransfield MT. Pulmonary artery enlargement is associated with cardiac injury during severe exacerbations of COPD. Chest. 2015. doi:10.1378/chest.15-1504.
22. Garcha DS, Thurston SJ, Patel AR, Mackay AJ, Goldring JJ, Donaldson GC, et al. Changes in prevalence and load of airway bacteria using quantitative PCR in stable and exacerbated COPD. Thorax. 2012;67:1075–80. doi:10.1136/thoraxjnl-2012-201924.
23. Soler N, Esperatti M, Ewig S, Huerta A, Agustí C, Torres A. Sputum purulence-guided antibiotic use in hospitalised patients with exacerbations of COPD. Eur Respir J. 2012;40:1344–53. doi:10.1183/09031936.00150211.
24. El Moussaoui R, Roede BM, Speelman P, Bresser P, Prins JM, Bossuyt PM. Short-course antibiotic treatment in acute exacerbations of chronic bronchitis and COPD: a meta-analysis of double-blind studies. Thorax. 2008;63:415–22. doi:10.1136/thx.2007.090613.
25. Barr RG, Rowe BH, Camargo Jr CA. Methylxanthines for exacerbations of chronic obstructive pulmonary disease: meta-analysis of randomised trials. BMJ. 2003;327(7416):643.
26. Walters JA, Gibson PG, Wood-Baker R, Hannay M, Walters EH. Systemic corticosteroids for acute exacerbations of chronic obstructive pulmonary disease. Cochrane Database Syst Rev. 2009;1, CD001288. doi:10.1002/14651858.CD001288.
27. Leuppi JD, Schuetz P, Bingisser R, Bodmer M, Briel M, Drescher T, et al. Short-term vs conventional glucocorticoid therapy in acute exacerbations of chronic obstructive pulmonary disease: the REDUCE randomized clinical trial. JAMA. 2013;309:2223–31. doi:10.1001/jama.2013.5023.
28. Walters JA, Wang W, Morley C, Soltani A, Wood-Baker R. Different durations of corticosteroid therapy for exacerbations of chronic obstructive pulmonary disease. Cochrane Database Syst Rev. 2011;10, CD006897. doi:10.1002/14651858.CD006897.
29. Kiser TH, Allen RR, Valuck RJ, Moss M, Vandivier RW. Outcomes associated with corticosteroid dosage in critically ill patients with acute exacerbations of chronic obstructive pulmonary disease. Am J Respir Crit Care Med. 2014;189:1052–64. doi:10.1164/rccm.201401-0058OC.
30. Frat JP, Thille AW, Mercat A, Girault C, Ragot S, Perbet S, et al. High-flow oxygen through nasal cannula in acute hypoxemic respiratory failure. N Engl J Med. 2015;372(23):2185–96. doi:10.1056/NEJMoa1503326.
31. Rittayamai N, Tscheikuna J, Praphruetkit N, Kijpinyochai S. Use of high-flow nasal cannula for acute dyspnea and hypoxemia in the emergency department. Respir Care. 2015;60(10):1377–82. doi:10.4187/respcare.03837.
32. Brochard L, Mancebo J, Wysocki M, Lofaso F, Conti G, Rauss A, et al. Noninvasive ventilation for acute exacerbations of chronic obstructive pulmonary disease. N Engl J Med. 1997;336:817–22.
33. Esteban A, Anzueto A, Frutos F, Alía I, Brochard L, Stewart TE, et al. Characteristics and outcomes in adult patients receiving mechanical ventilation: a 28-day international study. JAMA. 2002;287:345–55.
34. Gunen H, Hacievliyagil SS, Kosar F, Mutlu LC, Gulbas G, Pehlivan E, et al. Factors affecting survival of hospitalised patients with COPD. Eur Respir J. 2005;26:234–41.
35. Seymour JM, Moore L, Jolley CJ, Ward K, Creasey J, Steier JS, et al. Outpatient pulmonary rehabilitation following acute exacerbations of COPD. Thorax. 2010;65:423–8. doi:10.1136/thx.2009.124164.
36. Spruit MA, Singh SJ, Garvey C, ZuWallack R, Nici L, Rochester C, et al. An official American Thoracic Society/European Respiratory Society statement: key concepts and advances in pulmonary rehabilitation. Am J Respir Crit Care Med. 2013;188:e13–64. doi:10.1164/rccm.201309-1634ST.
37. Maddocks M, Kon SS, Singh SJ, Man WD. Rehabilitation following hospitalization in patients with COPD: can it reduce readmissions? Respirology. 2015;20:395–404. doi:10.1111/resp.12454.

38. Greening NJ, Williams JE, Hussain SF, Harvey-Dunstan TC, Bankart MJ, Chaplin EJ, et al. An early rehabilitation intervention to enhance recovery during hospital admission for an exacerbation of chronic respiratory disease: randomised controlled trial. BMJ. 2014;349:g4315. doi:10.1136/bmj.g4315.
39. Echevarria C, Steer J, Heslop-Marshall K, Stenton SC, Hickey PM, Hughes R, et al. Validation of the DECAF score to predict hospital mortality in acute exacerbations of COPD. Thorax. 2016;71(2):133–40. doi:10.1136/thoraxjnl-2015-207775.
40. Walters JA, Smith S, Poole P, Granger RH, Wood-Baker R. Injectable vaccines preventing Pneumococcal infection in patients with chronic obstructive pulmonary disease. Cochrane Database Syst Rev. 2010;11, CD001390. doi:10.1002/14651858.CD001390.
41. Aaron SD. Management and prevention of exacerbations of COPD. BMJ. 2014;349:g5237. doi:10.1136/bmj.g5237.
42. Wedzicha JA, Decramer M, Ficker JH, Niewoehner DE, Sandström T, Taylor AF, et al. Analysis of chronic obstructive pulmonary disease exacerbations with the dual bronchodilator QVA149 compared with glycopyrronium and tiotropium (SPARK): a randomised, double-blind, parallel-group study. Lancet Respir Med. 2013;1:199–209. doi:10.1016/S2213-2600(13)70052-3.
43. Magnussen H, Disse B, Rodriguez-Roisin R, Kirsten A, Watz H, Tetzlaff K, et al. Withdrawal of inhaled glucocorticoids and exacerbations of COPD. N Engl J Med. 2014;371:1285–94. doi:10.1056/NEJMoa1407154.
44. Calverley PM, Rabe KF, Goehring UM, Kristiansen S, Fabbri LM, Martinez FJ. Roflumilast in symptomatic chronic obstructive pulmonary disease: two randomised clinical trials. Lancet. 2009;374:685–94. doi:10.1016/S0140-6736(09)61255-1.
45. Martinez FJ, Calverley PM, Goehring UM, Brose M, Fabbri LM, Rabe KF. Effect of roflumilast on exacerbations in patients with severe chronic obstructive pulmonary disease uncontrolled by combination therapy (REACT): a multicentre randomised controlled trial. Lancet. 2015;385:857–66. doi:10.1016/S0140-6736(14)62410-7.
46. Albert RK, Connett J, Bailey WC, Casaburi R, Cooper Jr JA, Criner GJ, et al. Azithromycin for prevention of exacerbations of COPD. N Engl J Med. 2011;365:689–98. doi:10.1056/NEJMoa1104623.
47. Uzun S, Djamin RS, Kluytmans JA, Mulder PG, van't Veer NE, Ermens AA, et al. Azithromycin maintenance treatment in patients with frequent exacerbations of chronic obstructive pulmonary disease (COLUMBUS): a randomised, double-blind, placebo-controlled trial. Lancet Respir Med. 2014;2:361–8. doi:10.1016/S2213-2600(14)70019-0.
48. Zheng JP, Wen FQ, Bai CX, Wan HY, Kang J, Chen P, et al. Twice daily N-acetylcysteine 600 mg for exacerbations of chronic obstructive pulmonary disease (PANTHEON): a randomised, double-blind placebo-controlled trial. Lancet Respir Med. 2014;2:187–94. doi:10.1016/S2213-2600(13)70286-8.
49. Bhatt SP, Wells JM, Kinney GL, Washko GR Jr, Budoff M, Kim YI, et al. β-blockers are associated with a reduction in COPD exacerbations. Thorax. 2016;71:8–14. doi: 10.1136/thoraxjnl-2015-207251.
50. Fan VS, Gaziano JM, Lew R, Bourbeau J, Adams SG, Leatherman S, et al. A comprehensive care management program to prevent chronic obstructive pulmonary disease hospitalizations: a randomized, controlled trial. Ann Intern Med. 2012;156:673–83. doi:10.7326/0003-4819-156-10-201205150-00003.
51. Spencer S, Jones PW, GLOBE Study Group. Time course of recovery of health status following an infective exacerbation of chronic bronchitis. Thorax. 2003;58:589–93.
52. O'Donnell DE, Parker CM. COPD exacerbations.3: pathophysiology. Thorax. 2006;61:354–61.
53. Tanabe N, Muro S, Hirai T, Oguma T, Terada K, Marumo S, et al. Impact of exacerbations on emphysema progression in chronic obstructive pulmonary disease. Am J Respir Crit Care Med. 2011;183:1653–9. doi:10.1164/rccm.201009-1535OC.

54. Freixa X, Portillo K, Paré C, Garcia-Aymerich J, Gomez FP, Benet M, et al. Echocardiographic abnormalities in patients with COPD at their first hospital admission. Eur Respir J. 2013;41:784–91. doi:10.1183/09031936.00222511.
55. Matsuoka S, Washko GR, Yamashiro T, Estepar RS, Diaz A, Silverman EK, et al. Pulmonary hypertension and computed tomography measurement of small pulmonary vessels in severe emphysema. Am J Respir Crit Care Med. 2010;181(3):218–25. doi:10.1164/rccm.200908-1189OC.
56. Hartl S, Lopez-Campos JL, Pozo-Rodriguez F, Castro-Acosta A, Studnicka M, Kaiser B, et al. Risk of death and readmission of hospital-admitted COPD exacerbations: European COPD Audit. Eur Respir J. 2016;47:113–21. doi:10.1183/13993003.01391-2014.
57. Suissa S, Dell'Aniello S, Ernst P. Long-term natural history of chronic obstructive pulmonary disease: severe exacerbations and mortality. Thorax. 2012;67:957–63. doi:10.1136/thoraxjnl-2011-201518.

Part V
Associations with Other Respiratory Diseases

Chapter 16
The Asthma–COPD Overlap Syndrome (ACOS): What Is the Significance COPD Associated with Asthma?

Hidehiro Watanabe

Abstract Asthma is characterized by inflammation involving eosinophils and Th2 cytokines of the central to peripheral airways, with high reversibility of the airflow obstruction (hereafter simply, airflow reversibility). On the other hand, chronic obstructive pulmonary disease (COPD) is characterized by inflammation involving neutrophils and inflammatory cytokines of the peripheral airways to the alveoli, with low or no airflow reversibility. The asthma-COPD overlap syndrome (ACOS) is characterized by features of both and associated with moderate airflow reversibility. ACOS does not uniformly have the features of asthma or COPD, and its features depend on the type and major site of airway inflammation. The medical costs of ACOS are higher than those of either asthma or COPD. Under such circumstances, the Global Initiative for Asthma (GINA) and Global Initiative for Chronic Obstructive Lung Disease (GOLD) have provided guidelines for the management of ACOS. It is important to combine treatments for both COPD and asthma and not use treatment for either alone in patients with AOCS.

Keywords Juvenile asthma • Asthma – COPD overlap syndrome: ACOS • Airflow limitation

16.1 Introduction

Allergy is a major cause of asthma. Lesions of asthma are extensive, extending from the central to peripheral airways, and are histologically characterized by eosinophilic inflammation [1] and Th2 cytokine-associated inflammation [2, 3]. Therefore, inhaled corticosteroids (ICS) are effective in patients with asthma. On the other hand, chronic obstructive pulmonary disease (COPD) is etiologically diverse, being associated with genetic causes, air pollution, and/or smoking, the

---

H. Watanabe (✉)
Department of Infectious Diseases and Prevention, Tokyo Medical University, 6-7-1 Nishishinjuku, Shinjuku-ku, Tokyo 160-0023, Japan
e-mail: hw-nabe4@tokyo-med.ac.jp

H. Nakamura, K. Aoshiba (eds.), *Chronic Obstructive Pulmonary Disease*, Respiratory Disease Series: Diagnostic Tools and Disease Managements, DOI 10.1007/978-981-10-0839-9_16

etiological profile differing among countries and regions [4]. Tissues, including bronchioles and alveolar walls, are destroyed in COPD lesions, which are characterized by neutrophilic inflammation and inflammation involving cluster of differentiation (CD) 8 lymphocytes. The disease shows gradual progression, but the symptoms can be controlled in the early stages with bronchodilators. Asthma and COPD are diseases that occur frequently and are estimated to affect 1 in 12 people in the world [5]. The two diseases have been proposed as independent concepts, but belong to the high-prevalence disease groups and can exacerbate each other. Patients with asthma tend to develop COPD, and patients with COPD tend to develop asthma. Actually, this clinical situation has long been pointed out. In 1961, Orie et al. [6] proposed the "Dutch hypothesis" that these diseases may be different phenotypes of a single pathological condition [7]. However, thereafter, clinical studies of asthma have been performed only in patients with definitively diagnosed asthma (excluding those with pulmonary emphysematous changes on imaging) [8, 9], and clinical studies of COPD have excluded patients with asthma-like symptoms [10]. Therefore, no studies have been conducted in patients in whom these two diseases cannot be distinguished, and sufficient data have not been collected on this overlap condition. Under such circumstances, a joint meeting of the Global Initiative for Asthma (GINA) and Global Initiative for Chronic Obstructive Lung Disease (GOLD) expressed a consensus opinion in a report in 2014 and 2015, Diagnosis of Diseases of Chronic Airflow Limitation: Asthma COPD and asthma-COPD overlap syndrome (ACOS) (www.goldcopd.org/uploads/users/files/GOLD_ACOS_2015.pdf) [11]. The definition and concept of ACOS has been established worldwide, and diagnostic steps for this condition have been established. This chapter outlines the background of ACOS as the main subject, followed by its diagnosis and treatment.

16.2 Pathogenetic Mechanism of ACOS

There are three major hypotheses for the pathogenesis of ACOS.

16.2.1 First Mechanism (Dutch Hypothesis)

According to this hypothesis, the clinical pictures become difficult to distinguish when a common pathophysiologic process (e.g., airway hyperresponsiveness) leads to separate disease entities of asthma and COPD under the influence of different environmental factors (e.g., allergens, air pollution, and smoking), as described in Introduction [6, 7]. Smokers with greatly reduced respiratory function over time have asthma-like pathological manifestations, such as airway hyperresponsiveness, elevated peripheral blood eosinophil count, and elevated immunoglobulin E (IgE) levels [12, 13]. It has been reported that the peripheral blood eosinophil count is correlated with deterioration of the respiratory function [12]. The clinical pictures of asthma and COPD are difficult to distinguish, probably because they share common aggravating factors (airway hyperresponsiveness, tobacco smoke, lung growth impairment, viral infection, aging, and repeated exacerbations) during progression of the disease over time.

16.2.2 *Second Mechanism (British Hypothesis)*

This hypothesis was proposed by Reid et al. [14] in 1965. According to this hypothesis, in a process in which individual causes, such as allergy for asthma and tobacco smoke for COPD, lead to the development of the clinical pictures of asthma and COPD, the element of infection, including viral infection, is added, and the resultant airway hypersecretion leads to chronic airway narrowing, resulting in partial overlapping of the two clinical pictures. In this process, T helper (Th) cytokines induced by infection are thought to cause alveolar destruction-irreversible tissue damage [15].

16.2.3 *Third Mechanism (Hypothesis of Progression of Asthma)*

According to this hypothesis, in patients with long-term asthma, asthma progresses to COPD, resulting in the clinical picture of ACOS. This seems to be the case in clinically so-called elderly patients with asthma. For example, it is reported that 30 % of patients diagnosed as having COPD by clinicians have a history of asthma, while 30 % of patients diagnosed as having asthma have irreversible airflow obstruction [16]. Patients with asthma are reported to be at a 10-fold higher risk of developing COPD. Patients with severe asthma have reduced pulmonary elasticity and develop COPD [17]. Lung growth impairment and reduced elastic lung recoil (pseudo-emphysema) in childhood, in addition to airway remodeling, are involved in the development of irreversible airflow obstruction in patients with asthma. Furthermore, particularly in elderly patients, asthma and COPD are clinically similar to each other. In asthmatic patients with airway remodeling, irreversible airway obstruction develops over time, resulting in COPD-like symptoms. Similarly, COPD patients with reversible airway obstruction develop asthma-like symptoms. Consideration of these hypotheses makes it easier to understand ACOS as described in the guidelines (Tables 16.1 and 16.2) [11].

Table 16.1 Usual features of asthma, COPD and ACOS

Feature	Asthma	COPD	ACOS
Age of onset	Usually childhood onset but can commence at any age.	Usually > 40 years of age	Usually age ≥40 years, but may have had symptoms in childhood or early adulthood
Pattern of respiratory symptoms	Symptoms may vary over time (day to day, or over longer periods), often limiting activity. Often triggered by exercise, emotions including laughter, dust or exposure to allergens	Chronic usually continuous symptoms, particularly during exercise, with 'better' and 'worse' days	Respiratory symptoms including exertional dyspnea are persistent but variability may be prominent
Lung function	Current and/or historical variable airflow limitation, e.g. BD reversibility, AHR	FEV_1 may be improved by therapy, but post-BD $FEV_1/FVC < 0.7$ persists	Airflow limitation not fully reversible, but often with current or historical variability
Lung function between symptoms	May be normal between symptoms	Persistent airflow limitation	Persistent airflow limitation
Past history or family history	Many patients have allergies and a personal history of asthma in childhood, and/or family history of asthma	History of exposure to noxious particles and gases (mainly tobacco smoking and biomass fuels)	Frequently a history of doctor- diagnosed asthma (current or previous), allergies and a family history of asthma, and/or a history of noxious exposures
Time course	Often improves spontaneously or with treatment, but may result in fixed airflow limitation	Generally, slowly progressive over years despite treatment	Symptoms are partly but significantly reduced by treatment. Progression is usual and treatment needs are high
Chest X-ray	Usually normal	Severe hyperinflation & other changes of COPD	Similar to COPD
Exacerbations	Exacerbations occur, but the risk of exacerbations can be considerably reduced by treatment	Exacerbations can be reduced by treatment. If present, comorbidities contribute to impairment	Exacerbations may be more common than in COPD but are reduced by treatment. Comorbidities can contribute to impairment
Airway inflammation	Eosinophils and/or neutrophils	Neutrophils ± eosinophils in sputum, lymphocytes in airways, may have systemic inflammation	Eosinophils and/or neutrophils in sputum.

Table 16.2 Features that if present favor asthma or COPD

More likely to be asthma if several of ...[a]	More likely to be COPD if several of...[a]
☐ *Onset before age 20 years*	☐ *Onset after age 40 years*
☐ *Variation in symptoms over minutes, hours or days*	☐ *Persistence of symptoms despite treatment*
☐ *Symptoms worse during the night or early morning*	☐ *Good and bad days but always daily symptoms and exertional dyspnea*
☐ *Symptoms triggered by exercise, emotions including laughter, dust or exposure to allergens*	☐ *Chronic cough and sputum preceded onset of dyspnea, unrelated to triggers*
☐ *Record of variable airflow limitation (spirometry, peak flow)*	☐ *Record of persistent airflow limitation (post-bronchodilator $FEV_1/FVC < 0.7$)*
☐ *Lung function normal between symptoms*	☐ *Lung function abnormal between symptoms*
☐ *Previous doctor diagnosis of asthma*	☐ *Previous doctor diagnosis of COPD, chronic bronchitis or emphysema*
☐ *Family history of asthma, and other allergic conditions (allergic rhinitis or eczema)*	☐ *Heavy exposure to a risk factor: tobacco smoke, biomass fuels*
☐ *No worsening of symptoms over time. Symptoms vary either seasonally, or from year to year*	☐ *Symptoms slowly worsening over time (progressive course over years)*
☐ *May improve spontaneously or have an immediate response to BD or to ICS over weeks*	☐ *Rapid-acting bronchodilator treatment provides only limited relief.*
☐ *Normal*	☐ *Severe hyperinflation*

[a]***Syndromic diagnosis of airways disease: how to use Table 16.2***
Entries in italics list features that, when present, best identify patients with typical asthma and COPD. For a patient, count the number of check boxes in each column. If three or more boxes are checked for either asthma or COPD, the patient is likely to have that disease. If there are similar numbers of checked boxes in each column, the diagnosis of ACOS should be considered. See Step 2 for more details.

16.3 Epidemiology of ACOS

In elderly patients, it is not easy to accurately diagnose ACOS, because of the confounding influence of airway remodeling due to aging, long-term illness, etc. In an epidemiological study based on a population survey, the incidences of asthma, COPD, and ACOS were reported to be 2 %, 8.4 %, and 0.9 %, respectively [18], and according to reports based on the International Statistical Classification of Diseases and Related Health Problems (ICD10), the incidence was in the range of approximately 0.9–16.1 % [19–21]. Thus, the results of epidemiological studies are varied. The incidence tends to be higher in patients referred to specialists on account of possible difficulty in management. According to a cohort study by Cosio BG et al. [22], 15 % of 831 patients with COPD had ACOS, and in a study by Hardin M et al. [23], 13 % of 915 patients with COPD had ACOS. A review of the literature revealed that 12.1–55.2 % of patients with COPD had ACOS [24]. Furthermore, according to a publication by the GINA [11], 15 % of patients with COPD have ACOS. In general, approximately 10–20 % of patients with COPD are thought to have an asthmatic component [25]. The incidence is higher in elderly patients: it has been reported that approximately a half of all COPD patients aged 65 years or older have ACOS [26].

On the other hand, patients diagnosed as having asthma appear to develop irreversible airflow obstruction, namely, COPD, with age, because approximately 5 % have severe asthma and some are smokers. Milanese M et al. [27] reported that 29 % of 350 asthmatic patients aged 65 years or older had COPD. According to another report, 13.3–61.0 % of all asthmatic patients had ACOS [24, 28]. In humans, lung growth continues until early adulthood and is completed by the age of 30 years. Lung volume increases and pulmonary function measured in terms of the forced expiratory volume in 1.0 s (FEV1) is maintained. Even normal individuals show progressive airway obstruction with time, i.e., the FEV1 deceases by 25–50 mL each year even during early adulthood. The FEV1 has been shown to decrease by 80 and 150 mL per year in patients with asthma and COPD, respectively. There is limited evidence to suggest whether the annual rate of reduction of the FEV1 can be used to differentiate between asthma and COPD. With the increasing longevity of the population, an increase in the number of patients with long-term asthma, such as those developing asthma in childhood, and those with severe asthma may affect the epidemiology of ACOS. Development of COPD in patients with asthma can be diagnosed based on a history of smoking, findings on imaging (e.g., computed tomography [CT]), pulmonary function testing to determine the pulmonary diffusing capacity, etc. On the other hand, it is not easy to diagnose the development of asthma in patients with COPD. In specialized medical institutions, fractional exhaled nitric oxide (FeNO) and serum IgE levels can be measured; however, in nonspecialized institutions, these cannot be measured, and the diagnosis has to be made on the basis of the clinical findings. In particular, in elderly patients, differentiation based on clinical findings has to be carefully made.

16.4 Importance of ACOS (Table 16.3)

Table 16.3 The importance factors of ACOS (compared with asthma and COPD)

Factors	Reference
(1) High exacerbation frequency	[22, 24]
Low health-related quality of life	[22, 30, 31]
(2) High medical cost	[31–33]
High medical service requirement	
(High hospitalization frequency)	
(3) Association with asthmatic death	[26, 29]

16.4.1 High Incidence of Exacerbations and Low Health-Related Quality of Life (HRQoL)

The reported percentage of patients with ACOS experiencing frequently repeated exacerbations is 42.7 %, 2–3 times higher than that in patients with COPD (15 %) [21, 23]. The number of hospitalizations increases with repeated exacerbations and is reported to be the highest for patients with ACOS, followed by those with COPD and asthma (ACOS >> COPD > asthma). The HRQol is significantly lower in patients with ACOS than in those with asthma [21, 29, 30].

16.4.2 High Medical Costs and Medical Care

Because ACOS patients have a higher frequency of exacerbations than those with asthma or COPD alone, and ACOS is progressive, treatment and hospitalization costs are higher in ACOS patients. Gerhardsson de Verdier M et al. [31] conducted a comparison of the 12-month medical costs between 26,060 patients with asthma (without COPD) and 6505 patients with ACOS, which revealed twofold higher medical costs in ACOS patients than in asthmatic patients. In addition, Shaya FT et al. [32] performed a 2-year comparison between 3702 patients with asthma, 3455 patients with COPD, and 2064 patients with ACOS, which revealed that ACOS patients required nearly 5 times more medical services than patients with asthma or COPD. The overall patient profile has to be taken into account for the management of ACOS [30].

16.4.3 High Mortality (Relationship with Death from Asthma)

The mortality from ACOS is higher than that from asthma or COPD alone [25]. On the other hand, the number of deaths from asthma has shown a tendency to decrease over time, with elderly patients aged 65 years or older accounting for approximately 90 % of all deaths from asthma [28]. Considering that elderly patients with asthma show a high frequency of complication by COPD, deaths from ACOS may account for nearly 40 % of all deaths from asthma.

16.5 Diagnosis of ACOS (Table 16.4)

Five steps of a syndromic approach to the diagnosis of ACOS have been presented [summary of syndromic approach to diseases of chronic airflow limitation].

Table 16.4 Summary of syndromic approach to diseases of chronic airflow limitation

STEP 1 DIAGNOSE CHRONIC AIRWAYS DISEASE
Do symptoms suggest chronic airways disease?

Yes | No → Consider other diseases first

STEP 2 SYNDROMIC DIAGNOSIS IN ADULTS
(i) Assemble the features for asthma and for COPD that best describe the patient.
(ii) Compare number of features in favor of each diagnosis and select a diagnosis

Features: if present suggest	ASTHMA	COPD
Age of onset	❑ Before age 20 years	❑ After age 40 years
Pattern of symptoms	❑ Variation over minutes, hours or days ❑ Worse during the night or early morning ❑ Triggered by exercise, emotions including laughter, dust or exposure to allergens	❑ Persistent despite treatment ❑ Good and bad days but always daily symptoms and exertional dyspnea ❑ Chronic cough & sputum preceded onset of dyspnea, unrelated to triggers
Lung function	❑ Record of variable airflow limitation (spirometry or peak flow)	❑ Record of persistent airflow limitation ($FEV_1/FVC < 0.7$ post-BD)
Lung function between symptoms	❑ Normal	❑ Abnormal
Past history or family history	❑ Previous doctor diagnosis of asthma ❑ Family history of asthma, and other allergic conditions (allergic rhinitis or eczema)	❑ Previous doctor diagnosis of COPD, chronic bronchitis or emphysema ❑ Heavy exposure to risk factor: tobacco smoke, biomass fuels
Time course	❑ No worsening of symptoms over time. Variation in symptoms either seasonally, or from year to year ❑ May improve spontaneously or have an immediate response to bronchodilators or to ICS over weeks	❑ Symptoms slowly worsening over time (progressive course over years) ❑ Rapid-acting bronchodilator treatment provides only limited relief
Chest X-ray	❑ Normal	❑ Severe hyperinflation

NOTE: • These features, if present, best distinguish between asthma and COPD. • Several positive features (3 or more) for either asthma or COPD suggest that diagnosis. • If there are a similar number for both asthma and COPD, consider diagnosis of ACOS

DIAGNOSIS	Asthma	Some features of asthma	Features of both	Some features of COPD	COPD
CONFIDENCE IN DIAGNOSIS	Asthma	Possible asthma	Could be ACOS	Possibly COPD	COPD

STEP 3 PERFORM SPIROMETRY

Marked reversible airflow limitation (pre-post bronchodilator) or other proof of variable airflow limitation	$FEV_1/FVC < 0.7$ post-BD

STEP 4 INITIAL TREATMENT*

Asthma drugs No LABA monotherapy	Asthma drugs No LABA monotherapy	ICS, and usually LABA +/or LAMA	COPD drugs	COPD drugs

*Consult GINA and GOLD documents for recommended treatments.

STEP 5 SPECIALISED INVESTIGATIONS or REFER IF:

- Persistent symptoms and/or exacerbations despite treatment.
- Diagnostic uncertainty (e.g. suspected pulmonary hypertension, cardiovascular diseases and other causes of respiratory symptoms).
- Suspected asthma or COPD with atypical or additional symptoms or signs (e.g. haemoptysis, weight loss, night sweats, fever, signs of bronchiectasis or other structural lung disease).
- Few features of either asthma or COPD.
- Comorbidities present.
- Reasons for referral for either diagnosis as outlined in the GINA and GOLD strategy reports.

In Step 1, it is determined on the basis of the medical history and physical examination and imaging findings whether the patient has chronic airway disease. If the patient is determined to have chronic airway disease, in Step 2, the features and findings characteristic of asthma or COPD are listed. Respiratory symptoms tend to vary in asthma, while these symptoms persist chronically in COPD. The pulmonary function characteristics, such as variable airflow limitation in asthma and FEV1/forced vital capacity (FVC) of less than 70 % in COPD, are checked. As a result, each patient is characterized as having features "in favor of the diagnosis of asthma" and those "in favor of the diagnosis of COPD." According to the GINA, if 3 or more of the features of either asthma or COPD are present, the patient is likely to have the corresponding disease alone. In a patient with the same number of features of both asthma and COPD, diagnosis of ACOS should be considered. In Step 3, pulmonary function testing is carried out again to examine, in detail, the airflow reversibility in response to bronchodilators, etc. If the patient does not have the typical features of asthma or COPD alone, diagnosis of ACOS should be considered. If the patient has characteristics of both asthma and COPD based on these definitions, the patient can simply be diagnosed as having ACOS; however, if the patient has the clinical features of COPD associated with eosinophilic airway inflammation, etc., it is possible that the patient cannot be diagnosed as having ACOS. There might be cases in which features are inconsistent with the site of airway inflammation, and underreporting of features by the patients is likely to be involved in such cases. Therefore, it is desirable to make a diagnosis by combining the results of tests for the pulmonary diffusing capacity, concentration of nitric oxide in exhaled air, peripheral blood eosinophil count, serum IgE level, etc., with the results of spirometry.

16.6 Treatment of ACOS

Step 4 of the syndromic approach shows the initial treatment. The fundamental principles of the initial treatment are that asthma should not be treated with bronchodilators alone and COPD should not be treated with steroids alone.

Step 5 of the syndromic approach is instructing the patients to consult experts or undergo additional tests when the treatment fails to improve or worsens the clinical symptoms.

As described in the GINA and GOLD guidelines, ACOS should be basically treated with 3 drugs, namely, a long-acting muscarinic antagonist (LAMA) in addition to the two main drugs, ICS, and a long-acting β2 agonist (LABA). However, sufficient evidence has not been accumulated to rationalize the use of these 3 inhaled medications. This is because the element of smoking has been excluded in studies of inhaled treatments in patients with asthma and that of airflow reversibility has been excluded in studies of inhaled treatments in patients with COPD, resulting in little accumulation of data in patients with ACOS at present. It is speculated that ICS may be the mainstay of treatment from the standpoint of airway inflammation. Magnussen et al. [33] reported that addition of LAMA to the standard treatment with ICS was effective in asthma, and Yoshida et al. [34] reported that LAMA was effective in patients with severe asthma and COPD. These reports indicate that LAMA reduces the airway inflammation in ACOS and that treatment with 3 drugs, ICS + LABA + LAMA, is effective [35]. On the other hand, a study reported that treatment with ICS did not reduce the FEV1 decline over time or exacerbations in patients with ACOS and thereby drew a negative conclusion [36]. Other risk factors that are common to asthma and COPD include atopic dermatitis, smoking, air pollution, airway hyperresponsiveness, aging, and repeated exacerbations [37]. Roberto de Marco et al. [38] reported that development of asthma in childhood, i.e., early onset of asthma, is an important factor in the development of ACOS. Among other risk factors, smoking causes steroid resistance, which would make ICS less effective [39]. Therefore, abstinence from smoking is also important in patients with ACOS. In addition, low-dose theophylline therapy enhances the effects of ICS [40] and is considered as an adjuvant therapy. Actually, ICS + LABA, LAMA, leukotriene receptor antagonists (LTRAs), and theophylline are more commonly used for the treatment of ACOS than for the treatment of COPD [41, 42]. At present, treatment seems to be carried out mostly according to the guidelines. However, elderly patients have both COPD and asthma at a higher frequency [26], suggesting that early treatment with the combination of the 3 inhaled medications may prevent concomitant asthma and COPD and the development of ACOS. In the future, more data are expected to be accumulated from clinical studies.

16.7 Conclusion

Patients with ACOS, having the features of both asthma (atopic dermatitis, paroxysmal dyspnea, and airway hyperresponsiveness-airway reversibility) and COPD (history of smoking, dyspnea on exertion, and irreversible airflow obstruction), have a higher frequency of exacerbations, a lower HRQol, and higher mortality than those with asthma or COPD alone. Smoking, airway hyperresponsiveness, respiratory tract infection, aging, repeated exacerbations, etc., are aggravating factors for ACOS, as well as for asthma and COPD. Patients with early-onset asthma and those with a long history of asthma may develop ACOS in the future. Evidence of treatment is currently being gathered, but in patients with possible ACOS, it is important to avoid treatment with bronchodilators (LABA and LAMA) or ICS alone and to use all the three inhaled medications.

References

1. Saglani S, Lloyd CM. Eosinophils in the pathogenesis of paediatric severe asthma. Curr Opin Allergy Clin Immunol. 2014;14:143–8.
2. Koch S, Finotto S. Role of interferon-λ in allergic asthma. J Innate Immun. 2015;7:224–30.
3. Fahy JV. Type 2 inflammation in asthma–present in most, absent in many. Nat Rev Immunol. 2015;15:57–65.
4. Wang F, Ni SS, Liu H. Pollutional haze and COPD: etiology, epidemiology, pathogenesis, pathology, biological markers and therapy. J Thorac Dis. 2016;8:E20–30.
5. Papaiwannou A, Zarogoulidis P, Porpodis K, Spyratos D, Kioumis I, Pitsiou G, Pataka A, Tsakiridis K, Arikas S, Mpakas A, Tsiouda T, Katsikogiannis N, Kougioumtzi I, Machairiotis N, Siminelakis S, Kolettas A, Kessis G, Beleveslis T, Zarogoulidis K. Asthma-chronic obstructive pulmonary disease overlap syndrome (ACOS): current literature review. J Thorac Dis. 2014;6 Suppl 1:S146–51.
6. Orie NG, Slutter HJ, de Vries, Tammeling GJ. Chronic nonspecific respiratory diseases. Ned Tijdschr Geneeskd. 1961;105:2136–9. Article in Dutch.
7. Sluiter HJ, Koëter GH, de Monchy JG, Postma DS, de Vries K, Orie NG. The Dutch hypothesis (chronic non-specific lung disease) revisited. Eur Respir J. 1991;4:479–89.
8. Hernández G, Avila M, Pont A, Garin O, Alonso J, Laforest L, Cates CJ, Ferrer M, ASTRO-LAB group. Long-acting beta-agonists plus inhaled corticosteroids safety: a systematic review and meta-analysis of non-randomized studies. Respir Res. 2014;15:83.
9. Nelson HS, Gallegos CM, Silveira LJ, Newell JD, Gelfand EW. Effect of the inhaled corticosteroid mometasone on small airway patency in patients with asthma. Allergy Asthma Proc. 2009;30:284–92.
10. Tabberer M, Brooks J, Wilcox T. A meta-analysis of four randomized clinical trials to confirm the reliability and responsiveness of the Shortness of Breath with Daily Activities (SOBDA) questionnaire in chronic obstructive pulmonary disease. Health Qual Life Outcomes. 2015;13:177.
11. The Global Strategy for Asthma Management and Prevention, Global Initiative for Asthma (GINA) 2015. Diagnosis of Diseases of Chronic Airflow Limitation: Asthma COPD and Asthma-COPD Overlap Syndrome (ACOS) Available http://www.ginasthma.org/local/uploads/files/ACOS_2015.pdf. Accessed Jan 31 2016.
12. Burrows B, et al. Epidemiologic observations on eosinophilia and its relation to respiratory disorders. Am Rev Respir Dis. 1980;122:709–19.
13. Taylor RG, Gross E, Joyce H, Holland F, Pride NB. Smoking, allergy, and the differential white blood cell count. Thorax. 1985;40:17–22.
14. Reid L. The role of chronic bronchitis in the production of "chronic obstructive pulmonary emphysema". J Am Med Womens Assoc. 1965;20:633–8.
15. Elias JA, Kang MJ, Crothers K, Homer R, Lee CG. State of the art. Mechanistic heterogeneity in chronic obstructive pulmonary disease: insights from transgenic mice. Proc Am Thorac Soc. 2006;3:494–8.
16. Kesten S, Rebuck AS. Is the short-term response to inhaled β-adrenergic agonist sensitive or specific for distinguishing between asthma and COPD? Chest. 1994;105:1042–5.
17. Gelb AF, Zamel N. Unsuspected pseudophysiologic emphysema in chronic persistent asthma. Am J Respir Crit Care Med. 2000;162:1778–82.
18. Matsumoto K, Seki N, Fukuyama S, Moriwaki A, Kan-o K, Matsunaga Y, Noda N, Yoshida M, Koto H, Takata S, Nakanishi Y, Kiyohara Y, Inoue H, Hisayama Pulmonary Physiology Study Group. Prevalence of asthma with airflow limitation, COPD, and COPD with variable airflow limitation in older subjects in a general Japanese population: the Hisayama Study. Respir Investig. 2015;53:22–9.
19. Andersén H, Lampela P, Nevanlinna A, Säynäjäkangas O, Keistinen T. High hospital burden in overlap syndrome of asthma and COPD. Clin Respir J. 2013;7:342–6.

20. de Marco R, Pesce G, Marcon A, Accordini S, Antonicelli L, Bugiani M, Casali L, Ferrari M, Nicolini G, Panico MG, Pirina P, Zanolin ME, Cerveri I, Verlato G. The coexistence of asthma and chronic obstructive pulmonary disease (COPD): prevalence and risk factors in young, middle-aged and elderly people from the general population. PLoS One. 2013;8, e62985.
21. Menezes AM, Montes de Oca M, Pérez-Padilla R, Nadeau G, Wehrmeister FC, Lopez-Varela MV, Muiño A, Jardim JR, Valdivia G, Tálamo C, PLATINO Team. Increased risk of exacerbation and hospitalization in subjects with an overlap phenotype: COPD-asthma. Chest. 2014;145:297–304.
22. Cosio BG, Soriano JB, López-Campos JL, Calle-Rubio M, Soler-Cataluna JJ, de-Torres TP, Marín JM, Martínez-Gonzalez C, de Lucas P, Mir I, Peces-Barba G, Feu-Collado N, Solanes I, Alfageme I, Casanova C, CHAIN Study. Defining the asthma-COPD overlap syndrome in a COPD cohort. Chest. 2016;149:45–52.
23. Hardin M, Silverman EK, Barr RG, Hansel NN, Schroeder JD, Make BJ, Crapo JD, Hersh CP, COPDGene Investigators. The clinical features of the overlap between COPD and asthma. Respir Res. 2011;12:127.
24. Wurst KE, Kelly-Reif K, Bushnell GA, Pascoe S, Barnes N. Understanding asthma-chronic obstructive pulmonary disease overlap syndrome. Respir Med. 2016;110:1–11.
25. Gibson PG, McDonald VM. Asthma-COPD overlap 2015: now we are six. Thorax. 2015;70:683–91.
26. Soriano JB, Vestbo J, Pride NB, Kiri V, Maden C, Maier WC. Survival in COPD patients after regular use of fluticasone propionate and salmeterol in general practice. Eur Respir J. 2002;20:819–25.
27. Milanese M, Di Marco F, Corsico AG, Rolla G, Sposato B, Chieco-Bianchi F, Costantino MT, Crivellaro MA, Guarnieri G, Scichilone N, ELSA Study Group. Asthma control in elderly asthmatics. An Italian observational study. Respir Med. 2014;108:1091–9.
28. Ohta K, Ichinose M, Nagase H, Yamaguchi M, Sugiura H, Tohda Y, Yamauchi K, Adachi M, Akiyama K, Japanese Society of Allergology. Japanese guideline for adult asthma 2014. Allergol Int. 2014;63:293–333.
29. Kauppi P, Kupiainen H, Lindqvist A, Tammilehto L, Kilpeläinen M, Kinnula VL, Haahtela T, Laitinen T. Overlap syndrome of asthma and COPD predicts low quality of life. J Asthma. 2011;48:279–85.
30. Alshabanat A, Zafari Z, Albanyan O, Dairi M, FitzGerald JM. Asthma and COPD Overlap Syndrome (ACOS): a systematic review and meta analysis. PLoS One. 2015;10, e0136065.
31. Gerhardsson de Verdier M, Andersson M, Kern DM, Zhou S, Turnceli O. Asthma and chronic obstructive pulmonary disease overlap syndrome: doubled costs compared with patients with asthma alone. Value Health. 2015;18:759–66.
32. Shaya FT, Dongyi D, Akazawa MO, Blanchette CM, Wang J, Mapel DW, Dalal A, Scharf SM. Burden of concomitant asthma and COPD in a Medicaid population. Chest. 2008;134:14–9.
33. Magnussen H, Bugnas B, van Noord J, Schmidt P, Gerken F, Kesten S. Improvements with tiotropium in COPD patients with concomitant asthma. Respir Med. 2008;102:50–6.
34. Yoshida M, Nakano T, Fukuyama S, Matsumoto T, Eguchi M, Moriwaki A, Takata S, et al. Effects of tiotropium on lung function in severe asthmatics with or without emphysematous changes. Pulm Pharmacol Ther. 2013;26:159–66.
35. Alvarado-Gonzalez A, Arce I. Tiotropium bromide in chronic obstructive pulmonary disease and bronchial asthma. J Clin Med Res. 2015;7:831–9.
36. Lim HS, Choi SM, Lee J, Park YS, Lee SM, Yim JJ, Yoo CG, Kim YW, Han SK, Lee CH. Responsiveness to inhaled corticosteroid treatment in patients with asthma-chronic obstructive pulmonary disease overlap syndrome. Ann Allergy Asthma Immunol. 2014;113:652–7.
37. To T, Zhu J, Larsen K, Simatovic J, Feldman L, Ryckman K, Gershon A, Lougheed MD, Licskai C, Chen H, Villeneuve PJ, Crighton E, Su Y, Sadatsafavi M Williams D, Carlsten C, Canadian Respiratory Research Network. Progression from asthma to Chronic Obstructive

Pulmonary Disease (COPD): is air pollution a risk factor?. Am J Respir Crit Care Med. 2016 [Epub ahead of print].
38. de Marco R, Marcon A, Rossi A, Antó JM, Cerveri I, Gislason T, Heinrich J, Janson C, Jarvis D, Kuenzli N, Leynaert B, Probst-Hensch N, Svanes C, Wjst M, Burney P. Asthma, COPD and overlap syndrome: a longitudinal study in young European adults. Eur Respir J. 2015;46:671–9.
39. Spears M, McSharry C, Chaudhuri R, Weir CJ, de Wet C, Thomson NC. Smoking in asthma is associated with elevated levels of corticosteroid resistant sputum cytokines-an exploratory study. PLoS One. 2013;8, e71460.
40. Spears M, Donnelly I, Jolly L, Brannigan M, Ito K, McSharry C, Larfferty J, Chaudhuri R, Braganza G, Adcock IM, Barnes PJ, Wood S, Thomson NC. Effect of low-dose theophylline plus beclometasone on lung function in smokers with asthma: a pilot study. Eur Respir J. 2009;33:1010–7.
41. Rhee CK, Yoon HK, Yoo KH, Kim YS, Lee SW, Park YB, et al. Medical utilization and cost in patients with overlap syndrome of chronic obstructive pulmonary disease and asthma. COPD. 2013;11:163–70.
42. Izquierdo-Alonso JL, Rodriguez-Gonzálezmoro JM, de Lucas-Ramos P, Unzueta I, Ribera X, Antón E, et al. Prevalence and characteristics of three clinical phenotypes of chronic obstructive pulmonary disease (COPD). Respir Med. 2013;107:724–31.

Chapter 17
Combined Pulmonary Fibrosis and Emphysema (CPFE): Which Symptom, Fibrosis or Emphysema, Should Be Treated Preferentially? Or Should Both Be Treated Simultaneously?

Nariaki Kokuho, Shigeo Muro, and Arata Azuma

Abstract For a long time, emphysema and fibrosis occurred in the lung have been regarded as isolated disease entity. However, the synchronous occurrence of emphysema and lung fibrosis has been occasionally reported to date, and Cottin et al. organized the concept as combined pulmonary fibrosis and emphysema (CPFE) in 2005. The patients with CPFE are almost male smokers and presented severe breathlessness, and pulmonary function tests revealed preserved lung volumes and no evidence of obstruction but decrease of diffusing capacity for carbon monoxide. The amassed research evidence, which gathered through studies of many similar case reports of patients with CPFE, has revealed the pathophysiology and natural history. While at the same time, it have been revealed that there are no specific treatment for patients with CPFE, and the prognosis of these patents is quite poor. The authors will review the existing knowledge concerning patients with CPFE and present an overview of the current state of CPFE.

Keywords Combined pulmonary fibrosis and emphysema (CPFE) • Idiopathic pulmonary fibrosis (IPF) • Emphysema • Chronic obstructive pulmonary disease (COPD) • Review

---

N. Kokuho • A. Azuma (✉)
Department of Pulmonary Medicine and Oncology, Graduate School of Medicine, Nippon Medical School, 1-1-5 Sendagi, Bunkyo-ku, Tokyo 113-8603, Japan
e-mail: a-azuma@nms.ac.jp

S. Muro
Department of Respiratory Medicine, Graduate School of Medicine, Kyoto University, Kyoto 606-8507, Japan

H. Nakamura, K. Aoshiba (eds.), *Chronic Obstructive Pulmonary Disease*, Respiratory Disease Series: Diagnostic Tools and Disease Managements,
DOI 10.1007/978-981-10-0839-9_17

17.1 Introduction

Since early times, the presence of excess fibrosis has been thought to exclude the diagnosis of emphysema [1]. However, some reports have suggested that emphysema may be accompanied with fibrosis to some extent [2, 3].

In 1990, Wiggins et al. firstly reported a clinical condition of upper zone emphysema combined with cryptogenic fibrosing alveolitis in eight patients [4]. These patients were all smokers and presented severe breathlessness, and their pulmonary function tests revealed normal static lung volumes and no evidence of obstruction but decrease of diffusing capacity for carbon monoxide (DLCO). In Japan, the similar clinical condition was described as "chronic atypical (B group)" in the classification of the idiopathic interstitial pneumonia by the Ministry of Health and Welfare-specific disease study group of Japan in 1991 [5].

In 2005, Cottin et al. expanded awareness of the clinical entity as a well-defined termed, combined pulmonary fibrosis and emphysema (CPFE), which is typically characterized by upper lobe emphysema and pulmonary fibrosis of the lower lungs [6]. The authors conducted a retrospective study of 61 patients with CPFE and showed some clinical features (Table 17.1).

Whether the concept as CPFE represents a specific disease entity or a coincidence of two pulmonary diseases (emphysema and fibrosis) related to cigarette smoking is as yet unclear. And Cottin et al. proposed that a group of patients with its characteristic functional profile should be recognized as a certain type of distinct clinical entity related to smoking, that is to say, "CPFE syndrome." By contrast, the "idiopathic CPFE" is described in patients without etiology other than a history of smoking [7].

We will herein outline and review the comprehensive features of CPFE syndrome in diagnosis, epidemiology, physiology, complication, etiology, pathogenesis, management, prognosis, and future tasks.

Table 17.1 The clinical features of combined pulmonary fibrosis and emphysema by Cottin et al. [6]

I	Upper lobe emphysema and lower lobe fibrosis
II	All heavy smokers and almost all males, with a mean age of 65 years
III	Basal crackles were found numerously and finger clubbing in about half
IX	Pulmonary function is maintained at subnormal, diffusing capacity is reduced, and shortness of breath on exertion was present
X	Pulmonary hypertension was present in about half and determined a critical prognosis
XI	Survival was 54.6 % at 5 years, with a median of 6.1 years

17.2 Diagnosis

Radiological findings on chest high resolution computed tomography (HRCT) are the exclusive method for diagnosis of CPFE, which shows upper lobe emphysema and lower lobe fibrosis (Fig. 17.1). On a relevant note, various radiological and pathological features have been reported in recent years.

17.2.1 Radiologic Feature

Cottin et al. defined the following criteria as CPFE: a) presence of emphysema on CT scan, defined as well-demarcated areas of decreased attenuation in comparison with contiguous normal lung and marginated by a very thin (<1 mm) or no wall and/or multiple bullae (>1 cm) with upper zone predominance and b) presence of a diffuse parenchymal lung disease with significant pulmonary fibrosis on CT scan, defined as reticular opacities with peripheral and basal predominance,

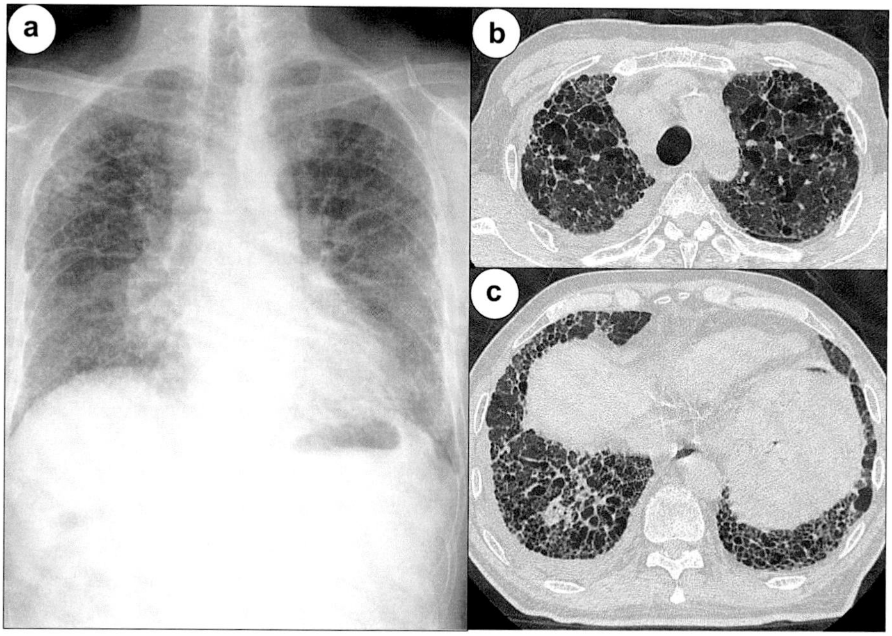

Fig. 17.1 Imaging of a typical case of combined pulmonary fibrosis and emphysema. (**a**) Chest X-ray showed the emphysema in the upper field and reticular shadow in the lower field. There were tumorlike shadows in the lower right lung field of mediastinum. Despite the existence of marked fibrosis, shrinkage of the lung was seemed to be relatively mild. (**b**) Chest high resolution computed tomography (HRCT) of the upper zones of the lungs showed paraseptal emphysema in bilateral lungs. (**c**) Chest HRCT of the lower zones of the lungs showed the typical honeycomb in the bottom, and a lung cancer was complicated in the right lower lobe (S^9)

honeycombing, architectural distortion, and/or traction bronchiectasis or bronchiolectasis. Focal ground-glass opacities and/or areas of alveolar condensation may be associated but should not be prominent [6]. And although chest X-ray is generally useful to evaluate the volume loss of the lung due to interstitial pneumonia, the lung volume is tend to be preserved by complicated with emphysema in CPFE.

The type of emphysema in CPFE was centrilobular emphysema, paraseptal emphysema, and bullae, whose prevalence was 97 %, 93 %, and 54 %, respectively [8]. Above all, paraseptal emphysema (low-attenuation areas in subpleural zone) has been described in almost all reports about CPFE, and Portillo et al. suggest that paraseptal emphysema is a typical feature of CPFE [9]. However, discrimination of the emphysema type in CPFE was very difficult because of the modification of the HRCT appearance by fibrosis [10]. And thick-walled large cysts (TWLCs), which are defined as cysts 2 cm or more in diameter and delimitated by a wall 1 mm or more thick in an area of the lung where reticulation is present, are also considered as one of the characteristic feature of CPFE [11, 12].

Matsuoka et al. evaluated the differences in 5-year morphological changes among the patients with CPFE, emphysema alone, and fibrosis alone [13]. The authors revealed that the mean change of the percentage of low attenuation area was higher in CPFE (7.4 ± 3.8 %) than in emphysema alone (4.5 ± 3.3 %). And the mean change of the percentage of destructed lung area was higher in CPFE (12.9 ± 5.8 %) than in emphysema alone (4.9 ± 2.8 %) and fibrosis alone (7.1 ± 5.7 %). So they concluded that the morphological progression of the patients with CPFE were different from the patients with emphysema alone or fibrosis alone.

Airspace enlargement with fibrosis (AEF) has been identified pathologically as a smoking-related change [14]. Watanabe et al. revealed that HRCT features of AEF were multiple thin-walled cysts (MTWCs) and/or reticular opacities. And the authors suggested the possibility that these changes had been confused with/interpreted as honeycombing and/or emphysema in the past [15].

The biggest problem in diagnostic criteria using CT findings is that there are no definitive criteria in the extent of emphysema or fibrosis. So this disease entity may include various phenotype because the diagnosis is arbitrary dependent on the physicians. Under such circumstances, some studies defined CPFE as the coexistence of "significant" emphysema that was the total percentage of low-attenuation area due to emphysema calculated from six lung fields (upper, middle, lower) on chest HRCT that is more than 5–25 % [16–20].

17.2.2 Pathologic Feature

Although the pathological features have not yet been fully studied, there were several reports of pathological consideration associated with CPFE, which were presented as the characteristic lung lesions in smokers (Fig. 17.2).

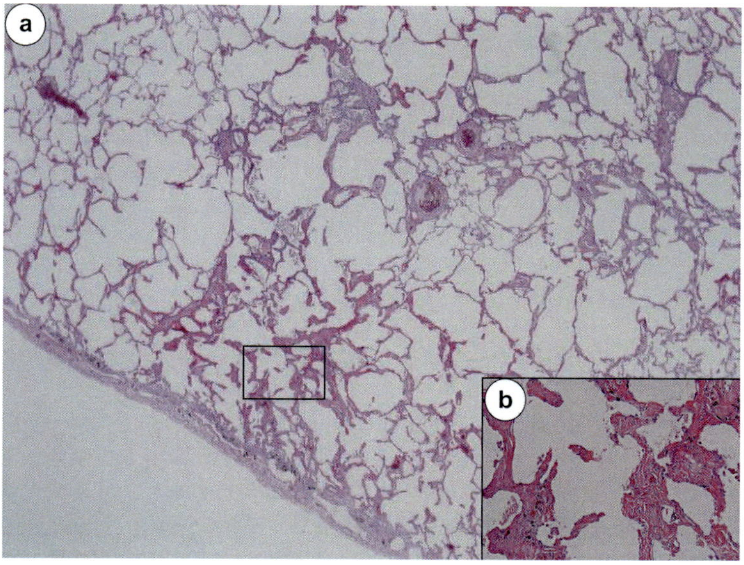

Fig. 17.2 Pathological imaging of combined pulmonary fibrosis and emphysema (airspace enlargement with fibrosis). (**a**) This area shows emphysematous change and reticular findings. (**b**) High-power view of the area in the box in (a) shows fibrous hyalinized interstitium with structural remodeling

In 2006, Yousem et al. reported respiratory bronchiolitis-associated interstitial lung disease with fibrosis, which was associated with a respiratory bronchiolitis having extensive paucicellular lamellar eosinophilic collagenous thickening of alveolar septa in a patchy, particularly subpleural distribution [21].

In 2008, Kawabata et al. examined the pathological findings of 587 smokers in lobectomy specimens for lung cancer and reported that AEF was an important smoking-related change in the lung [14] (Fig. 17.2). Macroscopically, AEF showed various sized thin-walled cysts (thinner than that of honeycombing) which was seen slightly apart from pleura in the basal areas of the lower lobe. And microscopically, AEF was characterized as (a) fibrous (frequently hyalinized) interstitium with structural remodeling, (b) emphysematous change, (c) frequent bronchiolocentric location, and (d) absence of fibroblast foci. The incidence of AEF was 6.5 % in mild smokers and 17.7 % in moderate smokers with lower lobe predominance, thus appeared to correlate with the smoking history.

In 2010, Katzenstein et al. also examined 20 smokers in lobectomy specimens excised for neoplasms and reported clinically occult interstitial fibrosis in smokers [22]. This lesion was characterized by varying degrees of alveolar septal thickening by collagen deposition along with emphysema and respiratory bronchiolitis. The fibrosis occurred both in subpleural and in deeper parenchyma and surrounded enlarged airspaces of emphysema, but it also involved non-emphysematous parenchyma. And the authors termed them smoking-related interstitial fibrosis.

In the study of an autopsy series of 22 CPFE patients, Inomata et al. described that thick-cystic lesions involving one or more acini with dense wall fibrosis and occasional fibroblastic foci surrounded by honeycombing and normal alveoli were confirmed as TWCL. And emphysematous destruction and enlargement of membranous and respiratory bronchioles with fibrosis were observed in the TWCLs. The prevalence of both radiological and pathological TWCLs was 72.7 % in CPFE patients, but nothing in patients with IPF or emphysema alone ($p = 0.001$). So the authors suggested that TWCLs would be considered the one of the feature in CPFE [12].

Various findings in the pathological features of CPFE have been reported as described above; however, Wright et al. concluded that smoking commonly produces a degree of fibrosis in the walls of the respiratory bronchioles (RB) and that this fibrosis might extend around the enlarged airspaces of centrilobular emphysema which is formed from damaged RB [23]. And the fibrosis can also extend in the interstitium away from the RB, typically toward the pleura.

17.3 Epidemiology

Although there is no specific data about the direct prevalence of CPFE, much attention has been paid to the fact that subclinical interstitial lung abnormality (ILA) is present in the smokers in recent years [24, 25]. According to a large cohort study of 2416 smokers who were performed with chest HRCT scans and spirometry, 1002 (41 %) met the GOLD criteria for COPD and 194 (8 %) showed interstitial lung abnormalities [25]. Jin et al. reported that the prevalence of ILA in current or former smokers enrolled in a lung cancer screening trial was 9.7 % (86 of 884 patients), and patients with fibrotic ILA progressed in 37 % at the 2-year follow-up [24].

In the retrospective study of 2016 male smokers who underwent chest CT at healthcare center, the prevalence of CPFE in asymptomatic smokers was 3.1 %, and CPFE progression on follow-up CT imaging was associated with current smoking [26]. On the other hand, there are some reports that the prevalence of CPFE in patients diagnosed with pulmonary fibrosis was 8–51 % [17, 19, 27, 28] and 21-33 % when it is limited in IPF [7]. This variation of prevalence in CPFE may depend on the evaluation of extent of emphysema by HRCT.

And most of the cohort studies are men and over 65 years of age who are heavy active/ex-smokers [9]. Jankowich et al. reviewed the published studies in CPFE and reported 90 % (529 of 587 patients) was men [29]. And they speculated that men were more susceptible to smoking-induced emphysema and pulmonary fibrosis because of greater vulnerability to abnormal lung aging. On the other hand, CPFE syndrome associated with connective tissue disease (CTD) was found in younger women and light smoker patients than in patients with idiopathic CPFE [11].

17.4 Physiology

17.4.1 Pulmonary Function

Cottin et al. demonstrated the physiological consequences of the coexistence of emphysema and fibrosis, which resulted in preserved lung volumes but a markedly decreased diffusing capacity [6]. More specifically, forced vital capacity (FVC), forced expiratory volume in the first second (FEV1), and total lung capacity (TLC) are usually within nearly normal ranges, unlike diffusing capacity for carbon monoxide (DLCO), which is significantly reduced. And almost all of the other reports have confirmed these physiological findings [6, 8, 11, 16, 17, 29–31, 34, 37, 59, 61, 62] (Table 17.2).

Portillo et al. discussed that although the hyperinflation and increase of pulmonary compliance due to the loss of elasticity in the areas with emphysema might compensate for the loss of volume caused by fibrosis, the overlapping of both pathologies might interact a negative synergic effect on gas exchange, resulting in a severe decrease in DLCO. Moreover, a decrease in DLCO will reflect not only the diffusion impairment of the lung but also disorders in the pulmonary vascular bed, specifically pulmonary hypertension, as it is a highly prevalent condition in this entity [9].

Akagi et al. reported the difference in pulmonary function between CPFE patients and IPF patients in a longitudinal study [32]. The authors revealed that the mean annual decrease of VC% pred was significantly less in CPFE patients than in IPF patients (−1.2 vs −8.0 %, $p < 0.001$). And the mean annual change of FEV1/FVC% in CPFE patients and IPF patients was −0.5 and +1.1 % ($p = 0.036$), respectively. The mean annual decrease of DLCO% pred was less severe in CPFE patients than in IPF patients (−3.7 vs −10.7 %, $p = 0.042$). This study revealed that ventilatory and gas exchange deterioration during the course of IPF would be mild when emphysema was coexistent.

Table 17.2 The summary of main case studies of patients with CPFE syndrome

Patients (number)	Age, years	Gender, M/F	Smoking, p-y (%)	TLC, %	FVC, %	FEV1/ FVC, %	DLCO, %	PH, %	Cancer, %	AE, %	5-y survival, %	Median survival, y	Annotation	Reference
61	65 ± 10	60/1	46 ± 27 (100)	88 ± 17	90 ± 18	69 ± 13	37 ± 16	55			55	6.1		Cottin et al. [6]
21	66 ± 10	20/1	25 ± 15 (100)	95 ± 25	77 ± 20	74 ± 18	48 ± 26							Mura et al. [20]
10	57–78	10/0	73(100)	82	82	70	31.4	33.3	20	10				Jankowich et al. [59]
11	71 ± 7	8/3	62 ± 44 (100)	65–124	72 ± 13	74 ± 11	28 ± 13	57						Silva et al. [30]
26	65 ± 9	23/3	60 ± 37 (89)	78 ± 17		77 ± 9	44 ± 15		23		50	5		Akagi et al. [32]
31	67 ± 7	30/1	5(77.4)		62 ± 16	91 ± 9		90				2.1		Mejía et al. [19]
14	62 ± 10	14/0	(93)		117 ± 14	69 ± 11	102 ± 31							Tsushima et al. [60]
20	69 ± 10	20/0	57 ± 29 (100)	76 ± 11	77 ± 14	67 ± 12	29 ± 11	42	15		35	4		Jankowich et al. [57]
47	70 ± 1	46/1	59 ± 4 (100)		95 ± 4	72 ± 2	40 ± 3		46.8					Kitaguchi et al. [16]
221	71 ± 8	209/12	55 ± 25 (100)	94 ± 17	87 ± 17	70 ± 12	65 ± 21		33.3	11.1	80	8.5		Kurashima et al. [61]
28	57	17/11	40(100)	64	60	81	27				>50	5.3		Todd et al. [58]
34	57 ± 11	23/11	39 ± 23 (88.2)	82 ± 17	85 ± 24	73 ± 15	46 ± 16	42	9	15	73		CTD	Cottin et al. [11]
42	64 ± 10	33/9	46 ± 28 (100)		76 ± 15	78 ± 7	42 ± 16							Schmidt et al. [28]

135	71 (50–97)	132/3	40(98.3)		89	73		48.3	35.8		>50			Lee et al. [62]
38	69 ± 1	35/3	52 ± 6 (100)			79 ± 2								Tasaka et al. [47]
46	67 ± 9	42/4	59 ± 34 (100)	91 ± 16	94 ± 17	78 ± 11	67 ± 17		52					Chiba et al. [37]
93	73	76/17	62(100)		64	80		39	13	24		2.6		Kishaba et al. [41]
29	70 ± 9	20/9	46 ± 15 (100)	79 ± 14	80 ± 16	74 ± 6	37 ± 14					2.8		Ryerson et al. [17]
61	65 ± 10	60/1	46 ± 27 (100)	88 ± 17	90 ± 18	69 ± 13	37 ± 16							Cottin et al. [8]
46	71 ± 7	43/3	60 ± 35 (98)	90 ± 16	94 ± 22	78 ± 12	50 ± 14		50	17.4		1.8		Sugino et al. [34]
63	64 ± 8		44 ± 18		94 ± 24	77 ± 5					89	7.3		Chae et al. [26]
42	70 ± 8	38/4	54 ± 26 (100)		92 ± 18	73 ± 11								Matsuoka et al. [13]
41	53 ± 15	18/74	(63)		77 ± 22	96	38 ± 13	24					SSc	Antoniou et al. [43]

Data are presented as mean ± SD or medians (range)

CPFE combined pulmonary fibrosis and emphysema, *TLC* total lung capacity, FVC forced vital capacity, *FEV1* forced expiratory volume in 1 s, *DLCO* diffusing capacity of the lung for carbon monoxide, *PH* pulmonary hypertension, *AE* acute exacerbation, *SSc* scleroderma

17.4.2 Oxygenation

The hypoxemia at rest and exertion is common in patients with CPFE. Cottin et al. reported that mean PaO2 at rest (room air) was 63 ± 14 Torr, average Alveolar-arterial difference was 41 ± 16 Torr, and average exertional desaturation was 8.9 ± 5.7 % during 6-min waking test. By contrast, hypercarbia does not appear in CPFE [6].

17.5 Complication

17.5.1 Pulmonary Hypertension

The patients with CPFE have a high probability of severe precapillary pulmonary hypertension (Table 17.2). In Cottin's original repot in 2005, the prevalence of pulmonary arterial hypertension (PAH) in 49 CPFE patients was 55 % during follow-up, and the mean estimated systolic pulmonary artery pressure (eSPAP) was 52 mmHg during follow-up [6].

The risk of the development of pulmonary hypertension is marked higher in CPFE patients than in IPF patients. In a cohort of 31 CPFE patients and 79 IPF patients, CPFE was highly associated with severe PAH (eSPAP; 82 ± 20 vs 57 ± 15 mmHg, $p = 0.0001$). There were a positive correlation between eSPAP and the extent of emphysema ($p = 0.0001$). Moreover 21 of 29 patients with CPFE had severe eSPAP (>75 mmHg) compared to 8 of 68 patients with IPF (OR 19.7; $p < 0.0001$), and severe eSPAP was associated with mortality [19].

In a retrospective multicenter cohort study of 40 CPFE patients with PAH confirmed by right heart catheterization, Cottin et al. described that the mean pulmonary artery pressure was 40 ± 9 mmHg, cardiac index was 2.5 L/min/m^2, and pulmonary vascular resistance was 521 dyn/s/cm^5. Moreover CPFE patients with pulmonary hypertension showed a poor prognosis, and the overall survival rate at 1 year from the date of right heart catheterization was only 60 %. The authors also showed that higher pulmonary vascular resistance (>485 dyn/s/cm^5), higher heart rate, and lower cardiac index (<2.4 L/min/m^2) were associated with shorter survival [33].

Sugino et al. reported that although there was no difference in eSPAP between CPFE and IPF at the time of diagnosis, eSPAP after 12 months was significantly increased in patients with CPFE than IPF (ΔeSPAP 11.3 vs 2.4 mmHg, $p < 0.0001$) [34].

17.5.2 Lung Cancer

There are many reports about the risk of the development of lung cancer in patients with CPFE [12, 16, 27, 35–37] (Table 17.2). And Jankowich et al. suggested that the development and progression of lung cancer in CPFE patients might be related to the "triple hit" effects of smoking, emphysema, and pulmonary fibrosis [29].

In a retrospective study of 47 CPFE patients, Kitaguchi et al. reported that 22 of 47 CPFE patients (46.8 %) had lung cancer, and squamous cell carcinoma was the most frequent (54.5 %) [16]. Usui et al. identified 101 (8.9 %) CPFE patients in the review of 1143 patients with lung cancer. And they also revealed that a high prevalence of smoking-related lung cancers, such as small cell lung cancer (18.8 %) and squamous cell lung cancer (30.7 %), was observed in patients with CPFE. The median overall survival (OS) of CPFE patients (10.8 months) was significantly less than that of normal patients (53.0 months) or that of patients with emphysema alone (21.9 months). Acute exacerbation (AE) of intestinal pneumonia occurred in 20 (19.8 %) CPFE patients with lung cancer, and the mortality rate and median survival time from onset of AE were 75 % and 22 days, respectively [35].

On the other hand, in the another review of 1536 patients with lung cancer, Minegishi et al. identified 88 (5.7 %) CPFE patients. The authors revealed that AE associated with initial treatment for lung cancer occurred in 22 (25.0 %) CPFE patients irrespective of treatment modality, and the median OS was 23.7 months, where the age (>68 years), PS (1-3), VC% (<80 %), and LDH (≧244 IU/L) were significant independent poor prognostic factors [27].

Fukui et al. reported that the risk of postoperative AE in CPFE patients was significantly higher than that of isolated idiopathic interstitial pneumonia (IIP) patients (CPFE 5.1 % vs IIP 0 %, $p = 0.032$). Therefore, the authors suggested that indications for surgical resection of lung cancer in CPFE patients should be considered carefully [36].

In the surgical outcomes of lung cancer in 233 patients with CPFE, CPFE patients with lung cancer had poor prognoses (six patients died within 30 postoperative days) and showed quite poor mortality rate in the 3-year postoperative overall survival (58.4 %). And the postoperative AE of interstitial pneumonia in the CPFE patients was 2 % [38].

17.5.3 Acute Exacerbation

AE of CPFE should be defined acute lung injury as with that of IPF, that is, unexplained worsening or development of dyspnea within 30 days and new bilateral ground-glass abnormality and/or consolidation on chest HRCT [39].

As presented above, CPFE may increase the risk of acute exacerbation after lung resection surgery and chemotherapy for lung cancer. Some Japanese reports described that AE occurred in 5–25 % CPFE patients with lung cancer [27, 35, 36]. Since AE of patients with IPF in natural course is considered to occur annually (approximately 5–10 %) [40], the CPFE patients with lung cancer should be observed carefully.

In the study of 93 CPFE patients, Kishaba et al. reported that baseline serum sialylated carbohydrate antigen Krebs von den Lungen-6 (KL-6) was a useful predictor of AE (cutoff =1050; AUC 0.7720), which occurred in 24 % (22/93) of the CPFE patients [41].

17.6 Etiology

Cigarette smoking has been suggested as the main etiologic factor in the majority of reported studies about CPFE, and 98 % of patients with CPFE is active/former smoker [29]. Cottin et al. speculated that both emphysema and fibrosis might be related to a common environmental trigger and/or genetic factor, with cigarette smoking playing a major role [6].

On the other hand, Cottin et al. reported 34 patients with CPFE syndrome in connective tissue disease (CTD) [11], and they showed that the CPFE syndrome was recognized within the spectrum of lung diseases associated with CTD, especially among patients with rheumatoid arthritis and systemic sclerosis, in current/former smokers. Furthermore, there were some reports about microscopic polyangiitis and other CTDs preceded by CPFE [42, 43].

Daniil et al. reported nine CPFE patients, who were farmers and had significant exposure to agrochemical compounds [44]. In the Japanese study, five of 47 CPFE patients (16.0 %) had a history of exposure to agrochemical compounds [16]. In addition, there were some reports of emphysema and fibrosis due to the mineral dust exposures such as asbestos, silica, coal dust, and talc [29]. Thus, CPFE might occur in tobacco-smoking individuals exposed to an environmental trigger.

There were some reports of the phenotype of CPFE syndrome in adult patients carrying mutation of the surfactant protein C (SFTPC) gene or ABCA3, which suggested the association of CPFE syndrome with the underlying genetic predisposition [45, 46]. These mutations are known to associate with diseases that involve the dysfunction of surfactant homeostasis, which cause injury or death of alveolar epithelial type 2 cells and myofibroblast proliferation. These case reports reflect that the coexistence of emphysema and pulmonary fibrosis might occur in a variety of clinical settings.

The mutation of telomerase, which is the enzyme that synthesizes telomere and repeats to the ends of chromosomes, are also considered to be risk factors for pulmonary fibrosis and emphysema [31].

17.7 Pathogenesis

Although little is known about the pathogenesis of CPFE, some animal experiments have suggested that the same lung injury might result in either fibrosis or emphysema. And the overexpression of inflammatory mediator, such as tumor necrosis factor-α (TNF-α), platelet-derived growth factor (PDGF), transforming growth factor-β1 (TGF-β1), and interleukin-13 (IL-13) in animal models, appears to relate to persisting lung damage characterized by CPFE [16, 31]. Furthermore, potential roles for surfactant protein D (SP-D), interleukin-1 beta (IL-1β), and neutrophil elastase in formation of both emphysema and fibrosis are also reported in various animal models [29].

In the study of the measurement of inflammatory mediators in bronchoalveolar lavage fluid (BALF) in patients with CPFE, the concentrations of CXC chemokines (interleukin-8 (IL-8/CXCL8) and epithelial neutrophil-activating peptide 78 (ENA-78/CXCL5)) were higher in the patients with CPFE than IPF alone. These inflammatory mediators were associated with the development of emphysematous changes, neutrophil accumulation in the alveolar space, and impaired diffusing capacity [47].

In the research of 178 smokers classified into fibrosis and/or emphysema, the serum concentration of club cell protein 16 (CC16) was highest in the CPFE (5.7 ± 0.4). And the serum concentration of combined testing for KL-6 and CC16 (AUC, 0.828) can effectively differentiate CPFE from emphysema alone [48]. The club cell activity decreases in emphysema, whereas the activity increase in fibrosis and inflammation, so the increased level of CC16 in CPFE might reflect the degree of lung inflammation and/or fibrosis. KL-6 reflected the hyperplasia and damage of type 2 alveolar epithelium, while CC16 reflected secretion from club cells resulting from bronchiolization associated with pulmonary fibrosis. So the combination of these biomarkers would be reasonable and helpful as a diagnostic tool in CPFE. Further investigation is needed to clarify the physiological basis for this phenomenon.

In investigation using immunohistochemistry, the expression of TNF-α, matrix metalloproteinase (MMP)-2, MMP-9, MMP-7, and membrane type 1 metalloproteinase (MT1-MMP) by fibroblastic foci has similar levels in CPFE and UIP patients, thus suggesting that the fibrotic lesions of CPFE and UIP display similar activation patterns of profibrotic gene. In contrast, fibroblasts in areas of parenchymal destruction of emphysema/UIP expressed MMP-2, MMP-9, MMP-7, and MT1-MMP at variable but significantly higher levels when compared to emphysema subjects, in the presence of similar levels of tissue inhibitor of metalloproteinase (TIMP)-1, TIMP-2, and TNF-α. MMP-10 is a novel biomarker in distinction of IPF and emphysema [49], the increased MMP expression may play a role in accelerating the process of destruction and remodeling of emphysema in CPFE patients [50].

Hanaoka et al. investigated the mechanism of CPFE regarding gene expressions by comparing the results of microarray sequences between fibrotic and emphysematous lesions in the lungs of CPFE patients [51]. In the fibrotic lesions, genes associated with the immune system are highly expressed, while genes related to the cellular fraction, membrane biology, and vascular biology are highly expressed in emphysematous lesions. Thus the authors speculated that the development of coexistent fibrotic and emphysematous lesions in CPFE is implemented by these different patterns of gene expression.

17.8 Management

Although the efficacy of drugs specifically indicated in patients with CPFE has not been demonstrated, several drugs was administered to fibrosis or emphysema. Treatment strategy for patients with CPFE is limited, and the clinicians may require treatment for both IPF and emphysema. Actually, it seems logical to base the treatment decisions on the guidelines for emphysema and pulmonary fibrosis.

According to a guideline released by the Global Initiative for Chronic Obstructive Lung Disease (GOLD), the patients with COPD should quit smoking, be vaccinated against influenza and pneumococcus, be offered rehabilitation, receive treatment of inhaled bronchodilators such as beta2 agonists and anticholinergics, and receive the long-term administration of oxygen to patients with severe resting hypoxemia [52]. Although whether patients with CPFE can benefit from bronchodilators or not remains unknown, the use of inhaled bronchodilators may be recommended for those who have obstructive pulmonary disorder [53].

And according to a guideline of an official ATS/ERS/JRS/ALAT clinical practice of IPF, the patients with IPF should be conditionally treated with nintedanib, pirfenidone, and antiacid therapy [54]. Nintedanib is an intracellular inhibitor of triple tyrosine kinases that target receptors of vascular endothelial growth factor, fibroblast growth factor, and PDGF. And pirfenidone, which is an antifibrotic drug with pleiotropic effects, has been shown to regulate important profibrotic and proinflammatory cytokine cascades while reducing fibroblast proliferation and collagen synthesis. And abnormal gastroesophageal reflux has been observed in about 90 % of patients with IPF and has been postulated to cause or worsen IPF. Thus antiacid treatments are expected to decrease this risk of microaspiration-associated lung injury or damage. However, the efficacy of these anti-COPD or antifibrosis drugs in patients with CPFE is still not well known. More prospective studies are needed to make a conclusion.

Although the treatments with corticosteroids and immunosuppressant in patients with IPF are not recommended [54], CPFE syndrome involves underlying disease such as CTD [7]. So the treatment with systemic corticosteroids and immunosuppressant in patients with CPFE syndrome associated with CTD should be considered. However, no randomized double-blind trials have been conducted.

Smoking cessation is a reasonable method that could suppress the progression of emphysema lesions, and the oxygen therapy is appropriate for management of hypoxemia. Lung transplantation should be considered for patients with CPFE, given the significant mortality associated with this disorder [29, 31].

In a prospective cohort study in a recent research in China, the efficacy of inhaled corticosteroids/long-acting beta2 agonists (ICS/LABA) in CPFE was reported [55]. Dong et al. studied the patients with CPFE which are divided into treated group (45 cases) and non-treated group (24 cases) and followed up for 12 months. And they described that compared with baseline levels, the FEV1%,

FVC%, and DLCO% levels were increased 11.2 %, 13.5 %, and 12.8 %, respectively, in treated group, but declined 14.2 %, 16.8 %, and 21.3 %, respectively, in non-treated group. Furthermore, the frequency of acute exacerbation of CPFE, which was defined as the reference standard for COPD or IPF, was 44.4 and 75 % in treated group and non-treated group, respectively ($p < 0.05$). And the incidence of adverse event was no significant difference. However, this study was a nonrandomized clinical research and the sample size was small, so further research is required to validate these results.

PAH is the most common complication in the CPFE patients, which is important to identify because of its association with the principal determinant of reduced survival. In the study of treatment of 40 patients with CPFE complicating pulmonary hypertension, 92 % of the patients received long-term oxygen therapy and 60 % of the patients received therapy with bosentan, sildenafil, or inhaled iloprost. However, no statistically significant effect of treatment was observed regarding NYHA class, 6-minute walk distance, or eSPAP [33]. Though CPFE dominated by PAH has a poor prognosis, there are currently no specific recommendations for the treatment of PAH in the setting of CPFE. The presence of PAH with CPFE may be associated with an imbalance in the ventilation/perfusion ratio. Although hypoxic vasoconstriction is one of the main mechanisms to avoid worsening arterial oxygenation, vasodilator drugs could worsen hypoxemia by inhibiting this mechanism [8]. Thus it is still unknown whether treating these components of disease influences clinical outcomes. One report demonstrated efficacy of long-term oxygen therapy or pulmonary vasodilator treatment specific for PAH by improving hemodynamics [56]; however, the potential clinical and survival benefit is unknown.

17.9 Prognosis

Many reports have showed that CPFE is associated with a poor prognosis, with a 5-year survival calculated by the Kaplan–Meier method of 35–89 % and a median survival of 1.8–8.5 years [6, 11, 17, 19, 26, 29, 32, 34, 41, 57, 58, 61, 62] (Table 17.2).

In a cohort of 31 CPFE patients and 79 IPF-alone patients, the variables of FVC < 50 % predicted (HR 2.6, $p = 0.016$) and eSPAP > 75 mmHg (HR 2.25, $p = 0.022$) were associated with mortality [19]. Cottin et al. reported that the presence of PAH in CPFE patients was an independent predictor of mortality (HR 4.03, $p = 0.03$), and the mean survival time in CPFE patients was worse from 6.1 to 3.9 years by the absence or presence of PAH [6].

In the longitudinal study of mortality associated with pulmonary function tests over 6 and 12 months in patients with CPFE, the 10 % decline in FEV1 predicted mortality (HR 3.7, $p = 0.046$) in patients with moderate/severe emphysema [28]. And Sugino et al., in the longitudinal study, demonstrated that the paraseptal type of emphysema (HR 4.2, $p = 0.097$) and high eSPAP (HR 7.9, $p = 0.0036$) were prognostic factors in the patients with CPFE [34].

Whether patients with CPFE have worse survival rate than patients with pulmonary fibrosis alone is controversial. And Jankowich et al. considered that the cases of these confliction might include the relative proportion of non-IPF pathology in patients with CPFE in individual studies, influence of emphysema subtypes, retrospective study design, inclusion and exclusion criteria, and control group selection [29].

17.10 Future Tasks

Diagnostic criteria of CPFE on chest HRCT are only upper lobe emphysema and lower lobe fibrosis and lack of specific quantitative methods to assess the extent of emphysema and fibrosis. Therefore, standard quantitative methods for diagnostic criteria in CPFE are required to establish.

The identification of molecular and genetic alterations involved in the etiology of CPFE through surgical lung biopsies might provide a more effective approach for elucidation of mechanism and identifying molecular targets for future therapies.

17.11 Conclusion

Because there are many variation in patients with CPFE syndrome, management is not homogeneous. So it is necessary to distinguish emphysema-dominant phenotype or fibrosis-dominant phenotype in clinical diagnosis. Therefore, patients with CPFE should receive individualized treatment according to each patient. However, there are no studies of randomized clinical trial about management of patients with CPFE, and further research is required to validate the efficacy of several drugs against emphysema and fibrosis.

Statement of Interest The authors declare no conflict of interest.

Acknowledgment The pathological images were provided through the courtesy of Yasuhiro Terasaki, MD. (Department of Analytic Human Pathology) of Nippon Medical School, Tokyo, Japan.

Reference

1. The definition of emphysema. Report of a National Heart, Lung, and Blood Institute, Division of Lung Diseases workshop. Am Rev Respir Dis. 1985;132(1):182–5.

2. Fukuda Y, Masuda Y, Ishizaki M, Masugi Y, Ferrans VJ. Morphogenesis of abnormal elastic fibers in lungs of patients with panacinar and centriacinar emphysema. Hum Pathol. 1989;20 (7):652–9.
3. Cardoso WV, Sekhon HS, Hyde DM, Thurlbeck WM. Collagen and elastin in human pulmonary emphysema. Am Rev Respir Dis. 1993;147(4):975–81.
4. Wiggins J, Strickland B, Turner-Warwick M. Combined cryptogenic fibrosing alveolitis and emphysema: the value of high resolution computed tomography in assessment. Respir Med. 1990;84(5):365–9.
5. Homma Y, Saiki S, Doi O, Yoneda R, Mikami R, Tamura M. Clinical criteria for definition of idiopathic interstitial pneumonia (IIP). Nihon Kyobu Shikkan Gakkai Zasshi. 1992;30 (7):1371–7.
6. Cottin V, Nunes H, Brillet PY, Delaval P, Devouassoux G, Tillie-Leblond I, et al. Combined pulmonary fibrosis and emphysema: a distinct underrecognised entity. Eur Respir J. 2005;26 (4):586–93.
7. Cottin V, Cordier JF. Combined pulmonary fibrosis and emphysema in connective tissue disease. Curr Opin Pulm Med. 2012;18(5):418–27.
8. Cottin V. The impact of emphysema in pulmonary fibrosis. Eur Respir Rev. 2013;22 (128):153–7.
9. Portillo K, Morera J. Combined pulmonary fibrosis and emphysema syndrome: a new phenotype within the spectrum of smoking-related interstitial lung disease. Pulmon Med. 2012;2012:867870.
10. Hansell DM. High-resolution computed tomography in the evaluation of fibrosing alveolitis. Clin Chest Med. 1999;20(4):739–60. viii.
11. Cottin V, Nunes H, Mouthon L, Gamondes D, Lazor R, Hachulla E, et al. Combined pulmonary fibrosis and emphysema syndrome in connective tissue disease. Arthritis Rheum. 2011;63 (1):295–304.
12. Inomata M, Ikushima S, Awano N, Kondoh K, Satake K, Masuo M, et al. An autopsy study of combined pulmonary fibrosis and emphysema: correlations among clinical, radiological, and pathological features. BMC Pulm Med. 2014;14:104.
13. Matsuoka S, Yamashiro T, Matsushita S, Fujikawa A, Kotoku A, Yagihashi K, et al. Morphological disease progression of combined pulmonary fibrosis and emphysema: comparison with emphysema alone and pulmonary fibrosis alone. J Comput Assist Tomogr. 2015;39(2):153–9.
14. Kawabata Y, Hoshi E, Murai K, Ikeya T, Takahashi N, Saitou Y, et al. Smoking-related changes in the background lung of specimens resected for lung cancer: a semiquantitative study with correlation to postoperative course. Histopathology. 2008;53(6):707–14.
15. Watanabe Y, Kawabata Y, Kanauchi T, Hoshi E, Kurashima K, Koyama S, et al. Multiple, thin-walled cysts are one of the HRCT features of airspace enlargement with fibrosis. Eur J Radiol. 2015;84(5):986–92.
16. Kitaguchi Y, Fujimoto K, Hanaoka M, Kawakami S, Honda T, Kubo K. Clinical characteristics of combined pulmonary fibrosis and emphysema. Respirology. 2010;15(2):265–71.
17. Ryerson CJ, Hartman T, Elicker BM, Ley B, Lee JS, Abbritti M, et al. Clinical features and outcomes in combined pulmonary fibrosis and emphysema in idiopathic pulmonary fibrosis. Chest. 2013;144(1):234–40.
18. Kitaguchi Y, Fujimoto K, Hanaoka M, Honda T, Hotta J, Hirayama J. Pulmonary function impairment in patients with combined pulmonary fibrosis and emphysema with and without airflow obstruction. Int J Chron Obstruct Pulmon Dis. 2014;9:805–11.
19. Mejía M, Carrillo G, Rojas-Serrano J, Estrada A, Suárez T, Alonso D, et al. Idiopathic pulmonary fibrosis and emphysema: decreased survival associated with severe pulmonary arterial hypertension. Chest. 2009;136(1):10–5.
20. Mura M, Zompatori M, Pacilli AM, Fasano L, Schiavina M, Fabbri M. The presence of emphysema further impairs physiologic function in patients with idiopathic pulmonary fibrosis. Respir Care. 2006;51(3):257–65.

21. Yousem SA. Respiratory bronchiolitis-associated interstitial lung disease with fibrosis is a lesion distinct from fibrotic nonspecific interstitial pneumonia: a proposal. Mod Pathol. 2006;19(11):1474–9.
22. Katzenstein AL, Mukhopadhyay S, Zanardi C, Dexter E. Clinically occult interstitial fibrosis in smokers: classification and significance of a surprisingly common finding in lobectomy specimens. Hum Pathol. 2010;41(3):316–25.
23. Wright JL, Tazelaar HD, Churg A. Fibrosis with emphysema. Histopathology. 2011;58 (4):517–24.
24. Jin GY, Lynch D, Chawla A, Garg K, Tammemagi MC, Sahin H, et al. Interstitial lung abnormalities in a CT lung cancer screening population: prevalence and progression rate. Radiology. 2013;268(2):563–71.
25. Washko GR, Hunninghake GM, Fernandez IE, Nishino M, Okajima Y, Yamashiro T, et al. Lung volumes and emphysema in smokers with interstitial lung abnormalities. N Engl J Med. 2011;364(10):897–906.
26. Chae KJ, Jin GY, Han YM, Kim YS, Chon SB, Lee YS, et al. Prevalence and progression of combined pulmonary fibrosis and emphysema in asymptomatic smokers: a case–control study. Eur Radiol. 2015;25(8):2326–34.
27. Minegishi Y, Kokuho N, Miura Y, Matsumoto M, Miyanaga A, Noro R, et al. Clinical features, anti-cancer treatments and outcomes of lung cancer patients with combined pulmonary fibrosis and emphysema. Lung Cancer. 2014;85(2):258–63.
28. Schmidt SL, Nambiar AM, Tayob N, Sundaram B, Han MK, Gross BH, et al. Pulmonary function measures predict mortality differently in IPF versus combined pulmonary fibrosis and emphysema. Eur Respir J. 2011;38(1):176–83.
29. Jankowich MD, Rounds SI. Combined pulmonary fibrosis and emphysema syndrome: a review. Chest. 2012;141(1):222–31.
30. Silva DR, Gazzana MB, Barreto SS, Knorst MM. Idiopathic pulmonary fibrosis and emphysema in smokers. J Bras Pneumol. 2008;34(10):779–86.
31. Papiris SA, Triantafillidou C, Manali ED, Kolilekas L, Baou K, Kagouridis K, et al. Combined pulmonary fibrosis and emphysema. Exp Rev Respir Med. 2013;7(1):19–31. quiz 2.
32. Akagi T, Matsumoto T, Harada T, Tanaka M, Kuraki T, Fujita M, et al. Coexistent emphysema delays the decrease of vital capacity in idiopathic pulmonary fibrosis. Respir Med. 2009;103 (8):1209–15.
33. Cottin V, Le Pavec J, Prévot G, Mal H, Humbert M, Simonneau G, et al. Pulmonary hypertension in patients with combined pulmonary fibrosis and emphysema syndrome. Eur Respir J. 2010;35(1):105–11.
34. Sugino K, Ishida F, Kikuchi N, Hirota N, Sano G, Sato K, et al. Comparison of clinical characteristics and prognostic factors of combined pulmonary fibrosis and emphysema versus idiopathic pulmonary fibrosis alone. Respirology. 2014;19(2):239–45.
35. Usui K, Tanai C, Tanaka Y, Noda H, Ishihara T. The prevalence of pulmonary fibrosis combined with emphysema in patients with lung cancer. Respirology. 2011;16(2):326–31.
36. Fukui M, Suzuki K, Matsunaga T, Oh S, Takamochi K. Outcomes of lung cancer resection for patients with combined pulmonary fibrosis and emphysema. Surg Today. 2015.
37. Chiba S, Ohta H, Abe K, Hisata S, Ohkouchi S, Hoshikawa Y, et al. The diagnostic value of the interstitial biomarkers KL-6 and SP-D for the degree of fibrosis in combined pulmonary fibrosis and emphysema. Pulmon Med. 2012;2012:492960.
38. Mimae T, Suzuki K, Tsuboi M, Nagai K, Ikeda N, Mitsudomi T, et al. Surgical outcomes of lung cancer in patients with combined pulmonary fibrosis and emphysema. Ann Surg Oncol. 2015;22 Suppl 3:1371–9.
39. Collard HR, Moore BB, Flaherty KR, Brown KK, Kaner RJ, King TE, et al. Acute exacerbations of idiopathic pulmonary fibrosis. Am J Respir Crit Care Med. 2007;176(7):636–43.
40. Raghu G, Collard HR, Egan JJ, Martinez FJ, Behr J, Brown KK, et al. An official ATS/ERS/JRS/ALAT statement: idiopathic pulmonary fibrosis: evidence-based guidelines for diagnosis and management. Am J Respir Crit Care Med. 2011;183(6):788–824.

41. Kishaba T, Shimaoka Y, Fukuyama H, Yoshida K, Tanaka M, Yamashiro S, et al. A cohort study of mortality predictors and characteristics of patients with combined pulmonary fibrosis and emphysema. BMJ Open. 2012;2(3).
42. Gocho K, Sugino K, Sato K, Hasegawa C, Uekusa T, Homma S. Microscopic polyangiitis preceded by combined pulmonary fibrosis and emphysema. Respir Med Case Rep. 2015;15:128–32.
43. Antoniou KM, Margaritopoulos GA, Goh NS, Karagiannis K, Desai SR, Nicholson AG, et al. Combined pulmonary fibrosis and emphysema in scleroderma lung disease has a major confounding effect on lung physiology and screening for pulmonary hypertension. Arthritis Rheumatol. 2015.
44. Daniil Z, Koutsokera A, Gourgoulianis K. Combined pulmonary fibrosis and emphysema in patients exposed to agrochemical compounds. Eur Respir J. 2006;27(2):434.
45. Cottin V, Reix P, Khouatra C, Thivolet-Béjui F, Feldmann D, Cordier JF. Combined pulmonary fibrosis and emphysema syndrome associated with familial SFTPC mutation. Thorax. 2011;66(10):918–9.
46. Epaud R, Delestrain C, Louha M, Simon S, Fanen P, Tazi A. Combined pulmonary fibrosis and emphysema syndrome associated with ABCA3 mutations. Eur Respir J. 2014;43(2):638–41.
47. Tasaka S, Mizoguchi K, Funatsu Y, Namkoong H, Yamasawa W, Ishii M, et al. Cytokine profile of bronchoalveolar lavage fluid in patients with combined pulmonary fibrosis and emphysema. Respirology. 2012;17(5):814–20.
48. Kokuho N, Ishii T, Kamio K, Hayashi H, Kurahara M, Hattori K, et al. Diagnostic values for club cell secretory protein (CC16) in serum of patients of combined pulmonary fibrosis and emphysema. COPD. 2014.
49. Sokai A, Handa T, Tanizawa K, Oga T, Uno K, Tsuruyama T, et al. Matrix metalloproteinase-10: a novel biomarker for idiopathic pulmonary fibrosis. Respir Res. 2015;16:120.
50. Rogliani P, Mura M, Mattia P, Ferlosio A, Farinelli G, Mariotta S, et al. HRCT and histopathological evaluation of fibrosis and tissue destruction in IPF associated with pulmonary emphysema. Respir Med. 2008;102(12):1753–61.
51. Hanaoka M, Ito M, Droma Y, Ushiki A, Kitaguchi Y, Yasuo M, et al. Comparison of gene expression profiling between lung fibrotic and emphysematous tissues sampled from patients with combined pulmonary fibrosis and emphysema. Fibrogenesis Tissue Repair. 2012;5(1):17.
52. Vestbo J, Hurd SS, Agustí AG, Jones PW, Vogelmeier C, Anzueto A, et al. Global strategy for the diagnosis, management, and prevention of chronic obstructive pulmonary disease: GOLD executive summary. Am J Respir Crit Care Med. 2013;187(4):347–65.
53. Lin H, Jiang S. Combined pulmonary fibrosis and emphysema (CPFE): an entity different from emphysema or pulmonary fibrosis alone. J Thorac Dis. 2015;7(4):767–79.
54. Raghu G, Rochwerg B, Zhang Y, Garcia CA, Azuma A, Behr J, et al. An official ATS/ERS/JRS/ALAT clinical practice guideline: treatment of idiopathic pulmonary fibrosis. An update of the 2011 clinical practice guideline. Am J Respir Crit Care Med. 2015;192(2):e3–19.
55. Dong F, Zhang Y, Chi F, Song Q, Zhang L, Wang Y, et al. Clinical efficacy and safety of ICS/LABA in patients with combined idiopathic pulmonary fibrosis and emphysema. Int J Clin Exp Med. 2015;8(6):8617–25.
56. Cottin V. Clinical case: combined pulmonary fibrosis and emphysema with pulmonary hypertension–clinical management. BMC Res Notes. 2013;6 Suppl 1:S2.
57. Jankowich MD, Rounds S. Combined pulmonary fibrosis and emphysema alters physiology but has similar mortality to pulmonary fibrosis without emphysema. Lung. 2010;188 (5):365–73.
58. Todd NW, Jeudy J, Lavania S, Franks TJ, Galvin JR, Deepak J, et al. Centrilobular emphysema combined with pulmonary fibrosis results in improved survival. Fibrogenesis Tissue Repair. 2011;4(1):6.
59. Jankowich MD, Polsky M, Klein M, Rounds S. Heterogeneity in combined pulmonary fibrosis and emphysema. Respiration. 2008;75(4):411–7.

60. Tsushima K, Sone S, Yoshikawa S, Yokoyama T, Suzuki T, Kubo K. The radiological patterns of interstitial change at an early phase: over a 4-year follow-up. Respir Med. 2010;104 (11):1712–21.
61. Kurashima K, Takayanagi N, Tsuchiya N, Kanauchi T, Ueda M, Hoshi T, et al. The effect of emphysema on lung function and survival in patients with idiopathic pulmonary fibrosis. Respirology. 2010;15(5):843–8.
62. Lee CH, Kim HJ, Park CM, Lim KY, Lee JY, Kim DJ, et al. The impact of combined pulmonary fibrosis and emphysema on mortality. Int J Tuberc Lung Dis. 2011;15(8):1111–6.

Chapter 18
Association of COPD and Lung Cancer: How Does COPD Management Change the Outcome of Treatment of Lung Cancer?

Shinsaku Togo, Yukiko Namba, and Kazuhisa Takahashi

Abstract Chronic obstructive pulmonary disease (COPD) and lung cancer are caused by cigarette smoking, and there is increasing evidence linking the two diseases beyond a common etiology. COPD is widely considered to be a preneoplastic condition of smoking-related lung cancer. However, COPD is an independent risk factor for lung cancer and suggests some selected COPD phenotype in high-risk patients associates the development of lung cancer. Lung cancer patients with COPD have a significantly worse outcome than those without COPD. Thus, screening of patients with COPD for early detection of lung cancer using biomarkers and computed tomography has been suggested to improve outcomes. However, this approach of increased surveillance is hampered by the lack of sensitivity of treatment and the resulting large number of false-positive diagnoses. Improved understanding of the links between COPD and lung cancer and biomarkers that are more reliable may make this approach viable. In future, it may be possible to treat COPD patients with targeted therapies to reduce the risk of development of lung cancer.

Keywords COPD-associated lung cancer • Lung cancer • Management

18.1 Introduction

The risk of lung cancer in patients with chronic obstructive pulmonary disease (COPD) is well established, and several mechanisms have been suggested to explain the strong association between emphysema and lung cancer. There are 55 carcinogens in cigarette smoke that have been evaluated by the International

S. Togo (✉) • Y. Namba • K. Takahashi
Department of Respiratory Medicine, Juntendo University School of Medicine & Graduate School of Medicine, 2-1-1 Hongo, Bunkyo-ku, Tokyo 113-8421, Japan

Research Institute for Diseases of Old Age, Juntendo University Graduate School of Medicine, 2-1-1 Hongo, Bunkyo-ku, Tokyo 113-8421, Japan
e-mail: shinsaku@juntendo.ac.jp

H. Nakamura, K. Aoshiba (eds.), *Chronic Obstructive Pulmonary Disease*,
Respiratory Disease Series: Diagnostic Tools and Disease Managements,
DOI 10.1007/978-981-10-0839-9_18

Agency for Research on Cancer (IARC) and for which there is "sufficient evidence for carcinogenicity" in laboratory animals or humans [1]. Thus, it is reasonable that both lung cancer and emphysema are associated with cigarette smoking, which, by generating reactive oxidant species (ROS), induces a chronic inflammatory state in the lung and results in DNA damage.

Typically, airway disease and smoking exposure are associated with proximal lung cancers, such as squamous cell carcinoma (SCC) and small cell lung carcinoma (SCLC), rather than adenocarcinoma. Squamous metaplasia is common in smokers and is associated with airway obstruction in COPD [2]. The function of bronchoalveolar stem cells (BASCs) is unknown, but these cells lead to Kras-induced lung adenocarcinoma in a mouse model [3]. Inflammatory mediators induced by cigarette smoke may promote growth of BASCs and stimulate nuclear factor-kB (NF-kB) and signal transducer and activator of transcription 3 (STAT3), which have key roles in development of lung cancer from COPD [4].

COPD is considered to be a preneoplastic condition of lung cancer, and about 2.2 % of COPD patients develop lung cancer per year [5]. The risk of lung cancer in patients with COPD is approximately fivefold greater than that of smokers without COPD, independent of age and amount of cigarette smoking [6]. Smoking is an independent risk factor for COPD. The genetic and biological characteristics of COPD are similar to those of lung cancer, but the mechanism of development of lung cancer in COPD is unknown. However, this mechanism seems to involve individual host susceptibility to cigarette smoke and features of heterogeneity between the two diseases. Further large cohort studies are needed in subjects with appropriate phenotypes to identify potential drivers and predict biomarkers for screening of COPD-associated lung cancer.

18.2 Screening for Early Detection of COPD-Associated Lung Cancer

18.2.1 Annual Computed Tomography (CT) for Lung Cancer Screening

It is unclear whether the degree of airflow limitation and alveolar destruction confers a regional or global risk of lung cancer. The incidence of lung cancer may be related to the severity of airspace destruction, as assessed by CT-based semiquantitative scoring of emphysema lesions in the lungs [7–9]. Emphysema lesions of $\geq$5 % on CT were found to be associated with a 3.8-fold increase in lung cancer risk among smokers [9]. An increased risk of lung cancer has also been found with more severe COPD, based on the percentage predicted forced expiratory volume in 1 s (FEV_1) [7, 10, 11].

Screening of COPD patients for development of lung cancer using annual CT scans has been suggested for early detection. Patients with COPD and those with >35 pack-years of smoking have a significantly increased risk of death due to lung cancer, but CT screening was reported to have no significant effects on lung cancer mortality [12]. However, the National Lung Screening Trial (NLST) showed that low-dose CT screening is associated with a decrease in mortality from lung cancer of 20 %. In screening of patients with spirometric COPD, there was a twofold increase in lung cancer incidence and a trend favoring greater detection of early-stage cancers and fewer late-stage cancers in CT screening compared with chest radiography screening [13]. However, this result was associated with 96.4 % false-positive findings, and 38.8 % of patients with lung cancer were false negatives that were missed by CT screening [14]. Therefore, these approaches of increased surveillance are hampered by the lack of sensitivity of treatment and the large number of false-positive diagnoses [13].

18.2.2 Screening Using Liquid Biomarkers

Early detection of lung cancer in high-risk individuals has been attempted using evaluation of serum tumor markers such as cancer antigen 19–9 (CA19-9) and CA125, which are increased in relation to the severity of COPD [15]. However, it is difficult to use markers to detect lung cancer in COPD, since the serum levels of carcinoembryonic antigen (CEA), neuron-specific enolase (NSE), and cytokeratin fragment 19 (CYFRA 21–1) do not differ between patients with lung cancer and those with nonneoplastic lung diseases such as acute pneumonia, COPD, and interstitial lung diseases [16, 17].

Methods used for early diagnosis of lung carcinoma, including biological tests of blood samples and multiplexed tumor-associated autoantibody-based blood tests, are inconclusive or require confirmation in larger cohorts [18]. A large prospective study of early detection of lung cancer in patients with lung impairment showed that serum p53Abs levels were associated with smoking level and lung function impairment, both of which are risk factors of cancer development. However, no occurrence of lung cancer was detected in follow-up of positive subjects [19].

Plasma cfDNA levels in patients with non-small cell lung cancer (NSCLC) are significantly higher than in patients with chronic respiratory inflammation and in healthy controls. The mechanism through which cfDNA is released into the bloodstream is unknown, but it is revealed that elevated plasma cfDNA levels in patients with NSCLC are primarily due to tumor development, which has clinical implications for lung cancer screening and early diagnosis [20]. Migration of circulating tumor cells (CTCs) into the bloodstream also seems to be an early event in carcinogenesis, based on data showing that tumors of size <1 mm are associated with the presence of CTCs in blood [21]. CTCs were detected in 3 % of COPD patients by the isolation by size of epithelial tumor cells (ISET) method in blood filtration size-based CTC selection. After a mean follow-up period of 3.2 years, a surveillance CT program revealed lung nodules with a mean size of 1.7 cm in diameter. All CTC-positive COPD patients had lung cancer of stage IA [22]. These results suggest that validation of liquid biomarkers for early detection of lung cancer in COPD patients is warranted in larger population-based studies in different ethnic groups.

18.2.3 Screening of Gene Mutations

Cigarette smoking is a major risk factor for COPD, but only a minority of smokers develop COPD, and this seems to depend on the host response against cigarette smoking [23]. A minor population of COPD patients with genetic susceptibility to COPD-associated lung cancer have DNA damage that results in occurrence of lung cancer. Genetic mapping has identified several single nucleotide polymorphisms (SNPs) that have been speculatively linked to COPD-associated lung cancer. In addition, genome-wide association studies (GWASs) have shown that lung cancer and COPD share some genetic mutations, independent of smoking. Genotypes with reduced α1-antitrypsin (A1AT) inhibitory capacity have an increased risk for lung cancer [24, 25]. Imbalance of oxidative stress and antioxidants is common in COPD and drives cancer onset through free radical-mediated DNA damage, repair of which may be impaired by mutations and polymorphisms. Mutation of antioxidant enzymes such as glutathione S-transferase μ1 (GSTM1) reduces lung tissue protection against damage-inducing substances in tobacco and increases the risk of lung cancer in patients with COPD compared to healthy subjects [26].

Epidemiological studies have consistently found associations between the chromosome 15q24–15q25.1 locus, which is linked to nicotine addiction, and lung cancer susceptibility in COPD [27]. The association with this locus encompasses four candidate genes (CHRNA3/CHRNA5, IREB2, PSMA4) and several functionally relevant SNPs in a region where the degree of linkage disequilibrium is still to be clarified. Genetic variation in the 15q25 locus, which encodes the nicotinic acetylcholine receptor subunits (CHRNA3/CHRNA5), has a strong association with tobacco consumption and is a risk factor for COPD and lung cancer [28]. Variants of *IREB2*, a mediator of iron homeostasis, have also been linked to COPD and lung cancer [29]. *PSMA4* encodes a structural protein of the 20S proteasome core and has recently been associated with in vitro lung cancer cell proliferation and apoptosis. *PSMA4* mRNA levels are increased in lung tumors compared with normal lung tissues [30]. The Hedgehog-interacting protein (HHIP), which mediates the epithelial response to smoking, including the epithelial-mesenchymal transition (EMT), is related to COPD and lung cancer, and genetic variants on the 4q31 (HHIP/glycophorin A (GYPA)) locus are also associated with lung cancer [31]. FAM13A protein has an N-terminal region containing a RhoGAP domain, which has tumor suppressor activity through inhibition of RhoA intracellular signal transduction. Genetic variants in *FAM13A* may determine susceptibility to COPD and lung cancer [32].

Smoking and oxidative stress can induce EMT-induced airway remodeling, which is related to the pathogenesis of COPD, and the occurrence of EMT in COPD may account for the high incidence of lung cancer in patients with COPD [33]. Recent GWASs have shown that germline variants in or close to EMT-related genes (e.g., *Snail*, *Slug*) are associated with a risk for lung cancer or COPD [31]. The functional germline variant c.353T>C (p.Val118Ala) of Snail confers decreased risks of lung cancer and COPD, and this variant affects lung cancer risk through a mediation effect on COPD [34].

Screening of gene mutations as susceptibility loci for COPD-associated lung cancer, particularly in the 15q24–15q25 region, should be considered after sensitivity is determined in future studies. Monitoring of mutation-positive COPD patients may allow early diagnosis of lung cancer at lower cost than noninvasive screening for inflammatory cells in blood or sputum, rather than lung tissues from invasive diagnostic modalities such as fine-needle aspiration, transbronchial biopsy, and thoracoscopic surgery. Genetic variants might be predictors for the risk of COPD and lung cancer separately, as well as for the risk of development of lung cancer in patients with COPD (Table 18.1).

18.2.4 Screening of Epigenetic Changes

Epigenetic changes in COPD include higher levels of methylation induced by cigarette smoking, while altered expression of numerous oncogenes and tumor

Table 18.1 Targets and effects of genetic mutations in COPD-associated lung cancer

Genetic mutations	Biological functions	Ref
Nicotinic acetylcholine receptor region on chromosome 15q25		
Cholinergic nicotinic acetylcholine receptor (CHRNA3/CHRNA5)	Associations with tobacco consumption and a risk factor for lung cancer	[28]
Family with sequence similarity 13, member A (FAM13A)	Dysfunction of tumor suppressor activity-mediated RhoA signaling	[32]
Iron-responsive element-binding protein 2 (IREB2)	Contains genes encoding CHRNA3/CHRNA5 and associated with lung cancer	[29]
Proteasome subunit alpha type 4 (PSMA4)	Lung cancer cell proliferation, apoptosis, and increased in lung tumors	[30]
Others		
Glutathione S-transferase μ1 (GSTM1)	Antioxidant-mediated DNA damage	[26]
Hedgehog-interacting protein (HHIP)	Epithelial response (EMT) to smoking	[31]
Snail	Powerful regulator of EMT	[34]

EMT Epithelial-mesenchymal transition

suppressor gene promoters is observed in most lung cancers. Methylation of *CDKN2A*, *MGMT*, *CCDC37*, and *MAP1B* is significantly associated with COPD and lung cancer. *CDKN2A*, which encodes tumor suppressors p16 (INK4A) and ARF, is a common methylation mark in COPD and lung cancer [35]. Such aberrant methylation of tumor suppressor genes in lung tissues and induced sputum may be a predictor for early diagnosis of COPD-associated lung cancer [36]. Epigenetic changes in noncoding RNAs, including microRNAs (miRNAs), which are small noncoding, single-stranded RNA molecules, may also be important. For example, *miR-1* has been linked to cigarette smoking-related conditions such as heart disease and cancer [37] and is related to atrophy of skeletal muscle in patients with COPD compared with non-smoking controls [37]. *miR-21* has roles in inflammation and carcinogenesis [38], whereas *miR-146a* suppresses inflammation and cancer cell proliferation [39]. However, the mechanisms of epigenetic biomarkers in COPD-associated lung cancer and their effects on prognosis remain poorly understood.

18.3 Management of Outcomes of COPD-Associated Lung Cancer

18.3.1 Management of Chronic Inflammation

Exposure to cigarette smoke causes inflammatory cells, particularly neutrophils and macrophages, to be recruited at the site of lung injury and activated to release neutrophil elastase (NE), serine and matrix metalloproteinases (MMPs), and ROS. A defect in A1AT contributes to degradation of elastin due to activation of NE and oxidative stress-mediated inflammation in the lung, resulting in development of emphysema and lung tumorigenesis [40, 41]. Many studies have shown that chronic inflammation in lung tissue and associated repair processes in COPD may initiate lung cancer [42, 43]. An excess of circulating inflammatory mediators such as IL-6, TNF-α, and IL-8 released from inflammatory cells maintains chronic systemic inflammation in patients with COPD and, thus, further contributes to carcinogenesis [44, 45]. Current therapies for COPD, including inhaled corticosteroids (ICS), long-acting muscarinic receptor antagonists (LAMAs), long-acting β2-agonists (LABAs), and theophylline, suppress inflammation in the lung and prevent spill-over of inflammatory mediators into the systemic circulation. Theophylline indirectly suppresses NF-kB, which is a cause of persistent airway inflammation, and may reduce the risk of tumorigenesis by activating histone deacetylase 2 (HDAC2), which restores sensitivity to ICS in patients with COPD [46]. Thus, patients with COPD who are treated with ICS have a reduced incidence of lung cancer and lower mortality, which suggests that inhibition of inflammation can slow lung tumor onset [47]. However, large prospective trials have failed to demonstrate a survival benefit in chronic use of ICS with or without LABAs [48].

18.3.2 Management of Oxidative Stress

The free radical hypothesis suggests that reactive nitrogen and oxygen species (RNOS) drive accumulation of cell and DNA damage, which results in mutations and cancer initiation if incorrectly repaired. RNOS can degrade proteins, including tumor suppressors, leading to cell division and decreased apoptosis and DNA repair [49], which results in cancer promotion and progression. Antioxidant therapy for reduction of the risk of lung cancer using vitamin C, vitamin E, or N-acetyl cysteine (NAC) may be of benefit for patients with COPD. However, supplementation with vitamins E or C was shown to have no significant effect on total cancer incidence in the USA [50, 51], and 2-year NAC supplementation resulted in no survival or event-free survival benefit in patients with lung cancer, most of whom were previous or current smokers [52].

18.3.3 Management of Angiogenesis

A recent study suggested that hypoxic regions of the lung may have a role in the association between COPD and lung cancer. The hypoxia-inducible factor (HIF) family, HIF-1α and HIF-2α, is well known as inducers of VEGF-mediated angiogenesis and is likely to play a role in the increased cancer risk in COPD [53, 54]. HIF-2α overexpression in a conditionally expressed mutant mouse model of lung carcinogenesis resulted in larger tumors [55]. However, HIF-2α deletion unexpectedly showed an increase in tumor burden, associated with a decrease in a candidate tumor suppressor gene.

Serum VEGF levels are significantly associated with clinical staging and lower survival of patients with NSCLC [56]. Bevacizumab is a recombinant, humanized, monoclonal antibody against VEGF that is approved as first-line treatment of NSCLC based on data from randomized phase III clinical trials [57]. In COPD pathogenesis, epithelial cell injury mediated by oxidative stress may induce a decrease in lung VEGF levels, resulting in promotion of COPD. Inhibition of VEGF receptors induces alveolar septal cell apoptosis and leads to enlargement of air spaces, indicative of emphysema [58]. These results suggest that bevacizumab-based chemotherapy for COPD-associated lung cancer may be disadvantageous for COPD management. However, some studies have linked COPD with increased expression of VEGF in bronchial tissue [59], and activation of NF-kB in COPD promotes HIF stabilization [60]. The significance of VEGF production in patients with COPD remains unclear, but inflammation and hypoxia regulation may have some impact on the prognosis of COPD-associated lung cancer. Thus, the response to specific treatment for tumors arising in a hypoxic lung-induced VEGF production might be exploitable in patients with underlying COPD.

18.3.4 Management of Extracellular Matrix Regulation

Neutrophil elastase (NE) has a well-known effect on elastin fiber degradation that results in emphysema and promotes lung tumor growth in a *Kras* mouse model of lung adenocarcinoma [61]. The relationship of NE activity with poor outcomes in human lung cancer has not been established, but drugs that inhibit NE activity might be of value as therapeutic prevention for COPD-associated lung cancer.

Members of the MMP family are matrix-degrading enzymes in emphysema and lung cancer and may be mechanistic links between COPD and lung cancer by contributing to lung tissue destruction in emphysema and promoting lung tumor growth and invasiveness. The activities of MMP9 (gelatinase B) in BAL fluid and serum correlate with COPD severity [62, 63], and MMP9 is essential for tumor angiogenesis in animal models [64]. MMP1 (collagenase I) contributes to growth of most solid tumors and promotes metastasis [65]. Overexpression of MMP1 in transgenic mice causes development of emphysema [66], and polymorphisms in the *MMP1* promoter predict disease severity in patients with COPD [67]. MMP12, a somewhat macrophage-specific proteinase, is a stimulator of emphysema, and its activity has been associated with disease severity in COPD [68]. Interestingly, MMP12 is known more as a tumor suppressor and not as a target for treatment of lung cancer [69] (Table 18.2).

The effects of AZD1236, a selective MMP9 and MMP12 inhibitor, on emphysematous lung tissue degradation were evaluated in patients with moderate-to-severe COPD, but AZD1236 and other MMP inhibitors do not improve lung function and symptoms [70]. Similarly, other MMP inhibitors, marimastat (BB2516) and BAY12-9566, failed to improve survival in patients with advanced NSCLC [71]. Clinical trials have yet to demonstrate significant increases in overall survival and toxicity remains an issue.

18.3.5 Drug Potency

Increasing intracellular levels of cAMP induce cancer cell death in vitro. Theophylline, which elevates intracellular cAMP, induces cancer cell apoptosis and thus may be a potential anticancer drug in combination with other chemotherapeutic agents [72]. COX2 generates prostaglandin E2 (PGE_2), which strongly elevates intracellular cAMP, but PGE_2 also promotes carcinogenesis in several ways, including increased resistance to apoptosis, increased angiogenesis, and enhanced invasion [73]. Celecoxib, a COX2-selective inhibitor, may reduce the cancer risk in a high-risk smoking population based on reduction of proliferation markers in the bronchial epithelium [74]. Celecoxib increased progression-free survival in combination treatment in patients with lung adenocarcinoma cancer with biomarkers for high metabolism of PGE_2 in urine [75] and reduced progression of cigarette smoke-

Table 18.2 Targets of proteinases in COPD-associated lung cancer

Proteinase	Source	Matrix substrate	LK	Ref	COPD	Ref
Neutrophil elastase	PMNs	Elastin, CI, CIII, CIV, laminin, fibronectin, and TIMPs	Promotion of lung tumor growth	[61]	Elastic fiber degradation resulting in emphysema	[40, 44]
MMP1	Stroma cells	CI, CIII, and A1AT	Promotion of solid tumor growth and metastasis	[65]	Polymorphisms related to disease severity	[66]
MMP9	Macrophages, PMNs, other cells	Elastin, CI, CIV, laminin, and A1AT	Induction of tumor angiogenesis	[64]	Associated with disease severity	[62, 63]
MMP12	Macrophages	Elastin, CI, CIV, fibronectin, laminin, and A1AT	Protective role as tumor suppressor	[69]	Associated with disease severity	[68]

CI collagen type 1, *CIII* collagen type 3, *CIV* collagen type 4, *MMP* matrix metalloproteinase, *PMNs* polymorphonuclear leukocytes induced pulmonary emphysema by suppression of NF-kB-regulated anti-inflammatory effects in an animal model [76]. Oral prostacyclin (iloprost) also has a tumor-suppressive effect and displays antiproliferative and antimetastatic properties [77]. However, the proven benefits of celecoxib and iloprost are limited to patients with established COPD. A nonselective COX inhibitor, indomethacin, and a nonselective PDE inhibitor, IBMX, significantly inhibit proliferation of SCLC cells with neuronal characteristics in vitro [78]. Beta-adrenergic receptors co-express COX2 in lung adenocarcinoma tissue [79], and indacaterol, an ultra-long-acting inhaled β2-agonist (LABA), inhibits NF-kB activity and reduces expression of NF-kB target genes related to COPD and lung cancer, including *MMP9* [80]. This suppresses tumor cell invasion and migration in vitro, but the effect on outcomes for lung cancer in human study is unknown.

Non-neuronal ACh activates downstream NF-kB signaling and acts as an autoparacrine growth factor to stimulate cell proliferation and promote epithelial-mesenchymal transition (EMT) in NSCLC via activation of the M2 muscarinic receptor (M2R) [81, 82]. Expression of another mAChR, M3R, is significantly increased in NSCLC and is correlated with tumor metastasis and poor survival. M3R enhances expression and activity of MMP9 through PI3K/Akt, which promotes migration and invasion of NSCLC cells, and blockade of M3R suppresses proliferation, invasion, and migration of NSCLC and SCLC cells [83–85]. R2HBJJ has high affinity to M3 and M1 AChRs and markedly suppresses growth of NSCLC cells [86]. These findings indicate that M2R and M3R antagonists may be beneficial therapy for COPD-associated lung cancer. Such compounds are currently used for COPD treatment, including LAMAs, LABAs, and theophylline, but they may be toxic at higher concentrations required for anticancer treatment according to the results from these in vitro experiments. There are currently no clinical trials of these drugs in lung cancer patients.

18.4 Treatment of COPD-Associated Lung Cancer

18.4.1 Thoracic Surgery

Severe airway obstruction, advanced clinical stage, and higher age are independent factors associated with an indication for thoracic surgery in COPD-associated lung cancer [87]. Comorbidities such as COPD can have a significant effect on long-term survival due to an influence on treatment indication, complication rate, and treatment efficacy. COPD and smoking are significant independent risk factors for postoperative pulmonary complications such as atelectasis and pneumonia and are associated with a poorer long-term outcome [88]. Patients receiving curative surgery for NSCLC who have co-existing COPD have worse survival than their counterparts with better pulmonary function. Notably, the treatment-naïve COPD patients who have improved preoperative symptoms and pulmonary function by

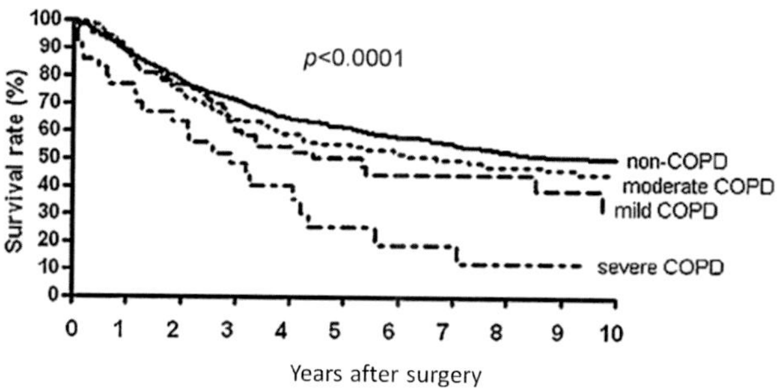

Fig. 18.1 Overall survival after pulmonary resection for lung cancer. The 5-year survival rates in the non-COPD, mild, moderate, and severe COPD groups were 61.5, 50.2, 55.3, and 25.1 %, respectively [90]

inhaled tiotropium starting 2 weeks prior to surgery demonstrated better postoperative pulmonary functions than expected [89].

Higher COPD grades have more postoperative pulmonary complications and poorer long-term survival because of higher rates of recurrence of lung cancer (Fig. 18.1) [90]. In patients with stage I resected NSCLC, COPD is an independent predictor of reduced recurrence-free survival, and these patients are at higher risk of recurrence than patients without COPD [91, 92]. Therefore, it is important to identify patients with early-stage NSCLC for more aggressive treatment. Clinical studies are needed in patients with lung cancer to determine how COPD promotes recurrence and affects the indication for adjuvant chemotherapy following curative resection.

18.4.2 Chemotherapy and Molecular Targeted Therapy

Although there is not yet strong evidence for specific difference in management for lung cancer comorbidity with COPD, the patients with high age, poor overall PS, and severe impaired lung function associated with COPD are generally restricted to receive the appropriate platinum-based standard chemotherapy for the high risk of adverse effects. Thus, they often receive single-agent chemotherapy or choose best supportive care due to rapid progression to death. The mild COPD patients with advanced metastatic disease who received chemotherapy can delayed progression, palliate symptom, and improved overall survival and did not find significant differences in improved treatment outcome between mild COPD and non-COPD [93]. However, COPD exacerbations by airway infections and other factors often prevent the chemotherapy, and once acute exacerbation has occurred, the mortality rate is high in patients with COPD-associated lung cancer during chemotherapy.

EGFR mutations and ALK rearrangements are major drivers in non-smoker lung adenocarcinoma, and these patients may be particularly responsive to molecular targeted therapy. In contrast, patients with COPD-associated NSCLC have a low prevalence of EGFR mutations and ALK rearrangements, but these are linked to COPD severity and more frequent poorly differentiated lung cancer with a poor prognosis [87, 94]. In a comparison of the molecular features of COPD-associated adenocarcinoma with those of smoke-related adenocarcinoma without COPD, Schiavon et al. found that EGFR mutation did not differ between the two groups, but KRAS mutation was higher in smokers than in COPD patients [95].

In contrast to idiopathic interstitial pneumonias, the presence of COPD is not recognized as a significant risk factor for drug-induced interstitial lung disease associated with lung cancer treatment. Expression of EGFR is higher in lung cancer patients and in COPD patients [96]. Thus, EGFR inhibition has been examined in COPD as a method to prevent stimulation of mucous hypersecretion, but the initial studies have produced negative findings [97].

18.4.3 Radiation Therapy

Stereotactic body radiotherapy (SBRT) is standard of care for early-stage non-small cell lung cancer at high risk of surgical complications and associated with excellent local control ($\sim$90 % at 3 years). In previous retrospective study, 32 % of stage I lung cancer patients with COPD who underwent SBRT had radiation pneumonitis, and COPD and the Brinkman index were statistically significant risk factors for the development of radiation pneumonitis. However, SBRT-mediated radiation pneumonitis did not associate OS, and thus SBRT can be tolerated in early lung cancer patients with COPD [98]. Severity of radiation pneumonitis associated higher in patients with a high V20 ($\geq$25 %) value and severe low-attenuation area (LAA) grade on CT scans [99]. In contrast, patients with severe emphysema had a low risk of radiation pneumonitis following SBRT rather than normal lung function and with mild emphysema. Furthermore, fewer pack-years smoked among COPD patients were the strongest predictor for severe radiation pneumonitis [100, 101].

SBRT can be considered as therapeutic option in patients with higher operative risks, such as the elderly and patients with severe COPD. However, previous studies still provide controversial results about the risk of radiation pneumonitis in severe COPD patients. Further follow-up study might be needed to evaluate the tolerability to SBRT in COPD-associated lung cancer patients.

18.4.4 Immunotherapy

Chronic inflammation is a common feature in COPD and lung cancer, but the characteristics of immune cells in COPD differ from those found in lung cancer. Immune cells in BAL fluid from COPD patients tend to shift toward the T helper 1 (T_H1) phenotype with interferon-γ (IFNγ) production [102]. In contrast, immune cells in most solid tumors show a trend for the T_H2 phenotype with infiltration of immunosuppressive cells in tumor tissue. These cells include myeloid-derived suppressor cells (MDSCs) and regulatory T cells (T_{Regs}) and express programmed cell death protein 1 (PD-1) on the cell surface, which results in suppression of cytotoxic T lymphocyte function and enhanced tumor viability [103, 104]. The use of PD-1- and PD-L1-blocking antibodies in therapy for NSCLC is focused on increasing cytotoxic T cell activity, which increases the cancer antigen-mediated immune response. Increasing PD-L1 expression in tumor tissue was observed in smokers and associated with more pack-years [105] and anti-PD-1/PD-L1 treatment prolonged OS in NSCLC patients with smoking history [106]. An increased proportion of CD8+ T cells in lung parenchyma in COPD patients has been described, and the PD-1 pathway has been suggested to be relevant in COPD pathogenesis. CD8+ T cells expressing PD-1 are present at higher levels in blood from COPD patients and are correlated with disease severity [107–109]. Furthermore, virus-induced expression of PD-L1, the ligand for PD-1, is decreased in COPD macrophages, with a corresponding increase in IFNγ release from infected COPD lungs resulting in increased severity of viral infection, prolonged viral shedding, and structural lung damage associated with exacerbations [110]. Although, anti-PD-1/PD-L1 treatment may associate better clinical outcome in smoking related lung cancers patients with COPD, we should note that the use of PD-1- and PD-L1-blocking antibodies may have indirect effects against chronic inflammation-mediated COPD development and aberrant immune regulation, especially during exacerbation of COPD. Aminophylline, which is often used as a bronchodilator for COPD patients, also has an unexpected effect on lymphocyte regulation and synergistically accelerates lymphocyte cell division in patients with lung cancer undergoing chemotherapy [111].

18.5 Conclusion

The incidence of COPD is a robust predictor of poor survival in lung cancer. Therefore, early detection of lung cancer is important in high-risk COPD sub-populations to prevent development of lung cancer. Although many approaches to predict the onset of lung cancer in patients with COPD have been proposed, most of them were still provided by experimental evidences (Table 18.3). Larger studies are needed to validate the potential of early diagnostic identification of COPD-associated lung cancer, along with further evidence of the efficacy of targeted therapies. Follow-up studies are also needed to evaluate the impact on patients with an increased risk of lung cancer and assess the predictive value of biomarkers for early detection of lung cancer in at-risk patients with COPD.

Table 18.3 Approach to early diagnosis and management of COPD-associated lung cancer

Approach to screening for early diagnosis of lung cancer
1. Annual low-dose CT screening
Follow-up of subjects with a strong emphysema lesion or low FEV_1
2. Liquid biomarker screening
Multiplexed tumor-associated autoantibody-based blood test: p53Ab
Circulating free DNA
Circulating tumor cells
3. Genetic and epigenetic susceptibility
Oxidative stress-regulated genes
Chromosome 15q24–15q25.1 locus
Epithelial-mesenchymal transition (EMT)-related genes
DNA methylation: CDKN2A, MGMT, CCDC37, and MAP1B
MicroRNAs: miR-1, miR-21, and miR-146a
Management of outcome of COPD-associated lung cancer
Management of chronic inflammation: theophylline, cyclooxygenase-2-selective inhibitors, long-acting inhaled β2-agonists (LABAs), and inhaled corticosteroids
Management of oxidative stress: vitamin C, vitamin E, and N-acetyl cysteine
Management of angiogenesis: bevacizumab and hypoxia-inducible factor-mediated VEGF dysregulation?
Management of extracellular matrix regulation: neutrophil elastase inhibitors and matrix metalloproteinase (MMP) inhibitors
Indirect effect of COPD medication on lung cancer
Theophylline, prostacyclin, LABAs, and phosphodiesterase 4 inhibitors: suppression of elevation of cAMP in cancer cells
LABAs: inhibition of NF-kB and MMP9 activity in cancer cells
Long-acting muscarinic receptor antagonists: suppression of EMT through muscarinic receptor 2 and suppression of cancer cell functions through muscarinic receptor 3

References

1. Hoffmann D, Hoffmann I. The changing cigarette, 1950–1995. J Toxicol Environ Health. 1997;50(4):307–64.
2. Araya J, Cambier S, Markovics JA, Wolters P, Jablons D, Hill A, et al. Squamous metaplasia amplifies pathologic epithelial-mesenchymal interactions in COPD patients. J Clin Invest. 2007;117(11):3551–62.
3. Kim CF, Jackson EL, Woolfenden AE, Lawrence S, Babar I, Vogel S, et al. Identification of bronchioalveolar stem cells in normal lung and lung cancer. Cell. 2005;121(6):823–35.
4. Houghton AM, Mouded M, Shapiro SD. Common origins of lung cancer and COPD. Nat Med. 2008;14(10):1023–4.
5. Rodriguez-Roisin R, Soriano JB. Chronic obstructive pulmonary disease with lung cancer and/or cardiovascular disease. Proc Am Thorac Soc. 2008;5(8):842–7.
6. Young RP, Hopkins RJ, Christmas T, Black PN, Metcalf P, Gamble GD. COPD prevalence is increased in lung cancer, independent of age, sex and smoking history. Eur Respir J. 2009;34 (2):380–6.

7. de Torres JP, Bastarrika G, Wisnivesky JP, Alcaide AB, Campo A, Seijo LM, et al. Assessing the relationship between lung cancer risk and emphysema detected on low-dose CT of the chest. Chest. 2007;132(6):1932–8.
8. Zulueta JJ, Wisnivesky JP, Henschke CI, Yip R, Farooqi AO, McCauley DI, et al. Emphysema scores predict death from COPD and lung cancer. Chest. 2012;141 (5):1216–23.
9. Li Y, Swensen SJ, Karabekmez LG, Marks RS, Stoddard SM, Jiang R, et al. Effect of emphysema on lung cancer risk in smokers: a computed tomography-based assessment. Cancer Prev Res (Phila). 2011;4(1):43–50.
10. Maldonado F, Bartholmai BJ, Swensen SJ, Midthun DE, Decker PA, Jett JR. Are airflow obstruction and radiographic evidence of emphysema risk factors for lung cancer? A nested case–control study using quantitative emphysema analysis. Chest. 2010;138(6):1295–302.
11. Wilson DO, Weissfeld JL, Balkan A, Schragin JG, Fuhrman CR, Fisher SN, et al. Association of radiographic emphysema and airflow obstruction with lung cancer. Am J Respir Crit Care Med. 2008;178(7):738–44.
12. Wille MM, Dirksen A, Ashraf H, Saghir Z, Bach KS, Brodersen J, et al. Results of the randomized Danish lung cancer screening trial with focus on high risk profiling. Am J Respir Crit Care Med. 2016;193(5):542–51.
13. Young RP, Duan F, Chiles C, Hopkins RJ, Gamble GD, Greco EM, et al. Airflow limitation and histology shift in the national lung screening trial. The NLST-ACRIN cohort substudy. Am J Respir Crit Care Med. 2015;192(9):1060–7.
14. National Lung Screening Trial Research T, Aberle DR, Berg CD, Black WC, Church TR, Fagerstrom RM, et al. The National Lung Screening Trial: overview and study design. Radiology. 2011;258(1):243–53.
15. Bulut I, Arbak P, Coskun A, Balbay O, Annakkaya AN, Yavuz O, et al. Comparison of serum CA 19.9, CA 125 and CEA levels with severity of chronic obstructive pulmonary disease. Med Princ Pract. 2009;18(4):289–93.
16. Hillas G, Moschos C, Dimakou K, Vlastos F, Avgeropoulou S, Christakopoulou I, et al. Carcinoembryonic antigen, neuron-specific enolase and cytokeratin fragment 19 (CYFRA 21–1) levels in induced sputum of lung cancer patients. Scand J Clin Lab Invest. 2008;68(7):542–7.
17. Sanguinetti CM, Riccioni G, Marchesani F, Pela R, Cecarini L. Bronchoalveolar lavage fluid level of carcinoembryonic antigen in the diagnosis of peripheral lung cancer. Monaldi Arch Chest Dis. 1995;50(3):177–82.
18. Farlow EC, Patel K, Basu S, Lee BS, Kim AW, Coon JS, et al. Development of a multiplexed tumor-associated autoantibody-based blood test for the detection of non-small cell lung cancer. Clin Cancer Res. 2010;16(13):3452–62.
19. Mattioni M, Chinzari P, Soddu S, Strigari L, Cilenti V, Mastropasqua E. Serum p53 antibody detection in patients with impaired lung function. BMC Cancer. 2013;13:62.
20. Szpechcinski A, Chorostowska-Wynimko J, Struniawski R, Kupis W, Rudzinski P, Langfort R, et al. Cell-free DNA levels in plasma of patients with non-small-cell lung cancer and inflammatory lung disease. Br J Cancer. 2015;113(3):476–83.
21. Pantel K, Brakenhoff RH, Brandt B. Detection, clinical relevance and specific biological properties of disseminating tumour cells. Nat Rev Cancer. 2008;8(5):329–40.
22. Ilie M, Hofman V, Long-Mira E, Selva E, Vignaud JM, Padovani B, et al. "Sentinel" circulating tumor cells allow early diagnosis of lung cancer in patients with chronic obstructive pulmonary disease. PLoS One. 2014;9(10):e111597.
23. Laniado-Laborin R. Smoking and chronic obstructive pulmonary disease (COPD). Parallel epidemics of the 21 century. Int J Environ Res Public Health. 2009;6(1):209–24.
24. Yang P, Sun Z, Krowka MJ, Aubry MC, Bamlet WR, Wampfler JA, et al. Alpha1-antitrypsin deficiency carriers, tobacco smoke, chronic obstructive pulmonary disease, and lung cancer risk. Arch Intern Med. 2008;168(10):1097–103.

25. Yang P, Bamlet WR, Sun Z, Ebbert JO, Aubry MC, Krowka MJ, et al. Alpha1-antitrypsin and neutrophil elastase imbalance and lung cancer risk. Chest. 2005;128(1):445–52.
26. Dialyna IA, Miyakis S, Georgatou N, Spandidos DA. Genetic polymorphisms of CYP1A1, GSTM1 and GSTT1 genes and lung cancer risk. Oncol Rep. 2003;10(6):1829–35.
27. Amos CI, Wu X, Broderick P, Gorlov IP, Gu J, Eisen T, et al. Genome-wide association scan of tag SNPs identifies a susceptibility locus for lung cancer at 15q25.1. Nat Genet. 2008;40 (5):616–22.
28. Hung RJ, McKay JD, Gaborieau V, Boffetta P, Hashibe M, Zaridze D, et al. A susceptibility locus for lung cancer maps to nicotinic acetylcholine receptor subunit genes on 15q25. Nature. 2008;452(7187):633–7.
29. Du Y, Xue Y, Xiao W. Association of IREB2 gene rs2568494 polymorphism with risk of chronic obstructive pulmonary disease: a meta-analysis. Med Sci Monit. 2016;22:177–82.
30. Liu Y, Liu P, Wen W, James MA, Wang Y, Bailey-Wilson JE, et al. Haplotype and cell proliferation analyses of candidate lung cancer susceptibility genes on chromosome 15q24-25.1. Cancer Res. 2009;69(19):7844–50.
31. Young RP, Whittington CF, Hopkins RJ, Hay BA, Epton MJ, Black PN, et al. Chromosome 4q31 locus in COPD is also associated with lung cancer. Eur Respir J. 2010;36(6):1375–82.
32. Young RP, Hopkins RJ, Hay BA, Whittington CF, Epton MJ, Gamble GD. FAM13A locus in COPD is independently associated with lung cancer – evidence of a molecular genetic link between COPD and lung cancer. Appl Clin Genet. 2011;4:1–10.
33. Walser T, Cui X, Yanagawa J, Lee JM, Heinrich E, Lee G, et al. Smoking and lung cancer: the role of inflammation. Proc Am Thorac Soc. 2008;5(8):811–5.
34. Yang L, Yang X, Ji W, Deng J, Qiu F, Yang R, et al. Effects of a functional variant c.353T > C in snai1 on risk of two contextual diseases. Chronic obstructive pulmonary disease and lung cancer. Am J Respir Crit Care Med. 2014;189(2):139–48.
35. Belinsky SA, Palmisano WA, Gilliland FD, Crooks LA, Divine KK, Winters SA, et al. Aberrant promoter methylation in bronchial epithelium and sputum from current and former smokers. Cancer Res. 2002;62(8):2370–7.
36. Guzman L, Depix MS, Salinas AM, Roldan R, Aguayo F, Silva A, et al. Analysis of aberrant methylation on promoter sequences of tumor suppressor genes and total DNA in sputum samples: a promising tool for early detection of COPD and lung cancer in smokers. Diagn Pathol. 2012;7:87.
37. Lewis A, Riddoch-Contreras J, Natanek SA, Donaldson A, Man WD, Moxham J, et al. Downregulation of the serum response factor/miR-1 axis in the quadriceps of patients with COPD. Thorax. 2012;67(1):26–34.
38. Schetter AJ, Heegaard NH, Harris CC. Inflammation and cancer: interweaving microRNA, free radical, cytokine and p53 pathways. Carcinogenesis. 2010;31(1):37–49.
39. Williams AE, Perry MM, Moschos SA, Larner-Svensson HM, Lindsay MA. Role of miRNA-146a in the regulation of the innate immune response and cancer. Biochem Soc Trans. 2008;36(Pt 6):1211–5.
40. Makita H, Nasuhara Y, Nagai K, Ito Y, Hasegawa M, Betsuyaku T, et al. Characterisation of phenotypes based on severity of emphysema in chronic obstructive pulmonary disease. Thorax. 2007;62(11):932–7.
41. Petrache I, Fijalkowska I, Zhen L, Medler TR, Brown E, Cruz P, et al. A novel antiapoptotic role for alpha1-antitrypsin in the prevention of pulmonary emphysema. Am J Respir Crit Care Med. 2006;173(11):1222–8.
42. de Torres JP, Marin JM, Casanova C, Cote C, Carrizo S, Cordoba-Lanus E, et al. Lung cancer in patients with chronic obstructive pulmonary disease– incidence and predicting factors. Am J Respir Crit Care Med. 2011;184(8):913–9.
43. Hanahan D, Weinberg RA. Hallmarks of cancer: the next generation. Cell. 2011;144 (5):646–74.

44. Gan WQ, Man SF, Senthilselvan A, Sin DD. Association between chronic obstructive pulmonary disease and systemic inflammation: a systematic review and a meta-analysis. Thorax. 2004;59(7):574–80.
45. Lee KY, Ho SC, Chan YF, Wang CH, Huang CD, Liu WT, et al. Reduced nuclear factor-kappaB repressing factor: a link toward systemic inflammation in COPD. Eur Respir J. 2012;40(4):863–73.
46. Ito K, Ito M, Elliott WM, Cosio B, Caramori G, Kon OM, et al. Decreased histone deacetylase activity in chronic obstructive pulmonary disease. N Engl J Med. 2005;352 (19):1967–76.
47. Parimon T, Chien JW, Bryson CL, McDonell MB, Udris EM, Au DH. Inhaled corticosteroids and risk of lung cancer among patients with chronic obstructive pulmonary disease. Am J Respir Crit Care Med. 2007;175(7):712–9.
48. Calverley PM, Anderson JA, Celli B, Ferguson GT, Jenkins C, Jones PW, et al. Salmeterol and fluticasone propionate and survival in chronic obstructive pulmonary disease. N Engl J Med. 2007;356(8):775–89.
49. Hussain SP, Hofseth LJ, Harris CC. Radical causes of cancer. Nat Rev Cancer. 2003;3 (4):276–85.
50. Gaziano JM, Glynn RJ, Christen WG, Kurth T, Belanger C, MacFadyen J, et al. Vitamins E and C in the prevention of prostate and total cancer in men: the Physicians' Health Study II randomized controlled trial. JAMA. 2009;301(1):52–62.
51. Lee IM, Cook NR, Gaziano JM, Gordon D, Ridker PM, Manson JE, et al. Vitamin E in the primary prevention of cardiovascular disease and cancer: the Women's Health Study: a randomized controlled trial. JAMA. 2005;294(1):56–65.
52. van Zandwijk N, Dalesio O, Pastorino U, de Vries N, van Tinteren H. EUROSCAN, a randomized trial of vitamin A and N-acetylcysteine in patients with head and neck cancer or lung cancer. For the EUropean Organization for Research and Treatment of Cancer Head and Neck and Lung Cancer Cooperative Groups. J Natl Cancer Inst. 2000;92(12):977–86.
53. Jackson AL, Zhou B, Kim WY. HIF, hypoxia and the role of angiogenesis in non-small cell lung cancer. Expert Opin Ther Targets. 2010;14(10):1047–57.
54. Giatromanolaki A, Koukourakis MI, Sivridis E, Turley H, Talks K, Pezzella F, et al. Relation of hypoxia inducible factor 1 alpha and 2 alpha in operable non-small cell lung cancer to angiogenic/molecular profile of tumours and survival. Br J Cancer. 2001;85(6):881–90.
55. Kim WY, Perera S, Zhou B, Carretero J, Yeh JJ, Heathcote SA, et al. HIF2alpha cooperates with RAS to promote lung tumorigenesis in mice. J Clin Invest. 2009;119(8):2160–70.
56. Kaya A, Ciledag A, Gulbay BE, Poyraz BM, Celik G, Sen E, et al. The prognostic significance of vascular endothelial growth factor levels in sera of non-small cell lung cancer patients. Respir Med. 2004;98(7):632–6.
57. Sandler A, Gray R, Perry MC, Brahmer J, Schiller JH, Dowlati A, et al. Paclitaxel-carboplatin alone or with bevacizumab for non-small-cell lung cancer. N Engl J Med. 2006;355 (24):2542–50.
58. Kasahara Y, Tuder RM, Taraseviciene-Stewart L, Le Cras TD, Abman S, Hirth PK, et al. Inhibition of VEGF receptors causes lung cell apoptosis and emphysema. J Clin Invest. 2000;106(11):1311–9.
59. Kranenburg AR, de Boer WI, Alagappan VK, Sterk PJ, Sharma HS. Enhanced bronchial expression of vascular endothelial growth factor and receptors (Flk-1 and Flt-1) in patients with chronic obstructive pulmonary disease. Thorax. 2005;60(2):106–13.
60. Punturieri A, Szabo E, Croxton TL, Shapiro SD, Dubinett SM. Lung cancer and chronic obstructive pulmonary disease: needs and opportunities for integrated research. J Natl Cancer Inst. 2009;101(8):554–9.
61. Houghton AM, Rzymkiewicz DM, Ji H, Gregory AD, Egea EE, Metz HE, et al. Neutrophil elastase-mediated degradation of IRS-1 accelerates lung tumor growth. Nat Med. 2010;16 (2):219–23.

62. Vignola AM, Riccobono L, Mirabella A, Profita M, Chanez P, Bellia V, et al. Sputum metalloproteinase-9/tissue inhibitor of metalloproteinase-1 ratio correlates with airflow obstruction in asthma and chronic bronchitis. Am J Respir Crit Care Med. 1998;158 (6):1945–50.
63. Linder R, Ronmark E, Pourazar J, Behndig A, Blomberg A, Lindberg A. Serum metalloproteinase-9 is related to COPD severity and symptoms – cross-sectional data from a population based cohort-study. Respir Res. 2015;16:28.
64. Nozawa H, Chiu C, Hanahan D. Infiltrating neutrophils mediate the initial angiogenic switch in a mouse model of multistage carcinogenesis. Proc Natl Acad Sci U S A. 2006;103 (33):12493–8.
65. Minn AJ, Gupta GP, Siegel PM, Bos PD, Shu W, Giri DD, et al. Genes that mediate breast cancer metastasis to lung. Nature. 2005;436(7050):518–24.
66. D'Armiento J, Dalal SS, Okada Y, Berg RA, Chada K. Collagenase expression in the lungs of transgenic mice causes pulmonary emphysema. Cell. 1992;71(6):955–61.
67. Joos L, He JQ, Shepherdson MB, Connett JE, Anthonisen NR, Pare PD, et al. The role of matrix metalloproteinase polymorphisms in the rate of decline in lung function. Hum Mol Genet. 2002;11(5):569–76.
68. Hunninghake GM, Cho MH, Tesfaigzi Y, Soto-Quiros ME, Avila L, Lasky-Su J, et al. MMP12, lung function, and COPD in high-risk populations. N Engl J Med. 2009;361 (27):2599–608.
69. Houghton AM, Grisolano JL, Baumann ML, Kobayashi DK, Hautamaki RD, Nehring LC, et al. Macrophage elastase (matrix metalloproteinase-12) suppresses growth of lung metastases. Cancer Res. 2006;66(12):6149–55.
70. Magnussen H, Watz H, Kirsten A, Wang M, Wray H, Samuelsson V, et al. Safety and tolerability of an oral MMP-9 and −12 inhibitor, AZD1236, in patients with moderate-to-severe COPD: a randomised controlled 6-week trial. Pulm Pharmacol Ther. 2011;24 (5):563–70.
71. Shepherd FA, Sridhar SS. Angiogenesis inhibitors under study for the treatment of lung cancer. Lung Cancer. 2003;41 Suppl 1:S63–72.
72. Hirsh L, Dantes A, Suh BS, Yoshida Y, Hosokawa K, Tajima K, et al. Phosphodiesterase inhibitors as anti-cancer drugs. Biochem Pharmacol. 2004;68(6):981–8.
73. Greenhough A, Smartt HJ, Moore AE, Roberts HR, Williams AC, Paraskeva C, et al. The COX-2/PGE2 pathway: key roles in the hallmarks of cancer and adaptation to the tumour microenvironment. Carcinogenesis. 2009;30(3):377–86.
74. Mao JT, Roth MD, Fishbein MC, Aberle DR, Zhang ZF, Rao JY, et al. Lung cancer chemoprevention with celecoxib in former smokers. Cancer Prev Res (Phila). 2011;4 (7):984–93.
75. Reckamp KL, Koczywas M, Cristea MC, Dowell JE, Wang HJ, Gardner BK, et al. Randomized phase 2 trial of erlotinib in combination with high-dose celecoxib or placebo in patients with advanced non-small cell lung cancer. Cancer. 2015;121 (18):3298–306.
76. Roh GS, Yi CO, Cho YJ, Jeon BT, Nizamudtinova IT, Kim HJ, et al. Anti-inflammatory effects of celecoxib in rat lungs with smoke-induced emphysema. Am J Physiol Lung Cell Mol Physiol. 2010;299(2):L184–91.
77. Keith RL, Miller YE, Hudish TM, Girod CE, Sotto-Santiago S, Franklin WA, et al. Pulmonary prostacyclin synthase overexpression chemoprevents tobacco smoke lung carcinogenesis in mice. Cancer Res. 2004;64(16):5897–904.
78. Lange A, Gustke H, Glassmeier G, Heine M, Zangemeister-Wittke U, Schwarz JR, et al. Neuronal differentiation by indomethacin and IBMX inhibits proliferation of small cell lung cancer cells in vitro. Lung Cancer. 2011;74(2):178–87.
79. Schuller HM, Plummer 3rd HK, Bochsler PN, Dudric P, Bell JL, Harris RE. Co-expression of beta-adrenergic receptors and cyclooxygenase-2 in pulmonary adenocarcinoma. Int J Oncol. 2001;19(3):445–9.

80. Lee SU, Ahn KS, Sung MH, Park JW, Ryu HW, Lee HJ, et al. Indacaterol inhibits tumor cell invasiveness and MMP-9 expression by suppressing IKK/NF-kappaB activation. Mol Cells. 2014;37(8):585–91.
81. Zhao Q, Gu X, Zhang C, Lu Q, Chen H, Xu L. Blocking M2 muscarinic receptor signaling inhibits tumor growth and reverses epithelial-mesenchymal transition (EMT) in non-small cell lung cancer (NSCLC). Cancer Biol Ther. 2015;16(4):634–43.
82. Zhao Q, Yue J, Zhang C, Gu X, Chen H, Xu L. Inactivation of M2 AChR/NF-kappaB signaling axis reverses epithelial-mesenchymal transition (EMT) and suppresses migration and invasion in non-small cell lung cancer (NSCLC). Oncotarget. 2015;6(30):29335–46.
83. Lin G, Sun L, Wang R, Guo Y, Xie C. Overexpression of muscarinic receptor 3 promotes metastasis and predicts poor prognosis in non-small-cell lung cancer. J Thorac Oncol. 2014;9(2):170–8.
84. Xu R, Shang C, Zhao J, Han Y, Liu J, Chen K, et al. Activation of M3 muscarinic receptor by acetylcholine promotes non-small cell lung cancer cell proliferation and invasion via EGFR/PI3K/AKT pathway. Tumour Biol. 2015;36(6):4091–100.
85. Zhang S, Togo S, Minakata K, Gu T, Ohashi R, Tajima K, et al. Distinct roles of cholinergic receptors in small cell lung cancer cells. Anticancer Res. 2010;30(1):97–106.
86. Hua N, Wei X, Liu X, Ma X, He X, Zhuo R, et al. A novel muscarinic antagonist R2HBJJ inhibits non-small cell lung cancer cell growth and arrests the cell cycle in G0/G1. PLoS One. 2012;7(12), e53170.
87. Hashimoto N, Matsuzaki A, Okada Y, Imai N, Iwano S, Wakai K, et al. Clinical impact of prevalence and severity of COPD on the decision-making process for therapeutic management of lung cancer patients. BMC Pulm Med. 2014;14:14.
88. Lugg ST, Agostini PJ, Tikka T, Kerr A, Adams K, Bishay E, et al. Long-term impact of developing a postoperative pulmonary complication after lung surgery. Thorax. 2016;71(2):171–6.
89. Kobayashi S, Suzuki S, Niikawa H, Sugawara T, Yanai M. Preoperative use of inhaled tiotropium in lung cancer patients with untreated COPD. Respirology. 2009;14(5):675–9.
90. Sekine Y, Suzuki H, Yamada Y, Koh E, Yoshino I. Severity of chronic obstructive pulmonary disease and its relationship to lung cancer prognosis after surgical resection. Thorac Cardiovasc Surg. 2013;61(2):124–30.
91. Kuo CH, Wu CY, Lee KY, Lin SM, Chung FT, Lo YL, et al. Chronic obstructive pulmonary disease in stage I non-small cell lung cancer that underwent anatomic resection: the role of a recurrence promoter. COPD. 2014;11(4):407–13.
92. Putila J, Guo NL. Combining COPD with clinical, pathological and demographic information refines prognosis and treatment response prediction of non-small cell lung cancer. PLoS One. 2014;9(6), e100994.
93. Izquierdo JL, Resano P, El Hachem A, Graziani D, Almonacid C, Sanchez IM. Impact of COPD in patients with lung cancer and advanced disease treated with chemotherapy and/or tyrosine kinase inhibitors. Int J Chron Obstruct Pulmon Dis. 2014;9:1053–8.
94. Lim JU, Yeo CD, Rhee CK, Kim YH, Park CK, Kim JS, et al. Chronic obstructive pulmonary disease-related non-small-cell lung cancer exhibits a low prevalence of EGFR and ALK driver mutations. PLoS One. 2015;10(11), e0142306.
95. Schiavon M, Marulli G, Nannini N, Pasello G, Lunardi F, Balestro E, et al. COPD-related adenocarcinoma presents low aggressiveness morphological and molecular features compared to smoker tumours. Lung Cancer. 2014;86(3):311–7.
96. de Boer WI, Hau CM, van Schadewijk A, Stolk J, van Krieken JH, Hiemstra PS. Expression of epidermal growth factors and their receptors in the bronchial epithelium of subjects with chronic obstructive pulmonary disease. Am J Clin Pathol. 2006;125(2):184–92.
97. Woodruff PG, Wolff M, Hohlfeld JM, Krug N, Dransfield MT, Sutherland ER, et al. Safety and efficacy of an inhaled epidermal growth factor receptor inhibitor (BIBW 2948 BS) in chronic obstructive pulmonary disease. Am J Respir Crit Care Med. 2010;181(5):438–45.

98. Inoue T, Shiomi H, Oh RJ. Stereotactic body radiotherapy for Stage I lung cancer with chronic obstructive pulmonary disease: special reference to survival and radiation-induced pneumonitis. J Radiat Res. 2015;56(4):727–34.
99. Kimura T, Togami T, Takashima H, Nishiyama Y, Ohkawa M, Nagata Y. Radiation pneumonitis in patients with lung and mediastinal tumours: a retrospective study of risk factors focused on pulmonary emphysema. Br J Radiol. 2012;85(1010):135–41.
100. Takeda A, Kunieda E, Ohashi T, Aoki Y, Oku Y, Enomoto T, et al. Severe COPD is correlated with mild radiation pneumonitis following stereotactic body radiotherapy. Chest. 2012;141(4):858–66.
101. Ishijima M, Nakayama H, Itonaga T, Tajima Y, Shiraishi S, Okubo M, et al. Patients with severe emphysema have a low risk of radiation pneumonitis following stereotactic body radiotherapy. Br J Radiol. 2015;88(1046):20140596.
102. Grumelli S, Corry DB, Song LZ, Song L, Green L, Huh J, et al. An immune basis for lung parenchymal destruction in chronic obstructive pulmonary disease and emphysema. PLoS Med. 2004;1(1), e8.
103. Mantovani A, Sozzani S, Locati M, Allavena P, Sica A. Macrophage polarization: tumor-associated macrophages as a paradigm for polarized M2 mononuclear phagocytes. Trends Immunol. 2002;23(11):549–55.
104. Whiteside TL. Immune suppression in cancer: effects on immune cells, mechanisms and future therapeutic intervention. Semin Cancer Biol. 2006;16(1):3–15.
105. Calles A, Liao X, Sholl LM, Rodig SJ, Freeman GJ, Butaney M, Lydon C, Dahlberg SE, Hodi FS, Oxnard GR, Jackman DM, Jänne PA. Expression of PD-1 and Its Ligands, PD-L1 and PD-L2, in smokers and never smokers with KRAS-Mutant Lung Cancer. J Thorac Oncol. 2015;10(12):1726–35. doi:10.1097/JTO.0000000000000687.
106. Yang Y, Pang Z, Ding N, Dong W, Ma W, Li Y, Du J, Liu Q. The efficacy and potential predictive factors of PD-1/PD-L1 blockades in epithelial carcinoma patients: a systematic review and meta analysis. Oncotarget. 2016. doi:10.18632/oncotarget.11291.
107. Kalathil SG, Lugade AA, Pradhan V, Miller A, Parameswaran GI, Sethi S, et al. T-regulatory cells and programmed death 1+ T cells contribute to effector T-cell dysfunction in patients with chronic obstructive pulmonary disease. Am J Respir Crit Care Med. 2014;190(1):40–50.
108. Yap KL, Ada GL, McKenzie IF. Transfer of specific cytotoxic T lymphocytes protects mice inoculated with influenza virus. Nature. 1978;273(5659):238–9.
109. Topham DJ, Tripp RA, Doherty PC. CD8+ T cells clear influenza virus by perforin or Fas-dependent processes. J Immunol. 1997;159(11):5197–200.
110. Diel R, Loddenkemper R, Meywald-Walter K, Niemann S, Nienhaus A. Predictive value of a whole blood IFN-gamma assay for the development of active tuberculosis disease after recent infection with Mycobacterium tuberculosis. Am J Respir Crit Care Med. 2008;177(10):1164–70.
111. Mylonaki E, Manika K, Zarogoulidis P, Domvri K, Voutsas V, Zarogoulidis K, et al. In vivo synergistic cytogenetic effects of aminophylline on lymphocyte cultures from patients with lung cancer undergoing chemotherapy. Mutat Res. 2012;740(1–2):1–5.